Penguin Health
Shopping for Health

After training as a journalist, Jar[...]
gional newspapers before joining [...]
Editor for five years. She is particularly interested in nutrition and the role diet has to play in preventing and curing illness and health problems. She has already written several books including *Slim Naturally*, *High-Fibre Cooking*, *The Wholefood Cookery Course* and *The Alternative Chocolate Book*.

JANETTE MARSHALL

SHOPPING FOR HEALTH

PENGUIN BOOKS

Penguin Books Ltd, Harmondsworth, Middlesex, England
Viking Penguin Inc., 40 West 23rd Street, New York, New York 10010, U.S.A.
Penguin Books Australia Ltd, Ringwood, Victoria, Australia
Penguin Books Canada Limited, 2801 John Street, Markham, Ontario, Canada L3R 1B4
Penguin Books (N.Z.) Ltd, 182–190 Wairau Road, Auckland 10, New Zealand

First published 1987

Copyright © Janette Marshall, 1987
All rights reserved

Made and printed in Great Britain by
Cox & Wyman Ltd, Reading
Filmset in Linotron Sabon by
Rowland Phototypesetting Ltd,
Bury St Edmunds, Suffolk

Except in the United States of America, this book is sold subject
to the condition that it shall not, by way of trade or otherwise,
be lent, re-sold, hired out, or otherwise circulated without the
publisher's prior consent in any form of binding or cover other than
that in which it is published and without a similar condition
including this condition being imposed on the subsequent purchaser

Contents

	Introduction	7
1.	Eating for Health	9
2.	Looking at Food Labels	31
3.	Finding Out about Food Additives	49
4.	Cooking for Health	120

THE SHOPPING LIST 135

Further Reading	436
References and Reports	437
Index	438

Introduction

This book is all about shopping for health. Its aim is to help you choose the healthiest foods for yourself and your family.

We all shop for food in one way or another. Most of us buy the raw ingredients in the supermarket, greengrocer's, butcher's, fishmonger's, delicatessen, health-food shop, grocer's or corner shop and take them home and prepare our meals with them. Sometimes we buy ready-made meals or convenience foods, fresh, chilled or frozen, canned or in Alutrays; perhaps for use in the microwave oven, or to store in the freezer. We may also buy food at a takeaway – Indian, Chinese, fish and chips, pizzas, fried chicken, burgers or pies. Most of us eat from time to time at cafés, wine bars, restaurants, pubs or clubs. Some people never cook for themselves, either eating out all the time, or having their meals cooked for them at home.

Whether you cook for yourself or not, this book aims to give you the information you need about the food you eat, so that you can eat healthily. In the Shopping List, the main section of this book, we go through each category of food, giving information on the health aspects, and then listing brand names or special products where appropriate. This gives you the key points to look out for, and tells you which brand names to ask for and where you are most likely to find them.

Before we proceed to the Shopping List, however, it will be helpful to look at how we arrive at the conclusion that some foods are 'better' than others. It is often said by nutritionists and the food industry that the modern Western diet, with its wide variety of foods, is bound to contain all the nutrients we need, and that no food is particularly bad for us. That is a statement with which I

Introduction

would disagree, as I shall explain in the chapters on food labelling and food additives.

The first chapter sets out some of the most recent ideas on healthy eating, as contained in the recent reports of the National Advisory Committee on Nutrition Education (NACNE) and the Committee on the Medical Aspects of Food Policy (COMA). It indicates which foods we should be eating less of, and suggests ways of cutting down on these foods. It also suggests ways of increasing the amount of fibre that we eat.

This is followed by a chapter on food labelling which will help you to read between the lines of the label. It will explain how to read and understand what the food label is really saying about the contents and – just as important – what it is *not* saying.

Chapter 3 discusses the use of additives. There are easy-to-follow charts which show which additives are considered 'safe', which 'suspect' and which 'harmful', and which additives are animal in origin, so that vegetarians and vegans can see at a glance which additives they should avoid. After reading this chapter you may find that certain foods that you buy no longer hold the same appeal.

Buying food, however, is not the end of the story; how we prepare the food is also important. We cannot improve poor-quality food and make it nutritionally better, but we can prepare our food so as to retain as many of the nutrients as possible. This is the subject of Chapter 4.

There is a bewildering variety of foods to choose from in our shops today, and many of them are low in nutritional value or potentially harmful to health. This book is a guide to foods which are good nutritional value for money.

1. Eating for Health

Why do we eat?

This may seem a daft question to ask, but it is worth going back to basics for a moment. To stay alive is the obvious answer, but there is more to it than just staying alive because the food we eat can directly affect the way we feel and the way we feel determines whether we are really enjoying life – to really buzz along in what we do, we need top-grade fuel. (You will, of course, meet some Flat Earthers who will disagree and deny the relationship between diet and health, but that is their problem.)

What are foods for?

Food is the fuel for the body, and is converted into energy to power all our activities. Food is also needed to build our bodies, fuel growth and repair and maintain us as we age. There are several basic types of food.

Carbohydrates

These are either sugars (the *simple carbohydrates*) or starches (the *complex carbohydrates*). They are converted into energy, and are sometimes called energy foods.

Some carbohydrates, which we have come to call dietary fibre, are indigestible – but none the less necessary for health. What is digested is converted by our bodies into fuel.

We also need to explain the terms 'refined carbohydrates' (the

Shopping for Health

baddies) and 'unrefined carbohydrates' (the goodies). *Unrefined carbohydrates* are as near to their original state as possible. They are the complex carbohydrates stored by plants when they turn sunlight and water into food starches, and they are found in roots and in grains and cereals. They go through a complicated process of digestion before their energy is released to the body. The fibre in them slows the digestion and regulates the rate of energy release (among other things). Foods like wholemeal bread and pasta, brown rice and porridge oats, whole-grain flours and crispbreads, and root vegetables provide a sustained, slow-release type of energy. They are also bulky and filling and difficult to eat too much of, so you feel fuller on fewer calories. Of course, if you eat too much of any type of carbohydrate you will end up with more calories than you need and this will be converted into fat, but if you stick to unrefined foods it is difficult to eat too much.

Refined carbohydrates – simple sugars and white flour, for example – have been subjected to processing which removes the dietary fibre, as well as many vitamins and minerals. They are absorbed too quickly into the bloodstream, causing the blood sugar levels to rise and then slump again soon afterwards, leading to a craving for yet more sugary foods. This hypoglycaemic (low blood sugar) reaction is typical of a diet high in refined carbohydrate foods like cakes and pastries, sweets and confectionery, and chocolate snacks.

Fats

Fats provide energy in a much more concentrated form than carbohydrates. Of all the macronutrients (carbohydrate, protein, fats) fats contain the highest number of calories per ounce – and if you eat too much fat then it will be deposited as fat, 'too much' being more calories than you are going to burn off as energy.

Fats are made up of fatty acids of which there are several types. The main ones that concern us as regards healthy eating are saturated fatty acids – called saturated fats for short – and unsaturated fats. Generally speaking animal fats (meat, dairy produce, lard and suet, butter) are saturated fats and vegetable fats are usually unsaturated. Some *unsaturated fats* are essential for our health and cannot be made by our bodies, so we have to eat them in our food. This is why one should never go on a totally fat-free diet. *Polyunsaturated fats*, such as good-quality vegetable oils (sunflower, safflower, corn and soya-bean oils), are the best, but not all vegetable oils are high in polyunsaturated fats – coconut and palm oils for example, are highly saturated. *Saturated fats* are not essential for health (as far as we know at the moment) and they are thought to be a contributory factor in heart disease, particularly arteriosclerosis, the hardening and narrowing of the arteries which makes it difficult for oxygenated blood to reach the heart and so increases the risk of heart attacks.

Because fats are so high in calories they are often responsible for weight problems; being overweight, or obese, will increase the risk of many other diseases as well as heart disease. We are therefore advised to cut down on the amount of fat in our diet and to make sure that the greater proportion of the fat we eat is polyunsaturated rather than saturated.

If we are to cut down on saturated fats, we must also avoid vegetable fats that have undergone processing – hydrogenation – to harden them. When you see the description '*hydrogenated vegetable fats*' on a packet of biscuits, for example, remember that the fat, although not derived from animals, will have the same effects in the body as saturated fats. *Trans fatty acids* are also equivalent to saturated fats once they are in the body.

Some fats such as olive oil, are *monounsaturated* and these appear to be neutral in the body, having neither the detrimental effects of saturated fats, nor the beneficial effects of polyunsaturated fats, with their essential fatty acids and their ability to help reduce the levels of harmful cholesterol in the body.

Cholesterol is an ingredient of animal fat. There are several types of cholesterol, but the ones which most concern us in healthy eating are *high-density lipoproteins* (HDL), *low-density lipoproteins* (LDL) and *very-low-density lipoproteins* (VLDL). The HDL cholesterols are 'good guys' that seem to work against the harmful types of cholesterol, LDL and VLDL, being deposited on damaged arteries, leading to increased risk of heart attacks. (Lipoprotein is just the scientific term for these fats.)

The latest research seems to indicate that we should reduce our intake of all saturated fats as much as possible, but that it is not necessary to single out cholesterol as being even more harmful than other saturated fats. In fact, the body does need some cholesterol, but it has the ability to manufacture it itself, so there is no necessity, as far as we know, to eat cholesterol in foods.

Fats also supply us with oil-soluble vitamins. Animal fats supply vitamins A and D and good-quality vegetable oils supply vitamin E. The vitamins A and D are well supplied in most Western diets (except those of some Asian groups) and vitamin D is made by exposure to sunlight, so we don't need to use animal fats to get these nutrients; they are, by law, added to margarine and are found in other foods. Vitamin E is often short in a typically highly refined diet so a good-quality vegetable oil is useful to supply this and the essential fatty acids.

Finally a word about fish oils. If you remember holding your nose to swallow cod liver oil, you should be grateful, for some fish oils, including cod liver oil, contain eicosapentanoic acid, a magic ingredient that stops our blood becoming sticky and too liable to clot, and so helps protect us against heart disease.

Protein

Protein is used for growth and repair. During digestion protein is broken down into amino acids, which are absorbed by the body to build its own protein. There are twenty-one amino acids and eight are called essential because the body cannot make them itself – they have to be eaten in food.

If we are ever short of carbohydrate foods in our diet – when we go on high-protein slimming diets (not a good idea!), for example – protein can be turned into energy, but this is a complex process and there are several by-products that are toxic and can aggravate

Eating for Health

conditions such as rheumatism, gout and joint problems. It also puts the body under strain and so you may feel below par (a common experience on high-protein slimming diets). Although we eat far more protein than we need in the typical British diet, excesses of protein will not have such disastrous effects on general health as excesses of sugar and fat (more of that on p. 15). So quantity is not a problem, but if you are a vegetarian or a vegan, then the quality of the protein might be of concern. Animal foods like meat, fish, eggs and milk (I have deliberately not mentioned cheese because this is now thought of as a fatty food rather than a protein food – see p. 203) contain amino acids in the right proportions for humans; vegetable protein foods don't. There are three basic groups of vegetable protein foods: cereal/grains, pulses, and nuts and seeds. Each of these groups is short of several amino acids, *but* by combining two of the groups at any one meal you can rectify the deficiencies of both and so eat protein which is as useful to the body as that from animal protein foods. In fact some people might consider vegetable proteins better because they have two advantages: first, they are low in fat (except nuts, which are quite oily and should be eaten in moderation, but you don't want many, anyway); and second, they are high in fibre – animal protein foods contain no fibre. Vegetable protein is easily digested and low in fats, and a higher proportion of the fat is unsaturated.

Combining dairy foods with vegetable protein foods will enhance their value even more (see BAKED BEANS,* p. 152), but vegetarians should be wary of relying too much on cheese and other dairy foods. (This is not a problem for vegans, who avoid all animal products.)

---

* Throughout the book, words in small capitals refer you to an article in the Shopping List section.

Vitamins and minerals

Vitamins and minerals are also essential to our diet, but they are needed in relatively small amounts. Different vitamins and minerals are obtained from different foods, which is why it is so important to have a varied diet. As well as keeping the body's chemical processes ticking over and helping to ward off infections, vitamins are needed in the digestion of food, to release the energy from carbohydrate foods. When we eat refined foods (white bread and anything else made from white flour, white rice, sugar, etc.), the body's own store of vitamins may be robbed in order to digest the food; unrefined foods have their store of vitamins intact, and do not deplete the body's supply of them.

Both vitamins and minerals are involved in a myriad of complex chemical processes of body metabolism, but minerals are required for body growth and repair rather than the direct absorption of food.

Water

Water is, of course, essential to life, like oxygen, and we cannot live without water. However, we might live without tap water, and we could certainly live without tea and coffee – it might be an idea to drink more plain water to quench thirst. (See the section on WATER in the Shopping List.)

Overfed and undernourished

Let's just take a quick look at the effects of the modern diet on our health and consider what happens if we eat too much of some foods and not enough of others.

Sugar

In our introduction to carbohydrates we saw that simple sugars, such as table sugar (sucrose), can cause swings in blood sugar and cravings for more sugary foods. Refined sugar is easy to eat and very high in calories. A spoonful of sugar will melt in the mouth, whereas eating your way through a stick of sugarcane or a sugar beet would take considerably longer – and it would also give you some fibre and vitamins and minerals in the process. Sugar can, therefore, easily lead to overweight because it is so simple to swallow far more calories than you need. It also develops a sweet tooth that is difficult, but far from impossible, to change, and it causes tooth decay (despite what the sweet industry may say).

Our sugar consumption, in Britain, is higher than almost anywhere else in the world and this is reflected in weight problems, poor teeth and poor health. The myth that sugar is needed for energy is perpetuated by the people selling and making sweets, ice-creams, cakes and pastries and so on. The body does not need *any* sugar in its refined (packet) form, whether brown or white, although all starches and sugars are broken down during digestion into simple sugars. Rather than eating sugar and sweets, we should get our supplies of carbohydrates from unrefined foods (complex carbohydrates). Brown sugar is less highly refined than white, but is almost equally harmful. Any sugar that is not burned off as energy will be deposited as fat in the body.

Eating too much sugar has also been linked with maturity-onset diabetes, because the pancreas has to produce more insulin to clear the bloodstream, so leading to a vicious circle of craving more sugar foods and to ups and downs in mood and energy. Excess sugar has also been linked with gallstones and kidney stones (in conjunction with too much fat) and with some cancers and heart disease.

Fat

Fat is probably the most problematic of our foods in the West. It has come under scrutiny mainly for its contribution to heart disease, but like sugar it is a high-calorie food (in all of its forms); many high-fat processed foods take up space in our diet that would be better given to more nutritionally valuable foods. Like sugar, fat is easy to eat. It makes food palatable, makes it slip down easily – you would not be tempted to eat too much dry bread or baked potato unless it had something to moisten it.

Most of us are not energetic enough to burn up all the calories we eat as fat and the extra will end up being deposited as fat. But it won't all be deposited as a spare tyre, or as a contribution to the typically pear-shaped British bottom. Much of it may be deposited inside our arteries where, from the pre-school milk to the grown-up chips with everything, it can gradually build up, narrowing and hardening the arteries.

Britain has one of the worst rates of heart attack in the world and the correlation between high-fat diets and high risk of heart disease is undeniable, whatever the actual mechanism that causes it. Excessive fat is also linked to certain cancers, especially breast cancer, and under investigation for its contribution to gallstones – the cholesterol link here is well known – and to heart disease among diabetics, who have traditionally been put on high-fat diets.

Salt

In Britain we also eat salt in excess; convenience foods – canned, packaged and processed foods – add large amounts of salt to our diet. As with sugar, a liking for salt is an acquired taste that can be unlearned. Cutting down will, at first, be difficult but you will soon find highly salted foods unpalatable if you persist. Unlike sugar, salt, or rather sodium, is essential for health, but sodium occurs naturally in many foods and, unless you use a lot of physical energy and so lose a lot of sodium, you do not need to take extra salt in your food. Too much salt has been linked with strokes and high blood pressure, and it is under investigation for its role in stomach cancer.

Fibre

Fibre, or rather the lack of it, is also associated with many of the health problems mentioned above, and is linked with excesses of fat and sugar. This is because many highly refined foods, which are vehicles for sugar, fat and salt, are also low in fibre. Eating natural, unprocessed foods with their fibre, vitamins and minerals intact, leaves less room in the diet for sugary and fat confectionery, cakes and pastries, etc.

Lack of fibre has been singled out as the main cause of constipation and related complications such as haemorrhoids, varicose veins, hiatus hernia and diverticulitis. Duodenal ulcers, appendicitis, gallstones, high blood pressure and cancers of the colon and breast have also been linked to lack of fibre and the interaction of fats and sugars.

Dietary conclusions

All these findings have been highlighted in recent reports by government-instigated groups like the National Advisory Committee on Nutrition Education (NACNE), the Committee on the Medical Aspects of Food Policy (COMA) and the Joint Advisory Committee on Nutrition Education (JACNE). The recommendations they make about the changes which should be made to the average British diet can be summarized as:

less fat, more of it polyunsaturated; reduce by 25 per cent
less sugar; reduce by 50 per cent
less salt; reduce by 25 per cent
more fibre; increase by 50 per cent
fewer calories from alcohol

This would result in the sensible sort of eating pattern that has been followed for many years by people on a wholefood diet and it is the basis of 'natural' diets used by naturopaths and others who have a nutritional approach to preventing illness or establishing good health.

Shopping for Health

You may want to add your own personal recommendations to the official ones given above. For example, I would add

eat fewer foods containing additives

This would automatically improve the quality of the food consumed, by placing greater reliance on fresher, more nutritious foods and on unrefined foods.

Alcohol, like sugar, consists purely of calories, without vitamins and minerals in any useful amount. Like sugar, it robs the body of the vitamins needed to keep us healthy. For example, the B vitamins are needed to metabolize alcohol, especially nicotinic acid or nicotinamide, thiamin (B_1), B_{12} and folic acid. The body's supply of the minerals zinc and magnesium are also depleted by alcohol, and vitamin C is needed to produce the enzyme that detoxifies alcohol.

In the NACNE Report, *Proposals for Nutritional Guidelines for Health Education in Britain*, 1983, both short-term and long-term goals were outlined:

Percentage of calories consumed	Long-term goals	Short-term goals	Present average
Fat	30	34	38
Saturated fat	10	15	18
Added sugar	10	12	18
Alcohol	4	5	6
Fibre (g per day)	30	25	20
Sodium (mg)*	3,600	4,300	4,700

*Average daily salt intake in the UK is 12 g, which corresponds to 4.7 g sodium.

It is probably easier to think about food in the amounts you eat each day and in these terms the table above translates into the following:

- A reduction from 128 g fat each day to 100 g
- A reduction from 59 g saturated fat each day to 32 g
- A reduction from 104 g sugar each day to 54 g
- A reduction from 12 g salt each day to 9 g.

It would not do any harm to aim for an even lower daily intake of fat – around 3 oz (85 g). Although the COMA Report on Diet and Cardiovascular Disease has recommended aiming for 0.45:1 ratio of polyunsaturates to saturates, some experts are saying we would do better to aim for 1:1 if we want to lower high blood fat profiles and reduce heart attack risks. However, government recommendations do not go this far because of the unknown effect of a long-term increased polyunsaturate intake, and also, no doubt, because of pressure from political lobbies such as the agricultural one and, to a certain extent, the food industry.

You would do better to do without any refined sugar at all, although this is very difficult to achieve without actually becoming a hermit or a diabetic, which allows you to refuse without offending! The calories 'lost' by reducing alcohol intake should be made up by eating more fruit, vegetables and cereals, says NACNE; this would also increase the intake of vitamins, minerals, fibre and essential fatty acids without producing a fall in protein intake.

How to do it

Here are some tips on how to make the changes recommended by NACNE.

How to cut down on sugar

- Choose the no-added-sugar versions of common foods such as jams and marmalades, breakfast cereals, baked beans, ketchups and sauces, cakes and ready-made foods. See the Shopping List, for where to find these foods and which brands to look for, and remember to read food labels before buying, in order to avoid sugar in processed foods.
- Reduce the amount of 'visible' sugar you use – the sugar from the sugar bowl that goes on to breakfast cereals and fruit salads and into tea and coffee and other drinks.

Shopping for Health

- Cut out coffee creamers and whiteners – they usually contain sugar. Use fresh skimmed milk or dried milk instead.
- Cut down on sweets, cakes and pastries; if you make cakes and biscuits at home adapt your recipes to use less sugar. In some recipes, you can substitute honey, 20 per cent of which is water, which equals fewer calories. See suggestions for alternative sweeteners under SUGAR in the Shopping List.

How to cut down on fat

- Choose the low-fat or no-added-fat versions of foods such as meat, cheese, milk, sausages (if you must!), snacks, etc. See the Shopping List for the brand names of these foods and where to find them. Remember to read food labels to discover the hidden fat in processed food products.
- Cut down on 'visible' fats such as the butter or margarine you spread on your bread, toast and vegetables. Use good-quality unsaturated cooking oil for salad dressings and cooking, and reduce the amount you use.
- Always measure fat or oil into the cooking pan if you have to use it; pouring from the bottle results in using more than you think.
- Buy an oil-well which has a brush that dips in the oil and squeezes out most of the oil as it leaves the well. This is handy for culinary use.
- Be aware of, and wary of, the invisible fats in foods such as pastry. Shortcrust pastry contains half as much fat as flour; puff pastry and flaky pastry contain more than half. There is also fat in cakes and biscuits and other baked foods.
- If you buy biscuits and baked goods, check the type of fat used. Read the label and avoid hydrogenated vegetable fats and unspecified animal fats or vegetable oils where possible.

Eating for Health

Fat in Our Food (national average)

	Percentage
Meat	15
Milk	15
Margarine	14
All other fats (ie. cooking oils, low-fat spreads, lard, suet, etc.)	13
Butter	10
Sausages/meat products	10
Miscellaneous (Cereal, bread, fruit, veg, other food)	7
Cakes/pastries/biscuits	6
Cheese	5
Eggs	3
Poultry	1
Fish	1

These figures show the percentage contribution of fat from different foods in the typical British diet. They have been rounded up to the nearest whole number and are based on Ministry of Agriculture, Fisheries and Food statistics for 1984, compiled from the National Food Survey.

- Switch from full-cream gold- or silver-top milk to skimmed or semi-skimmed milk. See the shopping list, under MILK.
- Remember cream is fat. Make use of 'creamy' strained yoghurts instead – see the Shopping List, under CREAM
- Remember that hard cheese and cream cheeses are very fatty. Don't nibble on them; take them 'seriously' and make them go further by adding them to cooked dishes where there are lots of other ingredients, so you are not tempted to eat too much.
- Reduce your meat consumption and choose the leanest types and cuts of meat. Free-range poultry and game have the least amount of fat on them; it is easy to remove because it is just under the skin and it is higher in polyunsaturates because animals that are active do not contain as much saturated fat as intensively reared, 'sedentary' animals. See also MEAT in the Shopping List.

Shopping for Health

- Cook food without added fat, i.e. grill, steam, poach, braise or roast it; when roasting meat, sit it on a tray in a pan so the fat can drain away. Skim fat off the top of stocks and casseroles.
- Trim all visible fat off meat (see illustration).

How to cut down on salt

- Choose the no-added-salt versions of popular foods like stock cubes, ketchups and sauces, peanut butter and spreads, margarine, canned vegetables, butter, etc.; see the Shopping List. Remember to read labels before buying.
- Avoid cured meat and fish and also those bottled or canned in brine.
- Smoked foods are often treated with salt before being smoked.
- Pickles and salad dressings are usually high in salt.
- Don't add salt during cooking – let people add as much as they want (or less!) at the table.
- Stop putting the salt mill or cruet on the table, or reduce the number of holes in it. Experiments have found this works well because shaking the cellar is often a matter of habit and does not have much to do with how much salt comes out.
- Avoid sodium-based food additives – listed on p. 118; this includes things like baking powder and bicarbonate of soda.
- Avoid obviously salty foods such as crisps and peanuts or savoury snacks, or buy the no-added-salt versions. See the Shopping List.

How to add more fibre

First, beware of the 'bran trap', especially in foods which are labelled 'high fibre' – these are often very high in fats and sugars too, to make the amount of bran added palatable. Many of these commercially prepared foods are as bad as highly refined foods that are low in fibre, being basically junk food with added bran. Adding fibre to a diet of refined carbohydrates will not solve anything; it will only mask any symptoms caused by fibreless diet.

Thickness of fat on chop after trimming (mm)	Percentage of fat in typical fat loin of pork (untrimmed thickness of fat over muscle, 17mm)	Percentage of fat in typical lean loin of pork (untrimmed thickness of fat over muscle, 8mm)
17	35·2	
12	26·9	
8	21·6	10·0
4	15·9	7·0
0	7·8	5·7

Source: Based on a diagram published by the Meat and Livestock Commission.

The Fat in a Loin Chop

Fat content by chemical analysis of edible part of chops after varying degrees of trimming of the external fat (percentage). Fat between the muscles was not trimmed before analysis, but could be trimmed on the plate.

Shopping for Health

Instead, choose foods as near to their natural state as possible. These are the unrefined foods such as cereal grains (not sugary, fatty, high-fibre breakfast cereals), fruits, vegetables, oats, and beans and other legumes that have not had the fibre and vitamins and minerals processed out of them.

Adding raw bran to foods can also cause a short-term problem because bran contains phytic acid which combines with minerals like zinc, making them unavailable to the body. Research has shown that the amounts present in natural foods such as wholemeal bread will not cause problems, especially as (*a*) the body will compensate in about six weeks for any increase in this substance and (*b*) cooked phytates in bread and wholemeal pasta, etc., are not as problematic as raw bran.

There are many better ways of increasing your fibre intake:

- Switch to 'natural' high-fibre products that are not high in fats and sugars. Specific products are mentioned in the Shopping List.
- Start using a mixture of white and wholemeal flour, aiming to switch entirely to wholemeal. It really is possible to make most things with wholemeal, except perhaps choux pastry, where 81 per cent extraction flour is used (see FLOUR).
- Switch to wholemeal bread, or other naturally high-fibre-grain breads, or at least include them as part of the diet along with white bread.
- Choose brown rice and wholemeal pasta instead of white.
- Increase the amount of beans, pulses, chick peas, lentils, etc., in your diet either to make meat dishes go further or to replace them entirely.
- Eat more fresh fruit and vegetables.
- Use dried fruits instead of sugary snacks.
- Four slices of wholemeal bread and two apples, and a Shredded Wheat for breakfast, should add up to about the right fibre intake for a day.

NB. Make any increase in fibre to your diet gradual. You may feel bloated or suffer flatulence if you make sudden switches to a new way of eating.

Eating for Health

Putting it all together

Having grasped the basics of a healthier way of eating, the next step is to translate the theory into 'food events'! Here are some suggestions for healthier meal times.

Breakfast

Having breakfast is a good habit to get into. It is important for several reasons. Firstly, as its name suggests, it is breaking a fast of nine hours or more. Blood sugar levels are low and fuel is needed for the morning's work. Children perform better in school if they have had a good breakfast. People at work can concentrate better and are less accident-prone if they have eaten breakfast. Breakfast should also fuel you safely past the elevenses – or 'half-past tenses' – cake-and-biscuit crisis . . .

Here are some suggestions for breakfast:

wholemeal toast with a little butter, unsalted, or polyunsaturated margarine
no-added-sugar jams or marmalades
no-added-sugar or -salt cereal (see BREAKFAST CEREALS)
porridge with porridge oats, oatmeal or rolled oats
fresh or dried fruits, with yoghurt or stewed
free-range eggs, boiled or scrambled, without fat or salt
no-added-sugar baked beans
mushrooms sweated without fat (in a non-stick or heavy-based pan)
fresh fruit juice
mineral water
skimmed milk or thin yoghurt.

Lunch or main meal

One meal a day should be based on salad, using as wide a variety of leaf and root vegetables as possible. If it is not based on a salad, then make sure it contains freshly cooked vegetables. If using potatoes, try to keep chips to a minimum because they are so high in fat. Try potatoes baked in their skins, or boiled potatoes which

Shopping for Health

can also be eaten with their skins on. Mashed potatoes can be 'creamed' with skimmed milk rather than butter and for a really creamy consistency finish them in the food processor or liquidizer after mashing by hand rather than add butter. Instead of potatoes, use brown rice or wholemeal pastas for some meals.

One meal a day should also contain some protein. We need only about 3–4 oz (85–115 g) a day, and this should consist of fish or lean meat if it is animal protein. Do not rely too much on eggs and cheese because they are high in fat. Vegetable protein should consist of a mixture either of beans and grains eaten together, or of nuts and grains, or of nuts and beans. Remember, however, that, like cheese, nuts are high in fats.

Many classic dishes supply protein, without using meat, for example, Indian food which combines chick-pea or bean curries with rice, or vegetable and chick-pea dishes with *naans* and other breads, thus combining legumes (the beans) and grains (the bread). Pitta breads with dips like *hummus* – a chick-pea and *tahini* (sesame seed) paste – pasta served with beans or nut roasts combining nuts and cereals also give non-meat protein. Even baked beans on toast gives the necessary combination of two types of vegetable protein.

If you make lunch your protein meal then the evening meal can be based on a pizza or a pasta dish which might have some protein in it, but not as its main ingredient. It could also include, or be based on, wholemeal quiche or flans, pies and/or salads. If you had salad vegetables at lunch then the evening meal should include cooked (lightly cooked) vegetables.

Of course you don't have to have two meals a day, and if you do they should not be large meals. A sandwich or a baked potato could be quite sufficient for lunch, especially if you have an office job which is not very active. Choose wholemeal bread and be mean with the butter, and use cottage cheese or a vegetable filling instead of butter with the potato. Fresh fruit and unsweetened yoghurts or a simple salad (preferably not swamped in high-calorie mayonnaise) would also be sufficient for lunch.

Here are some more specific suggestions for either lunch or evening meals:

wholemeal sandwiches – more salad filling, less meat/cheese
toasted wholemeal sandwiches – as above
salads – a mixture of root and leaf vegetables, plus fruit, dried fruits, nuts and seeds
wholemeal pizzas – they don't have to have cheese layer on top, especially if you are cutting down on fats
open sandwiches made from wholemeal rye breads, pumpernickel, etc.
cold pasta and cooked bean salads tossed in good-quality vegetable oil
risotto with brown rice, either hot or cold, with lots of vegetables and perhaps a few nuts or some chopped chicken
stir-fried vegetables cooked quickly at a high temperature with good-quality oil and possibly some shredded chicken or fish or nuts; serve with brown rice
wholemeal quiches – if making them yourself, use yeast dough rather than pastry, to cut down on fat. Use yoghurts, natural and strained natural, with a free-range egg rather than double or single cream for the filling
savoury scones made with wholemeal flour and flavoured with a little tasty cheese, such as mature Cheddar or Gruyère, or herbs
wholemeal breads/pitta breads/rolls, with dips like *hummus* or *taramasalata*
soups, with lots of vegetables and some wholemeal pasta or cooked beans
fish, grilled or poached, basted with lemon juice rather than oil or poached in a *court bouillon* or vegetable stock
poultry, grilled (as above) or roasted without added fat
baked and stuffed jacket potatoes with slimming fillings – not butter or sour cream with chives. Try, instead, ratatouille, stir-fried veg, baked beans, chilli con(or *sin*) carne, curried beans
bean and meat dishes like chilli con carne which contain a small amount of meat and plenty of fibre (in the beans)
rice dishes such as paella, risotto, curries, kedgerees, using brown rice
vegetables such as aubergine, tomatoes and courgettes stuffed with brown rice and vegetables with a few nuts
wholemeal pasta with low-calorie tomato-based sauces. Use also green pasta made with spinach and egg (not coloured, dyed pasta) or tomato pasta with fresh vegetable and fish sauces
shellfish in slimming vegetable *bouillon* or white-wine sauces with lots of herbs
wholemeal pancakes stuffed with vegetables, fish, beans, etc.
wholemeal pies – occasionally, because they are high in fat.

Desserts

Desserts can be a sticky problem! It is probably best to make them weekend treats only and to fill up on the main course. For everyday desserts fresh fruit, either whole or made into fruit salad, is a good idea. Natural yoghurts, with added fresh fruit, or strained yoghurts with fresh fruit or fresh fruit purées are not too high in fat. The yoghurt should be, ideally, unsweetened – the fruit will add sweetness. Other desserts like dried fruit compôtés are a good standby – any remainder can be eaten for breakfast. Pancakes with fruit purée fillings and cheesecakes made with low-fat soft white cheeses or sieved cottage cheese and topped with fruit purée can be made for weekends and special occasions. Grilled fruit is also a tasty dessert – try grapefruit, bananas, oranges.

If you are a pudding person try not to eat pudding at more than one meal a day and go carefully with the high-calorie puddings such as regular cheesecakes, baked and steamed puddings, pies and crumbles, meringues and gâteaux.

The cheese course is often offered in place of, or as well as, a pudding and this is where the calories and fats in particular really mount up. You may feel good if you have said no to the sugary puds, but the cheeseboard also has its pitfalls. If you really can't say no, leave out the butter or margarine on the cheese biscuits and just eat the cheese. You could also say no to the biscuits – most of which are low-fibre white biscuits; have fresh fruit with the cheese instead. Choose the lowest fat cheeses (see CHEESE).

Drinks

Drinks during the day and with meals can be vehicles for lots of calories in the form of sugar. Start by weaning yourself off the sugar added to tea and coffee. Replace tea and coffee with other drinks sometimes, or switch to decaffeinated coffee and drink it black. Try also the huge range of herb teas that are, in the main, non-stimulating and are drunk without milk. Try a slice of lemon instead of milk.

Mineral water and fruit and vegetable juices offer other alternatives to hot drinks, and these are preferable to soft drinks like cola drinks, which are high in either sugar or saccharin or other chemical additives. It is important to find a drink you like that does not contain sugar or saccharin because this will help you in the long term, not only to cut down on calories, but also to wean yourself off sugary foods altogether.

Alcoholic drinks are sometimes difficult to avoid, and indeed there are times when you don't want to avoid them. But on a daily basis it is best not to exceed two glasses of wine or spirits or 1½ pints (0.9 l) beer. Ideally we should be drinking less than this because alcohol replaces nutritious foods in our calorie intake; it is also habit forming.

Snacks

This is where the sweets and the chocolate confectionery usually creep into our diet. They are the between-meal snacks that cause us so many problems in terms of ruining our teeth and habituating us to sweet foods.

There are other things to have if you feel hungry. A sandwich is better than a bar of chocolate if you want something substantial. A scone is better than a cream cake or a fatty sponge cake or a Danish pastry. Yeasted teacakes and buns are much lower in fat and sugar than conventional sweets, cakes and pastries. A handful of dried fruit or a few nuts will give fibre and vitamins and minerals where sweets will not. Fresh fruit is also a better idea and an apple will help if you feel you can't last out until the next meal. Bananas, too, are filling, but they are also quite high in calories; they are still better than sweets and cakes, though.

If you must have a biscuit then digestive biscuits and oatmeal biscuits are lower in fats and sugars and higher in fibre than most biscuits; some cereal bars (see CEREAL BARS) make nutritious snacks.

For other snacks see the Shopping List, under SNACK FOODS.

Shopping for Health

Planning menus

We now have a wide range of suggestions from which to plan menus for healthier meals. When putting meals together there are a few basic pointers such as

- Include, as many different food varieties as possible, making the courses complement each other; for example, don't have pastry in more than one dish or course.
- Remember when planning and writing your shopping list that foods in season will usually be cheaper than those that have to be imported.
- Complement your vegetable ingredients if you are not using animal proteins.
- Watch the levels of fat and sugar in your meals.

Obviously you will not always be able to plan your own meals or make them yourself. Few of us have the time or the money to be able to do this every day. There will be many occasions when you will want to buy ready-made foods or shop for something that can be eaten as soon as you get home. Because most foods of this type contain additives, Chapter 3 gives information on food additives and how they are used, to help you decide which are harmless and which should be avoided.

Breaking the rules

Remember, too, that dietary advice is the basis of everyday eating. There will be times when you want to break the rules (although a healthy diet is an enjoyable diet). Don't feel guilty – it's the sum total that counts, and everyone can have their indulgences on high days and holidays. (That's what they're for!)

2. Looking at Food Labels

More than 80 per cent of our diet is now made up of processed foods – the kinds of foods that are wrapped and packed – so if you want to know what is in your food, you will have to get wise to the special language and jargon of the food labels. These are supposedly designed to give the customer information about the product, but some may seem more like advertising 'hype'; often the pictures on the packet bear little resemblance, especially on ready meals, to what is actually inside.

This chapter shows you how to interpret the small print – and also tells you what does *not* have to be stated clearly on the label.

The label is the only way you have of knowing what has gone into the food in your shopping basket, and the information that packaged foods display on their labels is strictly controlled by law. However, there are exemptions (see p. 38), and unwrapped foods like bread do not have to state what they contain.

Here is a checklist of the basic information on food labels which we will be looking at in more detail:

 the name of the food
 a list of ingredients
 the net quantity, either in weight or volume
 the datemark
 special storage conditions
 instructions for use, where necessary
 name and address of manufacturer, packed or importer
 in some cases, the place of origin

Take a look at the foods in your larder and discover what is really in them, what their main ingredients are and what additives

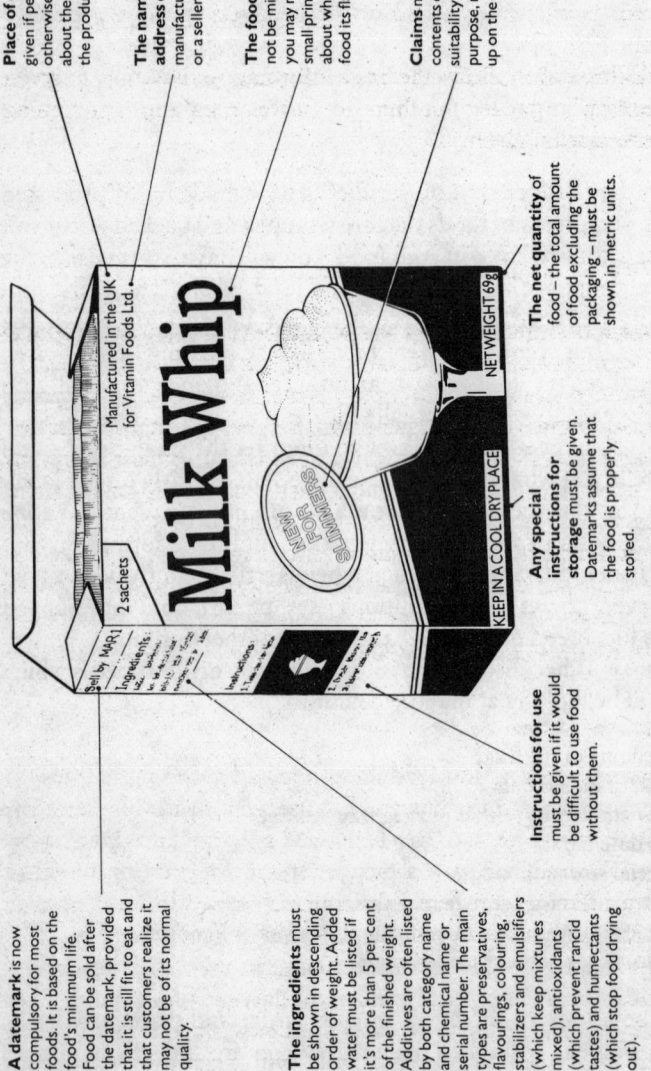

Place of origin must be given if people might otherwise be misled about the real origin of the product.

The name and address of the manufacturer or a packer or a seller must be given.

The food name must not be misleading. But you may need to read the small print to be clear about what gives the food its flavour.

Claims made about the contents of a food, or its suitability for a certain purpose, must be backed up on the label.

The net quantity of food – the total amount of food excluding the packaging – must be shown in metric units.

Any special instructions for storage must be given. Datemarks assume that the food is properly stored.

Instructions for use must be given if it would be difficult to use food without them.

The ingredients must be shown in descending order of weight. Added water must be listed if it's more than 5 per cent of the finished weight. Additives are often listed by both category name and chemical name or serial number. The main types are preservatives, flavourings, colouring, stabilizers and emulsifiers (which keep mixtures mixed), antioxidants (which prevent rancid tastes) and humectants (which stop food drying out).

A datemark is now compulsory for most foods. It is based on the food's minimum life. Food can be sold after the datemark, provided that it is still fit to eat and that customers realize it may not be of its normal quality.

Source: Based on an illustration in *Food for Thought*, Health Education Council.

have been used. Processed products often contain a surprising list of ingredients; sugar and fat are often at the top of the list in products where you thought you were getting something else. You may not want to buy some of the products in your cupboard again.

The illustration shows the basic information that must be given on the label or packet, but there are further regulations governing the information given.

Name

The name of the food may be covered by a legal definition in food regulations; examples are wholemeal bread (see p. 163), orange juice or yoghurt. Other foods may have a customary name for which there is no legal definition, for example muesli, pizza or Chelsea buns. If there is no prescribed or customary name the label must give a descriptive name distinguishing it from similar products. For example, malted milk drink as opposed to chocolate milk drink. Trade, brand or fancy names cannot be used in place of the actual name of the food. The name must also indicate any treatment that the food has undergone – for example, it should state if it is dried, frozen or smoked.

Misleading names

The names must not mislead the shopper. This applies especially to flavourings, and the law can be especially confusing here. For example, a yoghurt can only be named as 'strawberry' or 'strawberry-flavoured', or have a picture of strawberries on the lid or pot, if the flavour comes mainly from real strawberries. If it comes from flavouring it must be labelled 'strawberry flavour'.

This applies to other foods too. They can only have the name of the food in the title or description if the flavour comes mainly from that ingredient. Otherwise they must say 'flavour'; so 'cheese biscuit' or 'cheese-flavoured biscuit' will mean that the flavour comes mainly from real cheese. A 'cheese-flavour' biscuit will mean that the flavour is not mainly or wholly from cheese, but from some artificially created flavour.

Market research and polls have confirmed that most shoppers are not aware of such subtle distinctions; shoppers may, without realizing it, be sold products that do not contain the ingredients for which they bought them. The law which is designed to prevent consumers being mislead is in fact helping manufacturers to mislead them.

Datemark

The way in which the product is stored will determine how long it will keep. It is not illegal to sell food after its 'sell by' date, so long as it is still fit for human consumption and the shopper is told that the datemark has expired; often perishable goods are marked 'reduced for quick sale' when they reach expiry date. These are not always a good buy, however, because their nutritional value will probably have deteriorated, and you will not be getting good food value for your money.

There has been some criticism of the present system of datemarks; the *Egon Ronay Lucas Guide 1986 to Hotels, Restaurants, and Inns in Great Britain and Ireland,* for example, has called for a statutory date-stamping system, showing the actual freshness of food in addition to its supermarket 'sell-by' date. The *Guide* calls for a 'better, more foolproof, statutory date-stamping system of all fresh food. Our labelling laws should insist that the public is told more about freshness.'

In many cases the words 'best before' have taken over from the previous voluntary use of a 'sell by' date. The 'best before' is compulsory and it states that the words should be followed by the day, month and year up to which the food will be fresh. For foods that will be fresh for three months or less the date can be day and month only, and for those which are fresh for more than three months the month and year only need be given. For more perish-

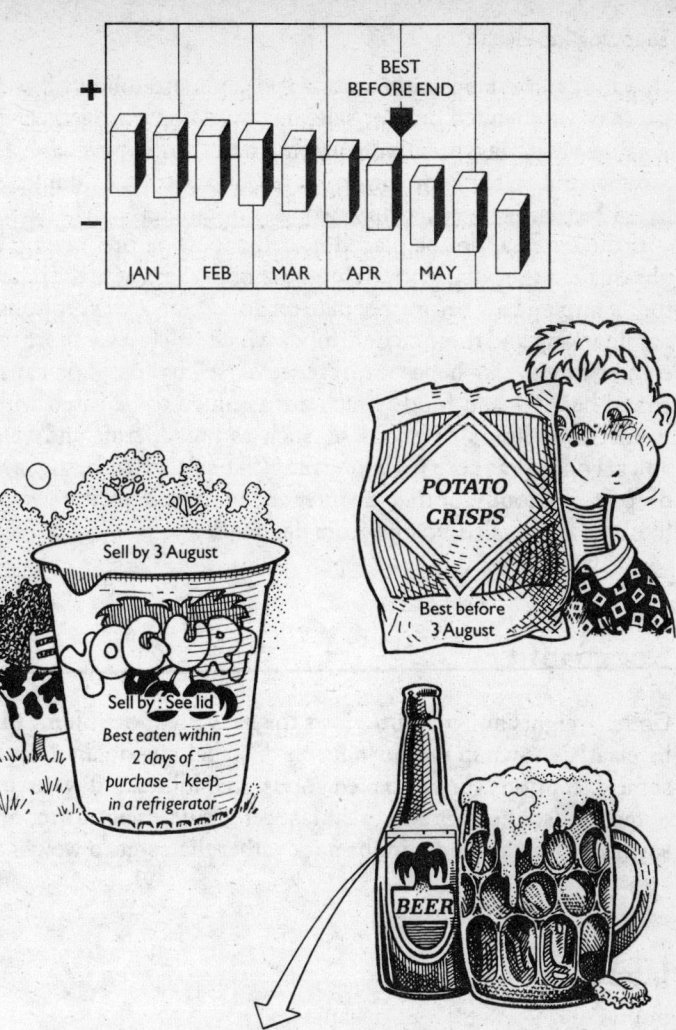

Source: Ministry of Agriculture Fisheries and Food, *Look at the Label,* HMSO.

Datemarks on Foods

able foods, the label must state a 'sell by' date followed by the latest recommended date of sale, day and month, together with the number of days the food will remain fresh after purchase. This is often seen on packs of yoghurt or ready meals; for example, 'sell by 14 November – eat within two days of purchase'.

If the date cannot be placed near the 'best before' or 'sell by' phrase then the pack has to refer the shopper to where the date is; for example, 'best before: see date on lid.' There are exceptions to datemarking and these include foods which will last for more than eighteen months – hence the absence of 'sell by' dates on cans of baked beans – and foods which are assumed to be eaten within twenty-four hours of purchase, such as bread, fruit and vegetables. Foods that keep for a long time, like salt, vinegar, sugar and deep-frozen foods, or that are intended to ripen in their packages, like cheese, are also exempt from datemarks.

Net quantity

Under weights and measures laws the net weight or volume must be clearly shown in metric units on the label, but again there are some exceptions such as baked goods, iced lollies and water ices. Some foods, like eggs and breakfast cereals in biscuit form, must say how many there are in the pack rather than state a weight.

Instructions for use

If a food needs special cooking instructions these must be given so that the 'appropriate use' can be made of the food. The pack must make it clear if ingredients other than water need to be added; for example, with rissole and burger mixes an egg is sometimes required. Cake mixes also need instructions, as do boil-in-the-bag foods which would be spoiled if they were taken out of the bag and fried.

Ingredients

For the health-conscious shopper this is probably the most important part of any label, because it is here that the food additives and the nutritional value of the product will be discovered. The ingredients must be listed in descending order of weight of what went into the foods. Most prepacked foods have contained a list of ingredients expressed in this way for some time and many people hoped that when the Food Labelling Regulations 1984 came into force, fuller information would be required (see p. 44). Added water must also be shown if it is more than 5 per cent of the weight of the finished product. However, frozen and deep-frozen poultry which comply with the EEC limits on water content do not have to declare added water on the label. The names given to the ingredients are covered by regulations, and the cases where it is necessary to be specific; for example, it is not enough to say 'fat', the label must also state 'animal' or 'vegetable' fat. Similarly oil must state whether it is animal or vegetable, and/or hydrogenated. (More about fat under 'Nutritional Labelling', p. 42.)

If manufacturers want to draw attention to special ingredients, the label may only state the minimum percentage contained in the food. Similarly, if emphasis is placed on the low or high content of the particular ingredient, such as polyunsaturates in margarine, the label must declare the minimum or maximum percentage to be found in the food. (See claims about polyunsaturates under the heading 'Nutritional Claims', p. 40.)

The missing additives

There are some ingredients which need not be named on labels and this is another area where the labelling regulations could mislead the shopper into thinking that a product is free from additives when traces might in fact remain. For example, an additive may be present because it was used to process a food, or sulphur dioxide might be used to preserve fruit which has been used to make jam. The maker of the jam would state on his ingredients panel that the jam contained fruit, but he would not

Shopping for Health

have to state that the fruit he used to make the jam contained sulphur dioxide. Similarly, although a lot of dried fruit is used in the baking and confectionery trades, baked goods do not have to state that the dried fruit used was sulphured. Other preservatives, apart from sulphur dioxide, may also be undeclared in food when used in the same way. Flour may contain many additives put in by the miller, but the ingredients panel of a cake made from the flour would list only the flour. And additives that are used as a solvent or carrier for another additive (for example, oils used to carry vitamins) can also remain undeclared on the label, as can a category of additives called processing aids (see p. 56).

Exemptions

If you have ever wondered why some foods do not contain a list of ingredients, it is probably because the law allows some exemptions where the ingredients need not be named. These include:

fresh fruit and vegetables
sparkling water
vinegar made by fermentation from one basic product without any other added ingredient
butter, fermented milk (i.e. yoghurt, buttermilk and smetana) and cream to which only lactic cultures and enzymes have been added
cheese (other than fresh, curd or processed) where only the amount of salt needed for manufacture is added
flavourings, because these are not yet covered by law (see pp. 53, 75)
single-ingredient foods, like flour, which includes nothing but the ingredients allowed by the Bread and Flour Regulations (see 'What the Labels Don't Say', p. 37)
alcoholic drinks of more than 1.2 per cent strength.

Although manufacturers and shops do not have to give the ingredients of these foods, if they do decide to provide an ingredients panels, they must comply with the general labelling regulations.

There are other groups of food that need only be labelled with their name and the broad category of any additives they contain.

Looking at Food Labels

These are unwrapped food, made and wrapped on the premises, or baked goods in crimp cases or transparent wrapping; these need only carry the name and indicate if they contain antioxidants, artificial sweeteners, colours, flavourings, flavour enhancers or preservatives.

Unwrapped bread and cakes and pastries, etc., and meat need not be labelled at all, but if the additives named above are used, there must be some sign in the shop to say that they are used. This can often be seen in butchers' shops, where notices state that artificial colourings, preservatives, etc., are used to make their sausages.

Other foods, such as sandwiches, rolls and hot food for immediate consumption, prepared meals and food from vending machines, can be either labelled with the name or go unmarked if a notice near the point of sale gives the name of the food. Food in miniature packs are also exempt from all except a 'best by' date and name.

Alcoholic drinks are also exempt from having to list their ingredients and thus any additives they may contain. In America consumers' groups are fighting for the compulsory introduction of ingredients listing in wine, beer and spirits. So far they have only won mandatory disclosure of sulphur additives, saccharin and tartrazine (E102), because the government agrees these may pose a health hazard. In Britain additives in wine are controlled by the EEC, which allows about twenty additives to be used and about fifteen substances to treat wine (i.e. to clarify it, etc.), but these substances do not have to be declared on the label.

In Britain there are no compositional regulations for beer and no specific laws on labelling; it is covered by general laws such as Preservatives in Food and Arsenic in Food regulations and other laws that state food and drink should be fit for human consumption. Similarly there are no specific laws about what may or may not be used in spirits or in liqueurs and vermouths, etc.; proposals before the EEC deal only with controlling type and strength of alcohol, flavourings and colourings. And there is resistance from the wine and liquor trade to the introduction of ingredients listing on the grounds that it would give away secret recipes and make the drinking public less enamoured of their favourite wines and beers, which are still enjoying a 'natural image'.

Nutritional claims

In July 1986, claims about vitamin content, fats, baby foods and low-calorie foods came under stricter food-labelling controls than previously. Restrictions on claims about vitamins have come in for some criticism, especially from the health-food trade, because the labelling laws allow claims to be made for 'scheduled' vitamins only. These are, at present: vitamins A, B_1, B_2, B_3, folic acid (a member of the B vitamin group), B_{12}, C and D. They are vitamins that the government considers may be deficient in the national diet. Foods that claim to be high in these vitamins must contain a least *half* the recommended daily amount (as recommended by the government, but these figures are also criticized by some as being too low). Foods that make general claims about their vitamin content must name the vitamin and can do so only if the food can reasonably provide *one sixth* of the daily requirement, 'reasonably' being interpreted to mean in one portion or serving or the amount normally eaten in one day.

The health-food industry and some nutritionists and doctors believe that other vitamins, especially vitamin B_6 and vitamin E, and the minerals selenium and zinc, should also be included as 'scheduled' vitamins, as they are either deficient in our diet, or are destroyed or our need for them increased by medications such as the contraceptive pill.

Other changes in the food-labelling laws which were brought into effect on July 1986 covered a ban on claims that a food is good for health because it contains polyunsaturated fatty acids or because of its low level of cholesterol. The claims 'low in saturates' and 'low in saturated fatty acids' now have to be accompanied by a label giving information about the amount of fat or oil in the food and the amount of polyunsaturated and saturated fatty acids.

Claims about *polyunsaturates* will only be allowed if the product contains at least 35 per cent fat by weight and at least 45 per cent of that is polyunsaturated; not more than 25 per cent may be saturated. Foods claiming to be *low in cholesterol* will have to comply with the standards for polyunsaturated foods and must contain as little as 0.005 per cent cholesterol. The lettering on the label making cholesterol claims must not be larger than the lettering making claims about polyunsaturates.

In slimmers' foods, a *reduced-calorie* claim can only be made where the food has not more than 75 per cent of the calories of similar food for which no claim is being made. A *low-calorie* food has to be a product where a 3½–4 oz (100 g) serving contains not more than 40 calories.

Foods that claim to be *high in protein* must contain at least 12 g of protein in a 'quantity of food that can reasonably be expected to be consumed in one day'.

Foods claiming to be *specially for diabetics* must contain no more calories and fat than similar non-diabetic food and they must also have only half the 'readily available carbohydrates' of similar non-diabetic food. Diabetic foods with more than 50 per cent of the readily absorbable carbohydrates of normal comparable foods must carry a statement that they are not suitable for overweight diabetics.

Claims that *food specifically for babies* are better than or as good as mother's milk have been banned under the Food Labelling Regulations 1984.

Manufacturers also make claims relating to what is *not* in their products. For example, an increasing number of canned foods proclaim 'no added sugar' on their labels, or 'no preservatives'. While this is a welcome move and good news, it is still worth reading the small print on the ingredients panel, as the product may still contain some other additives; for example, 'no preservatives' cans often contain colourings or flavourings.

Nutritional labelling

Despite the recent changes in food labelling as a result of the Food Labelling Regulations 1984, many people still think that the regulations do not go far enough in ensuring that we have all the information we need to make informed choices when shopping.

The NACNE Report, 1983, called for more detailed food labels which would make us more aware of what we are eating and make it easier to select foods that are low in fat, salt and sugar, and higher in fibre.

Clearer labelling on fats is on the way

Fat in particular was singled out by the COMA *Report on Diet and Cardiovascular Disease*, 1984, which recommended that shoppers should be told the percentage by weight of saturated, polyunsaturated or trans fatty acids found in high-fat foods like meat, milk, cakes, etc. COMA's recommendations for food processors and manufacturers, caterers and distributors were:

> The percentage by weight of fat and of saturated, polyunsaturated and trans fatty acids in butter, margarine, cooking fats and edible oils should be printed on the container or wrapping in which they are sold. Consideration should be given to providing *in addition* [my italics – J.M.] uniform and more simple labelling codes to enable the general public to distinguish easily between fats and oil with low or high contents of saturated fatty acids.

The COMA Report also said the same information should be given on all other foods with a fat content of more than 10 per cent by weight, or on foods that contribute a major proportion of our fat intake. If there is no food label, where food is not prepacked, the information should be displayed prominently at the point of sale. 'The foods in this category are mainly meats and meat products, milk and cream, cheese and cakes and biscuits. Equally, caterers should provide similar information in appropriate ways.'

The British government has accepted the need to cut down on fat in our diet to stem the epidemic of heart disease. The Joint

Committee on Nutrition Education (JACNE) was set up to translate the COMA findings into practical guidelines and everyday language, and has since produced a booklet, *Eating for a Healthier Heart*. In addition, the government has stated that fat-content labelling is to become statutory. Foods which make a significant contribution to fat in the diet, including butter, margarine and other spreads, cooking fats and oils, will be labelled. The saturated fat content and the trans fatty acid content will be given as a combined figure. (Trans fatty acids have the same effect in the body as saturated fats.) Both packaged and loose foods will be covered by the new law, but foods wrapped in individual servings will not, because there would not be enough room on the labels.

The government also plans to have discussions with the catering trade to find practical ways in which they can give information about the fat in food. A voluntary code is likely to be drawn up for restaurants, so that customers can tell how much fat is in various dishes.

Foods such as fruit and vegetables, cereals, bread and flour which do not make much fat contribution to the diet will not be affected by the new law.

Guidelines are also being drawn up to ensure that the nutritional information on labelling is given in a standard format. From the shopper's point of view, nutritional labelling at the moment can be very confusing because each manufacturer displays nutritional information in a different way. Many manufacturers and supermarket or high-street chains have given up waiting for the government's 'imminent' report and have committed themselves to full-scale nutritional labelling to their own designs.

There are many other interests at work, too. For example, the Dairy Trade Federation drew up a voluntary code on nutritional labelling, before the government announced theirs. Cynics would say this was a PR job, as the code suggests giving nutritional information along the following lines:

Shopping for Health

NUTRITIONAL INFORMATION
Average per 100 g of product

kilocalories	xxx
kilojoules	xxx
protein	xx g
fat	xx g
carbohydrate	xx g

This, obviously, would suit the dairy industry because it avoids the breakdown of fats into saturated, unsaturated, polyunsaturated or trans fatty acids.

The government's proposals recommend listing the nutrients in the following order:

> energy
> protein
> carbohydrate
> fat (with types identified)

followed by vitamins and minerals. Information would be given per 100 g or 100 ml and if the pack is for consumption by one person at a sitting that information is also recommended for inclusion. The first group of the big four 'macro nutrients' would be compulsory and the vitamins and minerals would be optional. The information would be given in a tabular form if there is enough space on the label.

What sort of labelling does the shopper want?

But what about the shopper? Research into consumer attitudes towards the understanding of nutrition and nutrition-labelling sponsored by the Ministry of Agriculture and undertaken by the National Consumer Council and the Consumers' Association show that shoppers are not satisfied with labels that just give information on fats or the 'big four'. Neither did they want labelling that told them what to eat or what not to eat.

The Consumers' Association says,

Looking at Food Labels

We don't think these proposals go far enough. Our survey on labelling showed a strong demand for nutrition information (nine out of ten people said they though nutrition labelling would be very or quite useful for themselves, their households or other people).

If nutrition labelling is really to serve its purpose, it should enable you to make sensible choices and ensure that what you lose in one area of your diet you gain in another. This means full nutrition labelling.

The people interviewed wanted labelling that gave information in plain, simple terms; they were put off by labels which contained unfamiliar technical terms – 'calories' was preferred to kilocalories or kilojoules. Practical labels with bar charts and pictorial devices were preferred because the information could then be seen at a glance. When shown these examples of nutritional labelling (see p. 46), the most popular was format B which 77 per cent of people thought others would find very or quite easy to understand. Next came E (68 per cent), D (60 per cent) and F (57 per cent); less than half thought A (47 per cent) and C (44 per cent) easy to understand. After they had actually used the labels, however, the selection was slightly different, with the first two choices still being B followed by E, and then C, followed by D, F and A in that order.

People in the survey were then given practical tests on identifying certain specific information from the labels and performing simple calculations using the labels. In these they performed best on E, followed by D, B and A in that order, and least well on C and F.

All of these examples give the information per 100 g, but how many people have a concept of 100 g of each food? Even though we have been metricated for some years there are still a great many people who could not even guess what 100 g of cornflakes or baked beans look like, and the situation may not improve because some school cookery classes still use imperial weights.

The information could be given in percentages, but if your cereal packet states 'dietary fibre 9.6 per cent' are you any the wiser as to how much fibre is in the bowl of cereal you eat for breakfast? Unless food is packed in 100 g packages we are not going to be able to work it out.

Shopping for Health

A

Nutrition information
100 grams of this product contain:
1579 kilojoules/375 kilocalories

27.0 g fat of which: 10.0 g are saturates
                    3.1 g are polyunsaturates

24.9 g carbohydrate
 9.8 g protein

B

Nutrition information
100 grams of this product contain

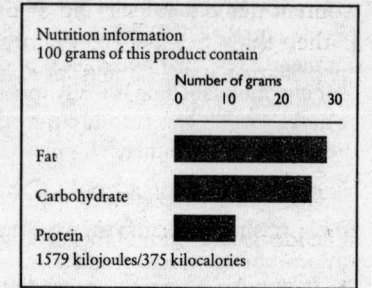

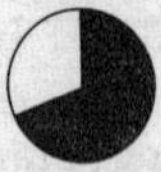

Number of grams
0   10   20   30

Fat

Carbohydrate

Protein

1579 kilojoules/375 kilocalories

C

Nutrition information
100 grams of this product contain:
1579 kilojoules/375 kilocalories

Fat		27.0 g
of which polyunsaturates	3.1 g	
and saturates	10.0 g	
Carbohydrate		24.9 g
of which sugars	0.0 g	
Protein		9.8 g
Dietary fibre		0.0 g
Salt		1.9 g

65% of calories from fat

D

Nutrition information
100 grams of this product contain:

Energy	1579 kJ/375 cal
Protein	9.8 g
Carbohydrate	24.9 g
Fat	27.0 g
(of which saturated fatty acids 10.0 g)	

E

Nutrition information
100 grams of this product contain:

27.0 g of fat	HIGH
of which 10.0 g are saturates	MEDIUM
3.1 g are poly unsaturates	MEDIUM
24.9 g of carboyhydrate	MEDIUM
9.8 g of protein	MEDIUM
1579 kilojoules/375 kilocalories	HIGH

F

Nutrition information

100 grams of this product contain:
1579 kilojoules/375 kilocalories: 27.0 g of fat:
24.9 g of carbohydrates: 9.8 g of protein

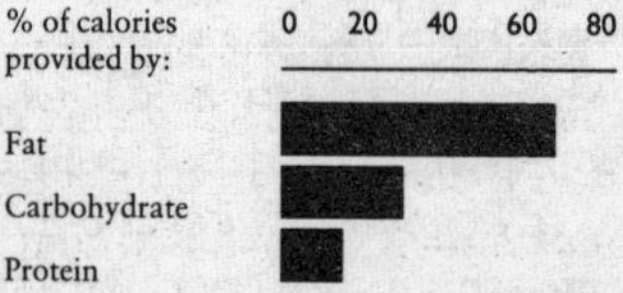

% of calories provided by:
0   20   40   60   80

Fat

Carbohydrate

Protein

Source: *Consumer Attitudes to and Understanding of Nutritional Labelling*, Consumers' Association/MAFF/National Consumers' Council.

Looking at Food Labels

It would be more useful if manufacturers stated the nutritional content per typical serving or portion; per biscuit, for example, rather than per packet of biscuits. Giving all the nutritional information (not only fat) per serving would make more sense.

The ideal nutritional label

The ideal nutritional label would give the following information.

- It would list all the ingredients, giving the percentage of the total weight.
- It would name each type of fat used, with its percentage content – not just state 'animal fat' or 'vegetable fat'.
- It would categorize additives by their function, followed by their E number, e.g. 'stabilizer (E412)'.
- It would give an at-a-glance nutritional guide, based on a nationally recognized symbol system. In the illustration on p. 48, filled squares indicate that a food is high in calories, fats, sodium or sugar; half-filled squares show that it contains a moderate amount of these substances and empty squares a low amount.
- The total number of calories and the amount of fats (saturated and unsaturated), sugars, sodium and fibre per portion or average serving, would be indicated.

Putting all this information together we would come up with something like the fictitious example illustrated on p. 48.

Research among shoppers has shown that there is mounting concern about the contents of our food. A Bradford University Food Policy Research briefing paper, *Who is Shaping the Nutritional Label?*, concluded that shoppers are 'switching to brands, and strengthening their allegiance to brands, providing a level of nutritional labelling which permits the selection of foods for a healthy diet'. The implication for those companies which fail to respond to the demand for better labelling, says the paper, is a fall in their share in the increasingly competitive food market.

Chocolate Cream Biscuits

Ingredients (% of total weight): animal fat 20%, wheat sugar 18%, hydrogenated vegetable fats 16% (soya oil 10%, palm kernel oil 6%), wheat flour 18%, whey powder 10%, glucose syrup 10%, fat-reduced cocoa 4%, cornflour 3%, modified starch 3%. Ingredients less than 1%: salt, colours (107, E150), antioxidant (E320), gelling agent (E413), flavourings.

Nutritional information per biscuit

Energy	85 cal	■
Fats: saturated	10.8 g	■
unsaturated	trace	☐
Sugars	6.7 g	■
Sodium	150 mg	◪
Fibre	0.2 g	☐

Warning: this product contains the following additives that may be harmful to your health: colours 107 (Yellow 2G), E150 (Caramel)*

Currently subject to safety review.

3. Finding Out about Food Additives

What is an additive?

Food additives are usually thought of as synthetic chemicals. They have also been described as anything added to food that has no nutritional value, but the term may also apply to vitamins and minerals added to enrich food.

It is probably more accurate to define a food additive as something that is not naturally (or normally) present in the food to which it is added. It can be substance of natural or synthetic origin. Some additives are synthetic items made from natural 'starters'. For example amidated pectin is pectin from citrus fruits or apples that has been treated with ammonium under alkali conditions to give 'mainly esters and amides ... and their ammonium, sodium, potassium and calcium salts', according to the British Food Manufacturers Industrial Research Association.

There is no legal definition of a food additive, apart from one in the Labelling Regulations 1980 which applies to labelling only, but the Food and Drugs Act 1955 makes it clear that additives are 'foods', although we would not normally think of them as such. Probably most people regard them as substances, either natural or synthetic, that are put in food for purposes other than nutrition – to preserve food or make it more attractive.

Shopping for Health

What are the functions of additives?

There are between 3,500 and 3,800 additives in use in Britain and they range from the well-understood preservatives to the more obscure items like mordants. Many categories are self-explanatory, but any one additive may perform several functions at once. Generally, they can be put into four broad categories: preservatives, texture modifiers, colours and flavours, and processing aids. A more detailed breakdown is shown in the table.

Categories of Additives

Category	Sub-group	Approximate number of additives in group
Preservatives	preservatives	43
	antioxidants	13
	sequestrants	7
		63
Texture modifiers	emulsifiers, stabilizers, thickeners	65
	others	5
		70
Colours and flavours	flavours	3,200+
	colours	34
	flavour enhancers	7
	sweeteners	13
		3,254
Processing aids	total	91
	TOTAL	3,478

Source: Melanie Millar, *Danger! Additives at Work*, London Food Commission.

These broad categories can be divided into the more familiar groups and names that we see on labels listing ingredients, or they may be more familiar to us by their E numbers (more about these

Finding Out about Food Additives

later). For those who want to know more about what these additives are *doing* in their food, here is an A–Z of additives and their functions.

Acids

Acids are used to give food sharpness or to free carbon dioxide gas in raising agents or to adjust acidity. They can also be used to dissolve food colours or as a preservative.

The most commonly used is citric acid, vitamin C, which is prepared commercially by the fermentation of molasses, but is found naturally in citrus fruit.

Anti-caking agents

These are added to food to prevent particles sticking together; they are found in products like table salt.

Anti-foaming agents

These help to prevent liquids boiling over during food processing by breaking down foams; they also reduce formation of scum.

Antioxidants

The chemical process of oxidation, which turns fats and oils rancid on contact with the air (oxygen) and destroys vitamins when they are exposed to the air after fruit and vegetables have been cut, can be slowed down by antioxidants. They prevent colour and flavour loss, thus protecting the taste and appearance of foods. Antioxidants include some of the most suspect additives, although some are innocent substances like vitamin E. Manufacturing processes such as vacuum packing serve the same purpose – but antioxidants are cheaper than expensive machinery and packing.

Shopping for Health

Bases

These have the opposite effect to acids – they lower acidity and increase alkalinity of foods. Like acids, they can also be used to dissolve colourings or react with acids to produce raising agents.

Bleaching and improving agents

Bleaches speed up the maturing of flour artificially, thus making bread dough quicker to process. They are added to flour and used in bread-, biscuit- and cake-baking.

Bulking aids

These give extra bulk to food and are commonly used in slimmers' foods to give substance without calories. They are made from plant fibres.

Colourings

Colours may be natural or artificial. Most artificial colours derive from coal tar or are azo dyes and were originally used to dye fabric. They are much cheaper than natural colours and are sold to food manufacturers ready mixed and under brand names. The majority of colours used in Britain are artificial colours. They are among the most suspect of food additives and, being entirely cosmetic, are considered by many to be the most easily dispensable.

Concentrates

Concentrates are ready-mixed blends of additives usually sold to a food manufacturer for a particular type of food product. They are not specifically covered by food regulations, and any permitted combination of additive may be used.

Emulsifiers and stabilizers

An emulsion is a mixture of oil and water – two substances that, under normal conditions, would not mix, but in the presence of an emulsifier they will. The emulsifiers bind or blend the oil-and-water-type mixtures and the stabilizers ensure that they do not separate out. Natural gums, lecithins and chemical food additives fall into this category.

Excipients

These are 'carriers' for other powdered additives, making them easier to handle. They occur in concentrates and can carry colours, flavours and preservatives in other foods.

Firming and crisping agents

These work by maintaining water pressure inside the cells of fruit and vegetables, stopping the cells collapsing.

Flavour enhancers

These intensify the flavour of other foods by stimulating the taste buds. The most common one is monosodium glutamate, often found in sauces, stocks, snack foods, canned products, packet and convenience foods. MSG can provoke allergic reactions.

Flavourings

This is the largest group of food additives. They are not covered by any permitted list or regulatory control other than the general provisions of the Food and Drugs Act. Flavours are often used as substitutes for the real ingredient because they are cheaper. Both natural and artificial flavours are in use and ingredients listing of synthetic flavours can be very complicated because they contain many chemicals. Natural flavours are also complicated substances, often containing more than hundred chemicals.

Shopping for Health

Freezants

These gases or liquids remove heat from foods, freezing them on contact. Liquified nitrogen is used to freeze fruit.

Glazing agents

Usually waxes and oils that give food such as dried fruit a shiny appearance and sometimes help preserve food.

Humectants

These prevent food drying out by holding moisture in the food.

Preservatives

These are added to food to slow down the natural process of decay caused by micro-organisms like bacteria, fungi and yeasts. Because some decay organisms contain or produce substances poisonous to humans, food processors claim this group of additives is essential; nevertheless, they are probably hazardous to man because they have to be toxic to the spoilage micro-organisms.

Propellants

These are gases or liquids used to expel foods from aerosol containers.

Release agents

Usually greases or powders which are used to stop food sticking to packaging, moulds, tins or machinery used in food processing.

Sequestrants

Sequestrants are substances that bind with trace metals, the presence of which speeds up the process of oxidation (see anti-oxidants), so slowing down the degeneration of fats and oils and other foods that are subject to oxidation.

Solvents

Solvents can be used to put things in food, or take them out. They can 'carry' flavours, colours and emulsifiers into food, or they can be used to extract substances like caffeine in the decaffeination of coffee by chemical-solvent methods. Regulations specifically to control them are pending; they are under investigation by the EEC and the UK's Food Advisory Committee.

Artificial sweeteners

Commonly used in slimmers' products because they have intense sweetness without calories. Saccharin, derived from coal tars, is the most common. More recently introduced sweeteners like Aspartame, produced from a combination of amino acids, are more 'natural'.

Thickeners

As the name suggests they thicken the texture of food; most are starches, gums and celluloses. In thickening food, they also stabilize it.

E numbers

When additives are used in food they must be declared on the ingredients panel on the label. All food products sold in Britain now (since July 1986) have to carry a description of ingredients, including the category of any food additive (e.g. preservative), and the E number (e.g. E220) or the name (e.g. sulphur dioxide). Some

Shopping for Health

additives used in Britain do not have an E number because they are not permitted for use by other EEC countries, so these substances will be described by category and name. Flavourings are not yet controlled by food regulations, other than by the general provisions of the Food and Drugs Act, and have not been given E numbers.

E numbers provide an international language for commonly used food additives and an economic way of labelling products.

E numbers start at E100 and continue to E483. There are gaps in the sequence to allow for new additives to be introduced, so the list can grow at various points. Numbers without an E indicate additives which are not permitted in other EEC countries. Generally they are arranged in major groups:

E100–E180   food colourings
E200–297   preservatives
E300–E321   antioxidants
E322–495   emulsifiers, stabilizers and thickeners (synthetic sweeteners appear in this group from E420 to 436)
500–529   acids, bases and others
530–578   anti-caking agents and others
620–637   flavour enhancers and sweeteners
900–907   glazing agents and others
920–927   improving and bleaching agents
928–   sweeteners, solvents, miscellaneous

Although most additives fit into these main categories, there are miscellaneous additives interspersed in each group; some additives can do more than one job, depending on the food in which they are used. Flavourings are not seen in the listing of E numbers because they are not yet regulated in that way. Some other additives will not be mentioned on food ingredients panels *because they are not used as additives*, but are used in processing food, although there may still be traces of them in food as residues of the manufacturing process. Examples are liquids used for contact freezing substances to stop food sticking to packaging and machinery and 'carriers' of added vitamins or minerals. The 'adjuncts' (or processing aids) used in brewing beer also go unlabelled and unlisted, as do all the additives and ingredients in alcoholic drinks.

Who controls food additives?

The Food and Drugs Act 1955 and its amendments, including the 1984 Food Act, which makes it an offence to sell or advertise 'any food rendered injurious to health by means of any operation' (including the use of food additives), is designed to make sure that the food we are presented with on the shop shelves is fit for human consumption and of the quality we demand. It covers all aspects of food from the manufacturing process to hygiene in the places where food is prepared and processed, and where it is sold. It also covers the rules laid down for the composition of foods, so it directly controls how much fruit, for example, goes into jam and how much of certain additives are permitted, although not all are subject to quantity control – much depends on 'good manufacturing practice'. The Food Labelling Regulations 1984 state that all additives must be individually identified by category and/or E number, except those which have no technological function, such as the processing aids just mentioned.

To help advise Ministers on food regulations the Food Standards Committee was set up in 1947 and the Food Additives and Contaminants Committee was established in 1965. In 1983 these were combined to form the Food Advisory Committee, which advises the Ministry of Agriculture, Fisheries and Food on matters relating to food additives.

Under this committee sits the one directly involved in additives, the DHSS Committee on Toxicity of Chemicals in Food, which also advises the Chief Medical Officer and the Committee on the Medical Aspects of Food Policy (COMA) on what is safe, as well as reporting back to the Food Advisory Committee. The Food Safety Research Committee was set up in September 1984 to advise on research and development needs relating to food safety.

Shopping for Health

Their reports form the bases of decision on whether additives are permitted or not.

The Food Safety Research Committee has identified the testing of food additives as an area needing more research, and has also called for more research into the effect of additives on allergies and for a review of the use of colourings in food. The FSRC has told the Priorities Board – which was set up to advise the UK Agriculture and Food Research Council on priority areas for food and agricultural research – that additives should be a priority for research.

The EEC also has a say in food additives and it is to the EEC that we owe the introduction of E numbers. Food regulations now have to take account of EEC regulations and directives, but UK food legislation does not always incorporate EEC requirements. Instead of cutting the number of food additives it uses, to conform with EEC regulations, the UK government won, through long court battles, exemption from food additive bans, so long as it does not export to the other EEC countries food containing additives which are banned there.

However, the Single European Act, which is commonly known as 'Harmonization' and is expected to be agreed by the British parliament in 1987, aims to set common standards for all member states, so that foods made in one country may be sold in another. The danger is that to gain consensus there may be a lowering of standards, with minimum regard to food health and safety.

The World Health Organization (WHO) and the Food and Agriculture Organization (FAO) also have a joint committee (JECFA) which advises on tolerable levels of additives in daily food intake (ADI). JECFA's reports are of most use to countries which do not have the resources for toxicological testing of additives, and Britain is free to accept or ignore JECFA reports and advice as it pleases.

Unintentional additives

Some substances find their way into food unintentionally. For instance, drugs and chemicals are given to animals being reared for meat and fish being grown on fish farms.

Farmers are paid by weight for the meat they produce. To put weight on the animal must eat, and foodstuff is expensive; so the farmer wants to use the system that is going to fatten his animals fastest, which usually means giving them feed concentrates – and it is very difficult to find a feed today that does not contain drugs.

It was first realized that antibiotics accelerated animal growth in the 1950s. Penicillin, chlortetracycline, oxytetracycline and tylosin were fed to animals until they were banned after the Swann Report in 1969, which showed that these antibiotics were becoming less effective in combating disease in humans; the bacteria which the drugs were supposed to kill were becoming resistant because of the continual low doses people were receiving in their food. Surveys showed that, at that time, 70 per cent of staphyloccoci in hospital patients were resistant to penicillin.

Antibiotics can still be used in animal feedstuff for young animals, but not the same antibiotics that are used in medicine for humans. However, recent investigative reports have suggested that antibiotics which should be reserved for medicinal use are still being used on the farm in drugs. The danger is that there will be no antibiotics which are effective in emergencies, because their routine use in animal feedstuffs used in the production of meat results in the bacteria developing resistance to them.

Feed for mature ruminants does not include antibiotics because they would kill the bacteria in the gut on which the animal's digestion relies, but it does contain other drugs, some designed to modify the digestive process so that the amount of methane produced during digestion is reduced and the animal puts on more weight. Hormones and anabolic steroids are used in animal feed to promote growth too, and animals may be given oestrogen, progesterone or thyroxine (the thyroid hormone) to encourage weight gain.

Shopping for Health

Modern methods of farming mean that the stock is bred by one farmer, who sells it to another to rear it – and it may then be sold to a third for fattening. It is easy to see how, in this situation, the animals may receive more than one hormone implant in their lifetime, which will be passed on to the butchers' customers. Neither hormones nor antibiotics should be administered for some time before slaughter, but contract farming makes it difficult to keep track of this. Checking for levels of antibiotics in meat at slaughterhouses is easier than checking for levels of hormones, because hormones are naturally present in the animal.*

In South America, in 1983, children developed sexual characteristics before puberty because of bad animal husbandry techniques resulting in excessive hormone levels (in poultry in particular).

The controversial additives BHA and BHT are used in animal feedstuff to prevent the destruction of vitamins A and E. Binders are used to make animal concentrate pellets and feed nuts, and colouring, flavouring and spices are added to give the food 'animal appeal'. (They can't be that effective because appetite stimulants are also allowed for animals!) Instead of grazing in meadows and pastures today's animals are fed synthetic proteins which are a byproduct of the petrol-refining industry – products that are not permitted in food for humans.

Milk suffers from the same problems as meat. Despite calls for stricter controls to stop antibiotics getting into milk, the Milk Marketing Boards tests take so long to come up with an answer that the milk has already been distributed by the time it has been discovered that it contains more than the permitted amount of antibiotic residue. Although it's too late from the consumer's point of view, the producer is paid less for it. Penicillin used to treat mastitis may also find its way into milk, causing problems for those allergic to it. Milk does not contain additives as such – but it can be affected by pesticide contamination, radioactive fallout and aflatoxin mould (from contaminated animal feedstuff).

---

* The health risks to humans from modern farming techniques are well documented in *Gluttons for Punishment* by James Erlichman (Penguin Books).

Finding Out about Food Additives

Animal feedstuff can also contain substances used to colour the flesh of fish pink and the yolks of eggs yellow (see pp. 80, 230). It is important to be aware of these if, for example, you are trying to deal with a hyperactive child – the colouring in egg yolks may be tartrazine, the yellow peril.

Shoppers and additives

Once you start taking an interest in food and your health you will find that shopping trips can turn into spot-the-additives outings! When you have become aware of additives they will leap out at you from the sides of packets in many weird and wonderful formulations. A lurid pack which does not illustrate any real food item is a good indication that the pack may contain an interesting collection of additives. Many shoppers will take new products from the shelves, willing to try them without too much thought of what they contain. However, shoppers are now becoming more wary of additives. Indeed it seems that concern about additives has caught the public imagination rather more than the campaign to promote healthier eating which was the subject of Chapter 1.

Do we care about additives?

A market-research report by the Food Policy Unit at Bradford University called *Does the Consumer Really Care?* (October 1985) supports this. It seemed that the people interviewed by the researchers did care about food additives.

'The negative attitude towards additives is clearly shown, with 91.7 per cent of the sample agreeing with the statement "If you can avoid preservatives then you might as well." Similarly 79.5 per cent of the respondents agreed with the statement, "I try to avoid food which contains additives, preservatives/colouring."' And in 1986 a Co-op survey into the most important factors avoided by shoppers in choosing food put additives at the top of the list, followed by preservatives, sugar, salt and fat. This appears to be quite a change of awareness, because in 1983 the Consumers' Association, publishers of *Which?*, found that only 38 per cent of respondents said they would not buy food because it contained additives.

The food industry might agree with the Bradford University hypothesis that 'The levels of apparent concern about the use of food additives appears to be linked with a lack of knowledge of various additives. The "image" of additives appears to be very poor.' The food industry itself actually fuels our fears, with its emphasis on 'natural' foods and its advertising campaigns which reiterate the popular belief that 'natural' foods are better for us. Manufacturer's decisions to market products on an 'additive-free', 'no preservatives', 'nothing added' ticket are reinforcing the negative attitudes to food additives.

There is, certainly, a deep-seated distrust of food that has been 'mucked about with'. It manifests itself in traditional and conservative eating patterns and a reluctance to change what we eat, even if it is harming us. It also manifests itself in our belief that natural is best and that all additives should be regarded with suspicion, although some are in fact 'natural' and harmless. There have even been spoof lists of 'dangerous' additives, such as the one purporting to be from a French hospital centre at Chousent, listing some additives which are actually safe, as 'cancerous', 'forbidden' and 'dangerous', while listing other safe ones as suspect, including vitamin C.

Is our fear justified?

Each year more and more common food additives come under suspicion of contributing to health problems as diverse as allergies and cancer. The 'wholefood' approach to healthy eating has always been that the right diet – one high in unprocessed and unrefined foods – combined with adequate rest and exercise, gives us the best chance of resisting disease, being healthy and making the most of our potential. Part of that approach includes avoiding cosmetic additives like colourings and flavourings. The presence of these food additives is a pretty good indication of 'junk food', food of lower nutritional value. When a food has to have preservatives to keep it fresh long after it would normally have gone off, and flavour enhancers, colourings and stabilizers to make it palatable, then the chances are that we would be nutritionally better off without it.

Are additives dressing up empty foods?

We have already seen that chocolate and sugar, confectionery, and cakes and pastries made from white flour are either 'empty' calories or pretty poor nutritional value for money. They give us only calories and rob the body of the vitamins and minerals which it needs. The same could be said of foods that consist of highly processed sugars, fats and starches made appealing with additives. Since 75−80 per cent of the food we eat today is processed, it obviously makes sense to review how much of your diet consists of these types of food.

For example, Birds Raspberry Flavour Trifle contains, according to its label:

Raspberry-flavour jelly crystals: sugar, gelling agents (carob gum, carrageen, E340, potassium chloride), adipic acid, acidity regulator (cream of tartar), flavourings, thickener (E466), artificial sweetener (soluble saccharin), colour (E123).

Raspberry-flavour custard powder: cornflour, salt, flavourings, colours (E124, E122).

Sponge, with preservative (E202), colours (E102, E110).

Decorations, with colours (E110, E132, E123, E127).

Trifle Topping Mix: palm-kernel and soya-bean oils (hydrogenated), sugar, emulsifiers (E477, lecithin), modified starch, whey powder, lactose, caseinate, thickener (E466), flavourings, antioxidant (E320), colour (beta-carotene).

Not all processed foods are that extreme, but there is a proliferation of novelty foods, especially packet foods, that offer little in the way of nutrition but a lot in what food manufacturers would call 'organoleptic experience' – that is colour, mouth feel and flavour.

In fact, 95 per cent of all food additives are organoleptic – they are cosmetic additions. At the extreme, they help to fool us into thinking we are eating good food when we are in fact getting a meal that is devoid of vitamins, minerals, fibre and all the other ingredients we need to keep us resilient against disease and feeling our best. Additives could, then, be contributing to the general malaise, the tiredness and listlessness that so many of us complain of. If that is the case, then we must ask who the additives are benefiting.

Who benefits?

A report on food additives and their control published by the London Food Commission states 'When the risks and benefits are analysed it becomes clear that the major benefits lie with the food industry and additive manufacturers.' More than £231m worth of food additives were bought in Britain by food manufacturers during 1984.

Improved profits result if expensive 'fresh' ingredients such as eggs in custard powder can be removed and replaced by a cheap chemical colouring and a thickener; if potatoes worth 1 p can be turned into potato crisps selling at 12 p; if the use of polyphosphates makes it possible to inject meat with water to increase its weight (*not* its food value).

Not only is the raw material sold at greater profit for the manufacturer, the makers of food additives and the makers of the sophisticated machinery used in food processing also benefit when food is 'mucked around with'. Mechanically recovered meat is a prime example of this. After the meat had been removed from the carcass, the dog used to get the bones, but not now. Now, a hydraulic or a centrifugal process can pressurize the meat off the carcass, producing a slurry of meat, connective tissue, sinew and

Finding Out about Food Additives

bone, which can also include intestines, lips, some hair and other previously unused parts of the carcass which, with a little help from texture improvers, colourings and flavourings can become 'meat' for use in sausages, meat pies and other meat products.

Practices like this are bound to polarize opinion. At one end, the food industry feels it is getting a bad press – that the media is giving the impression that the industry is using additives entirely for its own ends to maximize profits, without any regard for the consumers, who are acting as human guinea-pigs in a living experiment, the scale and scope of which has never before been seen – or allowed. At the other end the public thinks it not unreasonable to expect straight answers to questions such as 'If I eat sausages containing preservatives like nitrites and nitrates, what is going to happen to me? Will I get stomach cancer? How many can I eat before this happens? Or will I get asthma, or eczema, or an allergy from any of the other additives in my diet?'

Unfortunately, these questions cannot be answered with precision. Scientists can only deal in possibilities or probabilities, and even then, in the case of food additives, they are working with extrapolations of trials done on guinea-pigs or rats and making educated guesstimates about how this or that food additive will affect man (to say nothing of women and children, whose bodies are generally smaller and less able to cope with the same amount of a substance in food). We may want straight answers about the safety of additives in our food but we are a long way from getting them.

Who's looking after the shoppers' interests?

The government and the food industry encourage us to 'leave it to the experts'. We may, however, think that the implicit faith shown in the experts by many officials and members of government is foolhardy or lacking in responsibility to the people they represent. The government makes its decisions to permit or refuse the use of additives on the basis of information and scientific data provided by the food industry and given in secret at meetings which are covered by the Official Secrets Act. Companies' commercial interests are the reason for the secrecy – but what about us? Who is representing the interests of the consumer: on the relevant Food Advisory Committee there is one representative from the Consumers' Association, who is in a difficult position because the Association does no independent trials or assessments itself and so cannot give meaningful comments on the safety of additives.

An organization called FACT (Food Additives Campaign Team) has recently been launched with the aims of bringing food additives out of the realm of Official Secrets, reducing the number of additives used and tightening control on those in use. It hopes to represent the concern of all parties interested in food additives. Some MPs are backing FACT, as are trade unions and consumer organizations. (For a copy of the FACT manifesto write, enclosing a large sae, to Room W, 25 Horsell Road, London N5 1XL.)

Are safety tests good enough?

Most tests to determine if a proposed new additive is safe are done by the research laboratories of the company that wants to use the new substance, or in the labs of industrial organizations such as the British Industrial Biological Research Association (BIBRA). In America and Europe, governments conduct independent safety evaluations, where the emphasis is more on attempting to discover how the additive will affect humans, whereas British tests are designed to produce the animal test data needed to 'pass the test', so that the British government will allow a product to be used commercially.

In an article in *New Scientist*, Dr Erik Millstone,* lecturer in Science Studies at the University of Sussex, writes:

---

* Dr Millstone discusses the complex issue of food additives more thoroughly in his book *Food Additives* (Penguin Books).

Only recently has there been any attempt to establish a quantitative estimate of the correlation between toxicity tests within laboratory animals and human toxicology from chemicals that are believed to cause cancer. This analysis . . . suggests that the animal tests are successful in identifying carcinogens only some 37 per cent of the time. This means that the results of the tests are wrong more often than they are right, and that they are significantly worse than tossing a coin!

Yet regulations are determined by extrapolation from the results of animal tests. On account of possible differences between animals and humans and on account of differences within human populations, a safety factor of 100 is usually introduced between the no-effect-level in animals and the acceptable daily intake (ADI) for humans . . . There is, a however, wide-ranging disagreement on how to extrapolate from the results of tests on a small group of animals to a large group of human beings who do not live in laboratory conditions. There are at least twelve different competing statistical techniques for this extrapolation, and the results they produce may disagree by up to four orders of magnitude.

Additives (or drugs) cannot be tested on humans for ethical reasons: genetic changes could result or serious, irreversible illness such as cancer. Instead, laboratory trials are carried out on animals. These tests are conducted over a relatively short time, whereas man may consume additives over many years, making assumptions from tests on animals even more meaningless. In addition, good practice in laboratories has to be assumed – the results will be only as good as the staff.

Have all additives been tested?

There is, therefore, some concern over the adequacy of the tests. A cause for even more concern is the complete lack of testing of many additives. When the Food and Drugs Act, under which the use of additives is controlled, came into force in 1955 it was agreed to permit, *without testing*, many additives that had been in common use up to that time; subsequently many of these have come under suspicion and some have been banned in other countries.

Can additives interact in food?

Laboratory testing also fails to take into account what has become known as the 'cocktail effect'. For example, the ingredients panel of a typical soft drink, described as a 'whole orange drink', lists water, sugar, oranges, flavourings, citric acid, preservatives (E211, E223) artificial sweetener (saccharin), ascorbic acid (vitamin C), and the colours (E102, E110); faced with such a combination, we may well ask, 'Could any of these substances, harmless when taken by themselves, interact to create toxicity?'

It seems it is difficult enough to test one substance by itself, so tests to determine the interaction of additives in the human gut would be virtually impossible to undertake – and yet we are subjected daily to such cocktails in our food. The *Sunday Times* recently photographed four meals in a not-quite-typical day's eating and calculated the number of additives in each meal. The findings were:

Breakfast – fruit juice, muesli, bread, spread, milk and coffee – 53 additives;
Ploughman's lunch – bread, cheese, butter substitute, pickles, coleslaw, salami, pâté and brown ale – 42 additives;
High tea – burger, fishcake, peas, chips, packet cheesecake and cream, milk shake – 50 additives;
Dinner – canapés, smoked mackerel pâté and toast, chicken pie, salad and dessert of gâteau and wine – 72 additives.

This list does highlight the fact that even one meal can produce a surprisingly large harvest of additives. Testing their interaction would be virtually impossible. This example makes a nonsense of the government's guidelines on acceptable daily intake of additives (ADIs), where they exist. In one meal alone the acceptable intake of any one additive might be exceeded three or four times over – indeed, the consumer is not even told how much of each additive is used.

Finding Out about Food Additives

Can you prove that they have harmful effects?

A joint report of the Royal College of Physicians and the British Nutrition Foundation, *Food Intolerance and Food Aversion* (1984), says, 'Additives are widely used in the food industry to prevent microbial and chemical changes ... However, there seems to be a lack of evidence about the interaction between additives and the food itself, reaction which might occur during storage and give rise to substances capable of causing food intolerance.' The real worry, of course, is that they might produce something far worse than an allergic or intolerance reaction.

The amount of additives used has increased tenfold in the last thirty years. It is estimated that the average person now eats 8–11 lb (3.6–5 kg) of food additives a year; people who subsist almost entirely on additive-laden convenience foods will eat even more.

Despite rising concern about the increasing use of additives, it is difficult to prove in a scientific way that additives are actually responsible for particular health problems. Just as it is impossible to pinpoint the causes of cancer, which may be the cumulative effect of toxins or the result of one incident, it is equally impossible to prove many health hazards from additives. Indeed, there are still people and organizations that refuse to accept a link between smoking and cancer, although twenty-five years of epidemiological research has demonstrated that 25 per cent of smokers will die from their use of tobacco; it is not surprising, then, that the food industry does not accept the possible health hazards of additives.

What about the workers?

The risks have in fact been documented among food workers.

Consumers may be exposed to a mixture of up to sixty additives in one meal. Food workers may be exposed to a mixture of up to fifty additives at any one time. Food workers receive double exposure to additives, because they are also consumers! At work they can be exposed to additives by breathing them in or swallowing them from the surrounding air, and by skin contact with their dusts, fumes or splashes . . . although instances are rarely documented food workers are exposed to ill-health as a result.

Danger! Additives at Work (London Food Commission, 1985)

The same report gives examples of:

dermatitis among workers handling powdered mixture in the soft-drinks industry, despite protective clothing;
asthma and bronchitis brought on by exposure to the azo dye tartrazine — eating it and handling it produce the same effect;
respiratory problems among workers in fruit-processing factories due to exposure to sulphur dioxide, an irritating and corrosive gas.

(The sulphates are widespread in much of the British food industry as a preserver of colour in many fruit products, and as a straight preservative.)

At the 1985 TUC, Terry O'Neill, leader of the Baker's Union, won support for a year-long investigation into the health risks faced by workers in the food industry. The large number of food additives handled by workers in the baking industry were of particular concern to Mr O'Neill.

How do they affect hyperactive children?

Not many of us handle food additives in their raw state, but most of us eat them and it is not realistic or practical to say we will never again eat an additive. The risks are not 'proved', but there have been cases where certain health problems have been cured by avoiding additives. Probably the best publicized are the effects of additives on hyperactive children, particularly those of the colouring agent, tartrazine (E102). Most other colourings are also best avoided, says the Hyperactive Children's Support Group (HACSG).

HACSG also recommend avoidance of the benzoate preservatives E210 and 211, sulphur dioxide (E220), sodium nitrite (E250) and sodium nitrate (E251) see table, p. 117. As well as hyperactivity, this group of preservatives has been linked with allergic reactions, gastric irritation, nervous disorders and skin

Finding Out about Food Additives

reactions, and possibly wheezing. The suphites have been suspected of toxic cumulative effects and in 1985 they were banned from use in American restaurants and supermarkets where they were used to dress cut fruit and vegetables. Nitrites and nitrates are suspected of being chemically changed in the gut to produce nitrosamines, which are carcinogenic. Pollution of waterways by nitrates used as chemical fertilizers also adds to the amount we ingest (see ORGANIC FOODS).

The antioxidants E320, BHA, and E321, BHT, should also be avoided by hyperactive children; they are not permitted in foods for young children, yet they are used extensively in fatty products like nuts and crisps, which are often marketed to attract children. Because of their anti-rancidity powers, they are used in the manufacture of most fats and oils, and in almost all sections of the food industry.

Are babies allowed additives?

In fact there is a whole set of additives that is not permitted in food specifically for young children who, because of their small body mass, are more susceptible to reactions than adults (see table, p. 117). Babies have delicate and immature immune systems, which again means they have to be protected from certain additives. Even introducing certain types of foods to babies too soon can provoke reactions and allergies, so chemical food additives, for which the body has no inbuilt protection, are obviously a risk. Yet traces of the specially noxious BHA and BHT may be found in baby food, because residues of these from the manufacture of vitamin A are allowed in baby foods enriched with vitamin A.

The fact that a measure of protection from additives is given to babies and young children may reassure parents, but it also underlines the risk factor involved for the rest of us.

The medical profession has mainly limited its comments on food additives to their role in food allergy and intolerance, and it remains sceptical, generally, that there is more than a minor problem. 'When one considers that almost everyone in the population has probably been exposed to tartrazine at some time or other sensitivity to it is low,' says *Food Intolerance and Food Aversion*, which goes on to comment on hyperactivity:

> It is all too easy to collude with parents who cannot accept that psychological factors are to blame for their child's disruptive behaviour, by accepting their child is suffering from food intolerance. The use of the Feingold diet* has been extensively encouraged by lay organizations representing the parents of so-called hyperactive children. In the experience of a number of paediatricians, mood alterations in relation to food never occurs in isolation, but may be predominantly associated with other more obvious reactions such as diarrhoea, migraine, urticaria and eczema.

The experience of Dr Stephen Davies, medical adviser to HACSG, suggests more tangible evidence:

> Inability to adapt to artificial colouring and preservatives in almost all processed foods and drinks is one of the causes of behavioural symptoms of hyperactivity, due to the colourings intervening with brain chemistry. By excluding them from the diet of additive-sensitive children a 'problem child' can become a social, loving and well-behaved child.

The problem of reaction to additives is possibly more acute in the case of additives in drugs. For example, hyperactive children have been prescribed calming drugs which have contained exactly the artificial colourings that provoke attacks, yet the drugs industry is not obliged to label its products with an ingredient listing as the food industry is. The Association of the British Pharmaceutical Industry is 'interested' in the suggestion, which has been discussed in *Drugs and Therapeutics Bulletin*, published by the Consumer Association; the CA has forwarded the suggestion to the DHSS.

---

* The Feingold diet excludes food colourings and additives and salicytate-containing foods.

Common food additive problems

Food Intolerance and Food Aversion, the report published by the Royal College of Physicians and the British Nutrition Foundation, gives evidence of food additives which have been associated with urticaria (skin rashes and reactions). They are

Antioxidants
Butylated hydroxyanisole (E320)
Butylated hydroxytoluene (E321)

Colourings
Amaranth (E123)
Sunset Yellow (E110)
Tartrazine (E102)

Preservatives
Benzoates (E210 series)
Sodium metabisulphite (E223)
Sodium nitrite (E250)

Flavourings
Menthol
Quinine

Others
Papain (meat tenderizer)
Penicillin   (residues in meat from the
Tetracycline   veterinary treatment of animals)

The report also noted that it had been claimed that sodium nitrate and menthol had provoked certain types of rheumatic attack. Preservatives and artificial colourings were also among the doctors' top ten of the most common food allergens.

The report emphasizes the difficulty in assessing frequency of allergy or intolerance in respect of food additives, but it seems there is enough evidence from America to convince some authorities. According to Barbara Griggs, a journalist and author, some schizophrenic patients, when put on a wholefood diet which avoids stimulants like caffeine, refined foods and chemical food additives, have returned to normal behaviour patterns.

Additives and academic success

In 1986, after a four-year trial in which colourings and preservatives were removed from the diet of 800,000 New York schoolchildren and the sucrose (table sugar) intake in school breakfasts and lunches was reduced to a total of 11 per cent, there was a notable improvement in academic performance, reversing a ten-year decline in academic achievement and raising New York from its position 11 per cent below the national academic average to 5 per cent above it. More than 300 other variables were taken into consideration, but the evidence pointed to the change in diet as the vital factor.

The theory behind this is explained by Dr Alexander Schauss, World Health Organization expert on nutrition and behaviour, and also director of the American Institute of Biosocial Research. He argues that, although sugar and food additives are not directly responsible for poor performance in school, reducing overconsumption malnutrition, to which sugar and food additives contribute, was the primary cause of the improvements. This is because foods high in these substances tend to be high in calories but low in essential nutrients. The revised school diet replaced 'empty calorie' foods with wholefoods, which contribute a higher ratio of nutrients to calories, thus lowering any malnutrition present. This result is consistent with other studies showing that children's academic performance improves when the vitamins and minerals needed by the brain for the biochemical functions associated with learning are well supplied.

Why no controls on flavourings?

The additives already identified as being possibly problematic are among the 10 per cent of additives that are controlled by government regulations. The majority of additives are not yet subject to control by 'permitted' lists. As stated in *Danger! Additives at Work*:

Of the 3,500–3,800 additives available for use, less than 350 are covered by detailed legal controls. This means they have not been systematically and thoroughly tested for safety; permitted lists have not been established; and there are no legal limits set on their use. The additives that are not regulated are mainly flavours, but also include some solvents, processing aids, enzymes and modified starches.

Flavourings, many of them natural substances like herbs and spices, are the largest group of uncontrolled additives. In 1976 the Committee on Food Additives and Contaminants (now the Food Advisory Committee) produced a *Report on the Review of Flavourings in Food* which recommended that the use of flavours should be regulated, but this has not been implemented. An EEC Scientific Commission for Food is currently considering the ten-year-old report and we can expect a permitted list of flavourings, and regulations in their use . . . or can we?

How Britain got out of it

Although E numbers exist to provide a common language and a common set of regulations for all EEC countries, individual countries can opt out of the controls – and the British government (whether under the influence of powerful lobbying from the food and agriculture industries or not) does just this. In Britain we continue (after a hard-fought battle in the European courts) to use additives banned by many other European countries; these additives do not have E numbers and we are not allowed to export food containing them to other EEC countries.

We have far more food additives in use than other comparable countries. For example, the UK has nearly twenty approved artificial colourings; the rest of the EEC countries put together have a total of twelve and the USA has only seven. Not only do we use more but we allow each additive to be more widely used. In Britain a red dye – amaranth, E123, an azo dye, is used frequently in packet soups and sauces, canned and other preserved fruit, jams, ice cream, cake mixes, biscuits and yoghurt. In France and

Italy it is permitted only in red caviar. In Austria, Finland, Greece, Japan, Norway, Russia, Spain, the USA and Yugoslavia it is banned.

If the consumer complains that the controls in the UK are weak compared with other countries he is likely to be reminded by the food industry that the use of additives is for his benefit. The food industry is quick to point out that it is not possible to feed vast urban populations with fresh foods; that it is necessary to treat food so that it does not spoil between harvest or slaughter and consumption; that it has to survive transportation, processing and storage and that it must also have a long shelf-life under a variety of conditions.

But you like dyed food!

We are told that additives make for cheaper food by cutting down on waste. We are, also, apparently, hungry for new foods, for new flavours and new products, and additives allow the food industry to supply these demands. We are also reminded that we *like* brightly coloured and loudly flavoured foods because we buy them – don't we? Some manufacturers think we don't know what we do want. They cite examples of foods where the colourings were removed – canned peas and some jams – which sat on the shelves. (It took the manufacturers a year to recover financially.)

Yet in France, and other countries, canned peas are khaki and not bright green, and food is not dyed. People would recoil, '*Quelle horreur!*', at such a sight, so perhaps it is more a question of consumer education. Now that we know more about the subject, it seems we *are* asking for food without additives, since the supermarkets and food manufacturers are now making well-advertised efforts to produce it, working on removing them from their own-label products and encouraging their suppliers to do so too.

Most of the supermarket chains have been making woolly statements for some time about working towards removing chemical food additives wherever practicable, while the health-food trade has been finding it practicable for decades. It was Safeway who came out first and named a list of fifty-one 'contentious' additives which it was working to remove from its products, stressing that there is no conclusive medical evidence to suggest that they lead to serious health problems, but recognizing that they may cause symptoms such as stomach upsets, headaches, rashes or blurred vision.

Safeway's List of Additives Proposed for Removal from Their Own-label Products 'Where Possible and Practicable'

Colours

E102	Tartrazine
E104	Quinoline Yellow
107	Yellow 2G
E110	Sunset Yellow FCF
E120	Cochineal or carmine acid
E122	Carmoisine or Azorubine
E123	Amaranth
E124	Ponceau 4R
E127	Erthyrosine BS
128	Red 2G
E131	Patent Blue V
E132	Indigo Carmine or Indigotine
133	Brilliant Blue FCF
E142	Green S (Acid Brilliant Green)
E150	Caramel
E151	Black PN (Brilliant Black BN)
E153	Carbon Black (vegetable carbon)
154	Brown FK (Kipper Brown)
155	Brown HT
E180	Pigment Rubine (Lithol Rubine BK)

Flavour enhancers

Monosodium glutamate/sodium glutamate
621	Sodium hydrogen L-glutamate
622	Potassium hydrogen L-glutamate

Shopping for Health

623 Calcium dihydrogen di-L-glutamate
627 Guanosine 5'-(disodium phosphate)
631 Inosine 5'-(disodium phosphate)
635 Sodium 5'-ribonucleotide

Antioxidants

E320 Butylated hydroxyanisole (BHA)
E321 Butylated hydroxytoluene (BHT)
E310 Propyl gallate
E311 Octyl gallate
E312 Dodecyl gallate

Preservatives

E210 Benzoic acid
E211 Sodium benzoate
E220 Sulphur dioxide
E250 Sodium nitrite
E251 Sodium nitrate
E221 Sodium sulphite
E222 Sodium hydrogen sulphite
E223 Sodium metabisulphite
E224 Potassium metabisulphite
E226 Calcium sulphite
E227 Calcium bisulphite
E212 Potassium benzoate
E213 Calcium benzoate
E214 Ethyl 4-hydroxybenzoate
E215 Ethyl 4-hydroxybenzoate, sodium salt
E216 Propyl 4-hydroxybenzoate
E217 Propyl 4-hydroxybenzoate, sodium salt
E218 Methyl 4-hydroxybenzoate
E219 Methyl 4-hydroxybenzoate, sodium salt

What are supermarkets doing?

See also under SUPERMARKET in the Shopping List.

Finding Out about Food Additives

Safeway have embarked on consumer education with a planned series of twelve booklets to be given away free to customers, informing them on food, nutrition and healthy-eating-related topics. The first booklet was in response to customer's concern about additives – 'Additives – Why Do We Need Them?' Others on additives and labelling followed. Safeway was also the supermarket that pioneered the selling of organic fruit and vegetables (grown without artificial chemical fertilizers or sprays like pesticides, fungicides, herbicides, etc.) and has opened natural-food sections within its stores.

British Home Stores have also made positive moves to additive-free food, with the introduction of its Natural Foods sub-brand. Rather than adapt the piecemeal approach of introducing wholemeal and additive-free versions of regular foods alongside the existing products on its shelves, it has provided a separate section for whole foods within the stores – although some additives, such as the ubiquitous sulphur dioxide on dried fruit, remain.

Another high-street chain, Boots the Chemist, has chosen the same route, creating initially high-fibre range of additive-free foods under the Second Nature sub-brand. Like Safeway it is working towards removing as many additives as possible, particularly in food and drink for children. A wholemeal bakery range, vegetarian foods and fresh food in chill cabinets are other Boots innovations to meet public demand for food. They also promote consumer education through free postal diet analysis, in-store computer diet analysis, books and food fact sheets.

The Spar group of independent grocers has introduced a range of twenty-five Natural Spar products based on high-fibre foods that are free from additives.

Tesco was the 'first' with nutritional labelling (see Chapter 3); it has switched to natural colourings for its own-label biscuits and is removing all antioxidants from them. Its fish-finger range is being relaunched and is now additive-free.

The Co-op is introducing nutritional labelling on 'Consumer Care' panels on all its 1,500 own-brand foods; unlike others, the Co-op is not just highlighting the 'healthy' foods. A 'high',

Shopping for Health

'medium' and 'low' symbol system for protein, carbohydrate, fat, fibre and calories is being extended to other ingredients. In-store posters and leaflets are also part of their 'Eat Right Eat Well' campaign.

Bejam Freezer Food Centres have introduced additive-free sausages and state that all their frozen poultry is free from polyphosphates and colouring; they are reducing the use of artificial colouring in smoked fish.

Sainsbury's have for some time provided customers with lists of additive-free foods, foods free from artificial colourings and foods that are totally preservative-free.

Waitrose have taken great trouble to list foods suitable for vegetarian and vegan customers, and for some other special diet requirements. They also undertake extensive listing of food free from artificial colouring, preservatives and flavourings for those who are concerned about hyperactive children.

Although most large chains cannot guarantee that the fish in their wet-fish counters (such as salmon or trout) is free from artificial colouring added to the feed at the fish farms, Harrods do. They also offer additive-free foods in their in-store health-food section and sell free-range eggs.

Many high-street supermarket chains sell free-range eggs, not just because customers are sickened by the cruelty of battery-hen production, but because some object to the additives used in animal food (see ORGANIC FOODS) and especially the tartrazine used in some poultry food to colour the egg yolks deep yellow, disguising the pale yolks produced by the battery system.

Superdrug has introduced health-food sections with additive-free snacks and cereals, as well as some other lines, both proprietary brands and their own-label products.

In Ireland, the Superquinn chain sells organic fruit and vegetables whenever it can obtain supplies, and has in-store bakeries that produce additive-free breads (baked daily, with unsold bread going to local charities at the end of the day). Superquinn aims to sell wet fish which comes from farms that do not use colourings, and has a positive policy of preferring sea fish to fish-farmed fish.

Marks & Spencer avoid food additives as much as possible, and make a point of selling fresh produce, often from chill cabinets, with a very short shelf-life.

By removing the additives from their own-label products, supermarkets are reducing the shelf life of their products, but they are finding that, contrary to their expectations, this food does not have to be vastly more expensive. (Another food-industry claim for additives – cheapness – bites the dust!) Removing the preservatives from orange squash, for example, and using fresher ingredients, puts only ¼p on the cost of a bottle, says one supermarket chain. Health-food manufacturers have consistently produced food without additives and so have proved that business can exist without preservatives. Other techniques like vacuum packing, chilling and freezing can obviate the need for chemical preservatives.

Twisting the logic

Even if the economic argument for preservatives collapses, the food industry may remind us that additives enhance food safety, preventing horrors like botulism, and that there are many 'natural' substances that can do us much more harm than food additives. They are, of course, right in some respects – there are many natural poisons in food. Apart from deadly nightshade, we all know that if we eat green potatoes we are asking for trouble, because the solanine they contain will give us a nasty upset. Rhubarb leaves can cause oxalic poisoning; some people avoid rhubarb and spinach altogether because their oxalic-acid content may aggravate joint conditions or some kinds of kidney stones. If we eat too many bananas we risk upsets from naturally present toxins. *Food Intolerance and Food Allergy* lists forty-three natural foods which can cause an allergic reaction.

Experts think consumers should be more worried about the danger from naturally occurring food-spoilage organisms like mycotoxins (moulds), which are currently undergoing close scientific scrutiny; bacteria such as botulism, which is potentially lethal; or salmonella, which causes food poisoning in healthy individuals, and can be fatal for the sick.

Salmonella is on the increase and is associated with poor food hygiene, but – a fact overlooked by the food-additive proponents – it is probably becoming more common because of current farming practices, such as the overcrowding of animals. The use of low-dose antibiotics in animal feed to stimulate growth is making the bacteria resistant to drugs, so they are passed on to us from the meat, poultry and fish we eat, causing food poisoning. It is naïve of the food industry and some scientists to believe it is public ignorance of food-handling techniques and hygiene that is to blame for most cases of salmonella poisoning. Bacterial resistance to drugs is also dangerous if the drugs have to be used in life-and-death emergencies.

The argument that there is nothing 'natural' is yet another twist to logic applied by the food industry. Everything, they say, is chemical. Nevertheless, it is possible to distinguish between natural and synthetic food additives and to assess which we might wish to avoid.

Life might not be the same without additives, but it is easy to question the need for so many – especially when other Western nations manage with far fewer, and distribute food over far greater areas than the UK.

Go on, you can do it . . .

It takes more effort when shopping to avoid the products that contain additives – especially the most suspect sort of additives – but it is not impossible. It may not be realistic to say you will never eat another food containing additives, but it is certainly possible to cut down greatly the number of additives that you and your family eat. In the absence of government controls on the food industry, YOU can apply your own controls. The tables which follow will help you to decide which additives you should try to avoid.

Table 1
E Numbers: Natural or Synthetic? How Safe are They?

- N natural
- S synthetic
- U chemically or synthetically derived from a natural substance
- ! BEWARE
- ? query mark for SUSPECT
- ✓ tick for SAFE

		Natural or synthetic	Chemically or synthetically derived from a natural substance	Beware	Suspect	Safe	Comments
Colours							
E100	Curcumin	N					
E101	Riboflavin (Lactoflavin)	N	S			✓	
101(a)	Riboflavin-5'-phosphate	N	U			✓	
E102	Tartrazine		S	!			These artificial colours are implicated in hyperactivity, skin reactions, asthmatic attacks, runny noses, chest tightness and some adverse symptoms in people who are aspirin- and salicylate-sensitive
E104	Quinoline Yellow		S	!			
107	Yellow 2G		S	!			
E110	Sunset Yellow FCF (Orange Yellow S)		S	!			
E120	Cochineal (Carmine of Cochineal or Carminic acid)	N					
E122	Carmoisine (Azorubine)		S	!			
E123	Amaranth		S	!			
E124	Ponceau 4R (Cochineal Red A)		S	!			

Table 1 – continued

		Natural or synthetic	Chemically or synthetically derived from a natural substance	Beware	Suspect	Safe	Comments
E127	Erythrosine BS		S	—			E150 Caramel (not an azo dye) might cause vitamin B_6 deficiency; available in many forms, now reduced to six – research to find the safest is continuing
128	Red 2G		S	—			
E131	Patent Blue V		S	—			
E132	Indigo Carmine (Indigotine)		S	—			
133	Brilliant Blue FCF		S	—			
E140	Chlorophyll	N				✓	
E141	Copper complexes of chlorophyll and chlorophyllins		U			✓	
E142	Green S (Acid Brilliant Green BS or Lissamine Green)		S	—			
E150	Caramel		U				These azo dyes are especially problematic for hyperactive children, etc., as above
E151	Black PN (Brilliant Black BN)		S	—			
E153	Carbon Black (Vegetable Carbon)	N					
154	Brown FK		S	—			
155	Brown HT (Chocolate Brown HT)		S	—			
E160(a)	alpha-carotene, beta-carotene, gamma-carotene	N				✓	
E160(b)	Annatto, bixin, norbixin	N				✓	
E160(c)	Capsanthin (Capsorubin)	N				✓	
E160(d)	Lycopene	N				✓	
E160(e)	beta-apo-8'-carotenal (C_{30})	N				✓	

Code	Name			
E160(f)	Ethyl ester of beta-apo-8'-carotenoic acid (C_{30})	N		
E161(a)	Flavoxanthin	N		✓
E161(b)	Lutein	N		✓
E161(c)	Cryptoxanthin	N		✓
E161(d)	Rubixanthin	N		✓
E161(e)	Violaxanthin	N		✓
E161(f)	Rhodoxanthin	N		✓
E161(g)	Canthaxanthin	N		✓
E162	Beetroot Red (Betanin)	N		✓
E163	Anthocyanins	N		✓
E170	Calcium carbonate	N		✓
E171	Titanium dioxide	N		✓
E172	Iron oxides, iron hydroxides	N		✓
E173	Aluminium	N	!	Aluminium has been linked with Alzheimer's disease (premature senility)
E174	Silver	N	!	
E175	Gold	N	!	
E180	Pigment rubine (Lithol rubine B K)	S	?	

Preservatives

Code	Name			
E200	Sorbic acid	N		
E201	Sodium sorbate	S	?	
E202	Potassium sorbate	N		✓
E203	Calcium sorbate	N		✓

Table 1 – continued

		Natural or synthetic	Chemically or synthetically derived from a natural substance	Beware	Suspect	Safe	Comments
E210	Benzoic acid	N	S				Benzoates can cause problems for hyperactive children, asthmatics and those with skin problems; they trigger allergies more commonly than other additives and cause gastric irritation and nervous disorders
E211	Sodium benzoate	N	S				
E212	Potassium benzoate	N	S				
E213	Calcium benzoate	N	S				
E214	Ethyl 4-hydroxybenzoate (Ethyl para-hydroxybenzoate)		S				
E215	Ethyl 4-hydroxybenzoate, sodium salt (Sodium ethyl para-hydroxybenzoate)		S				
E216	Propyl 4-hydroxybenzoate (Propyl para-hydroxybenzoate)		S				
E217	Propyl 4-hydroxybenzoate, sodium salt (Sodium propyl para-hydroxybenzoate)		S				
E218	Methyl 4-hydroxybenzoate (Methyl para-hydroxybenzoate)		S				
E219	Methyl 4-hydroxybenzoate, sodium salt (Sodium methyl para-hydroxybenzoate)		S				
E220	Sulphur dioxide		S				Sulphates are banned in America for salad bar use; they can irritate the stomach and cause wheezing; thought to have
E221	Sodium sulphite		S				
E222	Sodium hydrogen sulphite (Sodium bisulphite)		S				
E223	Sodium metabisulphite		S				
E224	Potassium metabisulphite		S				

Code	Name				Notes
E226	Calcium sulphite		S		cumulative toxic effects and may destroy B vitamins. Also have to be declared on labels of wine and beer in USA
E227	Calcium hydrogen sulphite (Calcium bisulphite)		S		
E230	Biphenyl (Diphenyl)		S		
E231	2-Hydroxybiphenyl (Orthophenylphenol)		S		
E232	Sodium biphenyl-2-yl oxide (Sodium orthophenylphenate)		S		
E233	2-(Thiazol-4-yl) benzimidazole (Thiabendazole)		S		
234	Nisin		S	✓	
E236	Formic acid	N	S	✓	
E237	Sodium formate	N	S	?	
E238	Calcium formate		S	?	
E239	Hexamine (Hexamethylenetetramine)	N	S	?	E239. Thought to become Formaldehyde in the gut – irritant also to kidneys
E249	Potassium nitrite		S		Nitrites and nitrates are under suspicion of being carcinogenic; widely used in curing bacon and ham, nitrites are changed to nitrosamines in the gut which are known to cause cancer; effect worsened by nitrites and nitrates being widely used in chemical fertilizers and being washed from land to water; also used in beers and other drinks
E250	Sodium nitrite	N	S		
E251	Sodium nitrate	N	S		
E252	Potassium nitrate		S	✓[1]	
E260	Acetic acid		S		
E261	Potassium acetate		S	✓	
E262	Sodium hydrogen diacetate		S	✓	
262	Sodium acetate		S	✓	
E263	Calcium acetate	N	S	✓	
E270	Lactic acid	N	U	✓[2]	
E280	Propionic acid		S	✓	
E281	Sodium propionate		S	✓[3]	
E282	Calcium propionate		S	✓	
E283	Potassium propionate		S	✓	
E290	Carbon dioxide	N		✓[1]	

Table 1 – continued

		Natural or synthetic	Chemically or synthetically derived from a natural substance	Beware	Suspect	Safe	Comments
296	DL-malic acid, L-malic acid	N(L) S(DL)				✓	
297	Fumaric acid	N				✓	

Antioxidants

E300	L-ascorbic acid (vitamin C)	N				✓	
E301	Sodium L-ascorbate		S			✓	
E302	Calcium L-ascorbate		S			✓	
E304	6-O-palmitoyl-L-ascorbic acid (Ascorbyl palmitate)		S			✓	
E306	Extracts of natural origin rich in tocopherols (Vitamin E)	N				✓	
E307	Synthetic *alpha*-tocopherol		S			✓	
E308	Synthetic *gamma*-tocopherol		S			✓	
E309	Synthetic *delta*-tocopherol		S			✓	
E310	Propyl gallate		S	!			Gallates are not permitted in baby food and can also cause problems for the hyperactive, asthmatics, aspirin- and salcylate-sensitive subjects, causing gastric irritation and other symptoms
E311	Octyl gallate		S	!			
E312	Dodecyl gallate		S	!			

E320	Butylated hydroxyanisole (BHA)			S	⎫ BHA and BHT used widely in products containing fats; may interfere with blood fat metabolism and contribute to vitamin D deficiency
E321	Butylated hydroxytoluene (BHT)			S	⎭

Emulsifiers, stabilizers, thickeners

E322	Lecithins	N			
E325	Sodium lactate		U		>
E326	Potassium lactate		U		>
E327	Calcium lactate				
E330	Citric acid	N			>
E331	Sodium dihydrogen citrate (*monoSodium citrate*), *diSodium citrate*, *triSodium citrate*		U	?	>
E332	Potassium dihydrogen citrate (*monoPotassium citrate*), *triPotassium citrate*		U	?	>
E333	*mono*Calcium citrate, *di*Calcium citrate, *tri*Calcium citrate		U	?	>>
E334	L-(+)-tartaric acid	N			>
E335	*mono*Sodium L-(+)-tartrate, *di*Sodium L-(+)-tartrate				>>
E336	*mono*Potassium L-(+)-tartrate (Cream of tartar), *di*Potassium L-(+)-tartrate		U		>
E337	Potassium sodium L-(+)-tartrate		U		>>
E338	Orthophosphoric acid (Phosphoric acid)		U		>>>

Table 1 – continued

		Natural or synthetic	Chemically or synthetically derived from a natural substance	Beware	Suspect	Safe	Comments
E339	Sodium dihydrogen orthophosphate, *di*Sodium hydrogen orthophosphate, *tri*Sodium orthophosphate	S				✓	
E340	Potassium dihydrogen orthophosphate, *di*Potassium hydrogen orthophosphate, *tri*Potassium orthophosphate	S					
E341(a)	Acid calcium phosphate (ACP) dibasic	N				✓	
(b)	Calcium hydrogen orthophosphate		C			✓	
(c)	*tri*Calcium diorthophosphate		C			✓	
350	Sodium malate, sodium hydrogen malate		C			✓	
351	Potassium malate		C			✓	
352	Calcium malate, calcium hydrogen malate		C			✓	
353	Metatartaric acid		C			✓	
355	Adipic acid	N				✓	
363	Succinic acid	S				✓	
370	1,4-Heptonolactone	S			?		
375	Nicotinic acid (Vitamin B$_3$)	N				✓	
380	*tri*Ammonium citrate	S	C			✓	
381	Ammonium ferric citrate		C			✓	
385	Calcium disodium ethylenediamine – NNN'N' tetra-acetate (Calcium disodium EDTA)	S			?		
E400	Alginic acid	N				✓	

E401	Sodium alginate		U	✓	
E402	Potassium alginate		U	✓	
E403	Ammonium alginate		U	✓	
E404	Calcium alginate		U	✓	
E405	Propane-1,2-diol alginate (Propylene glycol alginate)		S		
E406	Agar	N		✓	
E407	Carrageenan	N		?	Gelling agent; although natural, under suspicion of being carcinogenic and implicated in bowel problems if taken in large amounts
E410	Locust bean gum (Carob gum)	N		✓	
E412	Guar gum	N		✓	
E413	Tragacanth	N		✓	
E414	Gum arabic (Acacia)	N		✓	
E415	Xanthan gum	N		✓	
416	Karaya gum	N		✓	

Synthetic Sweeteners

E420	Sorbitol, sorbitol syrup	S	U	?
E421	Mannitol	S	U	?
E422	Glycerol	S	U	?

Table I – continued

		Natural or synthetic	Chemically or synthetically derived from a natural substance	Beware	Suspect	Safe	Comments
430	Polyoxyethylene (8) stearate		U		?		Under consideration for E numbers; it is suggested they may cause kidney stones and affect gastrointestinal and urinary tracts; also skin allergies
431	Polyoxyethylene (40) stearate		U		?		
432	Polyoxyethylene (20) sorbitan monolaurate (Polysorbate 20)		U		?		
433	Polyoxyethylene (20) sorbitan mono-oleate (Polysorbate 80)		U		?		
434	Polyoxyethylene (20) sorbitan monopalmitate (Polysorbate 40)		U		?		
435	Polyoxyethylene (20) sorbitan monostearate (Polysorbate 60)		U		?		
436	Polyoxyethylene (20) sorbitan tristearate (Polysorbate 65)		U		?		

Emulsifiers, Stabilizers, Thickeners

E440(a)	Pectin	N				✓	
E440(b)	Amidated pectin		U			✓	
442	Ammonium phosphatides	S			?		
E450(a)	diSodium dihydrogen diphosphate, triSodium diphosphate, tetraSodium diphosphate, tetraPotassium diphosphate	S	U		?		

E450(b)	pentaSodium triphosphate, pentaPotassium triphosphate		S	?	
E450(c)	Sodium polyphosphates, Potassium polyphosphates		S	?	
E460	Microcrystalline cellulose, Alpha-cellulose (Powdered cellulose)				
E461	Methylcellulose	N		✓	
E463	Hydroxypropylcellulose		U	✓	
E464	Hydroxypropylmethylcellulose		U	✓	
E465	Ethylmethylcellulose		U	✓	
E466	Carboxymethylcellulose, sodium salt (CMC)		U	✓	
E470	Sodium, potassium and calcium salts of fatty acids	N	U	✓	
E471	Mono- and di-glycerides of fatty acids	N	U	✓	
E472(a)	Acetic acid esters of mono- and di-glycerides of fatty acids		U	✓	
E472(b)	Lactic acid esters of mono- and di-glycerides of fatty acids (Lactoglycerides)		U	?	Fats and soaps may, in quantity, interfere with intestinal function and absorption
E472(c)	Citric acid esters of mono- and di-glycerides of fatty acids (Citroglycerides)		U	?	
E472(d)	Tartaric acid esters of mono- and diglycerides of fatty acids		U	?	
E472(e)	Mono- and diacetyltartaric acid esters of mono- and di-glycerides of fatty acids		U	?	
E473	Sucrose esters of fatty acids	N	U	?	
E474	Sucroglycerides		U	?	
E475	Polyglycerol esters of fatty acids		S	?	
476	Polyglycerol esters of polycondensed fatty acids of castor oil (Polyglycerol polyricinoleate)		U	?	
E477	Propane-1,2-diol esters of fatty acids		S	?	
478	Lactylated fatty acid esters of glycerol and propane-1,2-diol		U	?	

Table 1 – continued

		Natural or synthetic	Chemically or synthetically derived from a natural substance	Beware	Suspect	Safe	Comments
E481	Sodium stearoyl-2-lactylate	S	U		?		Stearates and sorbitans may produce skin allergies and may increase gut absorption of irritant paraffins
E482	Calcium stearoyl-2-lactylate	S	U		?		
E483	Stearyl tartrate	S	U		?		
491	Sorbitan monostearate	S	U		?		
492	Sorbitan tristearate	S	U		?		
493	Sorbitan monolaurate	S	U		?		
494	Sorbitan mono-oleate	S	U		?		
495	Sorbitan monopalmitate	S	U		?		
500	Sodium carbonate, Sodium hydrogen carbonate (Bicarbonate of soda), Sodium sesquicarbonate	S	U			✓	

Acids, bases

501	Potassium carbonate, Potassium hydrogen carbonate	S				✓	
503	Ammonium carbonate, Ammonium hydrogen carbonate	S				✓	
504	Magnesium carbonate	N				✓	
507	Hydrochloric acid	S			?		

508	Potassium chloride	N			
509	Calcium chloride	N	S		
510	Ammonium chloride		S		
513	Sulphuric acid		S	?	
514	Sodium sulphate	N		?	
515	Potassium sulphate	N		?	
516	Calcium sulphate	N		?	
518	Magnesium sulphate	N		?	
524	Sodium hydroxide		S		
525	Potassium hydroxide		S	?	>
526	Calcium hydroxide		S	?	>
527	Ammonium hydroxide		S	U	
528	Magnesium hydroxide	N	S	?	>
529	Calcium oxide	N	S	U	>

Anti-caking agents

530	Magnesium oxide	N		?	
535	Sodium ferrocyanide (Sodium hexacyanoferrate II))		S	!	⎫ Cyanides have obvious
536	Potassium ferrocyanide (Potassium hexacyanoferrate II))		S	!	⎬ dangers
540	diCalcium diphosphate	N	S	!	> ⎭

Table I – continued

		Natural or synthetic	Chemically or synthetically derived from a natural substance	Beware	Suspect	Safe	Comments
541	Sodium aluminium phosphate		S	!			Aluminium-containing additives may add to the burden already high from other sources, e.g. cookware, deodorants, baking powders; implicated in Altzheimer's disease (premature senility)
542	Edible bone phosphate	N	S				
544	Calcium polyphosphates		S				
545	Ammonium polyphosphates		S				
551	Silicon dioxide (Silica)	N			?	✓✓	Silicates also contain aluminium (see above) and suspected carcinogens
552	Calcium silicate	N	S			✓	
535(a)	Magnesium silicate synthetic, Magnesium trisilicate	N	S				
553(b)	Talc	N		!	?		
554	Aluminium sodium silicate	N					
556	Aluminium calcium silicate	N		!			
558	Bentonite	N	U				
559	Kaolin	N			?		
570	Stearic acid	N				✓✓✓	
572	Magnesium stearate		S	U		✓✓	
575	D-glucono-1,5-lactone (Glucono delta-lactone)			U	?		

576	Sodium gluconate			S	
577	Potassium gluconate			S	
578	Calcium gluconate			S	

Flavour enhancers, sweeteners

620	L-glutamic acid	N	U	!	
621	Sodium hydrogen L-glutamate (*mono*Sodium glutamate or MSG)		U	!	Glutamates – not permitted in baby food – may cause very bad allergic reactions such as Kwok syndrome (Chinese-restaurant syndrome)
622	Potassium hydrogen L-glutamate (*mono*Potassium glutamate)		U	!	
623	Calcium dihydrogen di-L-glutamate (Calcium glutamate)		U	!	
627	Guanosine 5′-(disodium phosphate) (Sodium guanylate)		U	!	Purines in these additives could give gout sufferers and rheumatics problems and should be avoided for children
631	Inosine 5′-(disodium phosphate) (Sodium inosinate)		U	!	
635	Sodium 5′-ribonucleotide		U	!	?
636	Maltol	N	S		?
637	Ethyl maltol		U		?

Glazing agents

900	Dimethylpolysiloxane	N			?
901	Beeswax		S		✓

Table 1 – continued

		Natural or synthetic	Chemically or synthetically derived from a natural substance	Beware	Suspect	Safe	Comments
903	Carnauba wax	N				✓	
904	Shellac	N				✓	
905	Mineral hydrocarbons	S			?		Liquid paraffin – laxative effect
907	Refined microcrystalline wax	S				✓	

Improving and bleaching agents

920	L-cysteine hydrochloride		U			✓	
924	Potassium bromate	S	U	!			Bleaches may destroy vitamins, especially vitamin E, and may cause intestinal upset.
925	Chlorine	S	U	!			
926	Chlorine dioxide	S	U	!			
927	Azodicarbonamide (Azoformamide)	S	U	!			Improving agent – see E471

No E numbers

Sweeteners

—	Saccharin	S			Saccharin was formerly banned in the US, now carries US government health warning; coal tar based
—	Saccharin calcium	S			
—	Saccharin sodium	S			
—	Aspartame	S		U	
—	Acesulfame potassium	N		U	?
—	Thaumatin			U	?
—	Hydrogenated glucose syrup	S		U	?
—	Isomalt	S		U	?
—	Xylitol				?

Solvents

—	Ethyl alcohol	N			
—	Ethyl acetate	S		U	?
—	Diethyl ether	S			?
—	Glycerol monoacetate	S			?
—	Glycerol triacetate	S			?
—	Isopropyl alcohol	S			Suspected carcinogen
—	Propylene glycol	S			Suspected carcinogen

Table 1 – continued

	Natural or synthetic	Chemically or synthetically derived from a natural substance	Beware	Suspect	Safe	Comments
Miscellaneous						
— Ethoxyquin		S		?		
— Dioctyl sodium sulphosuccinate		S		?		
— Extract of quillaia	N		!			
— Dichlorodifluoromethane		S		?		
— Calcium phytate	N				✓	
— Glycine		S			✓	
— Sodium heptonate		S				⎫
— Calcium heptonate		S				⎬ Not known
— Hydrogen		S			✓	⎭
— Nitrogen	N				✓	
— Nitrous oxide		S		?		
— Oxygen	N				✓	
— Octadecyl ammonium acetate		S			✓	
— Oxystearin		S		?		

1. Except in cases of kidney failure.
2. Except for the very young.
3. Except for migraine sufferers.
4. Increases stomach acidity; may irritate an ulcer.

Table 2
Vegetarians and Vegans

Note: if there is more than one entry it means that the additive may be from either of the sources entered. If the exact source is not stated on the label, you could check it with the manufacturer.

A — animal – derived from animal source
V — vegetarian – animal-free, but may derive from dairy produce
√ — vegan – totally animal free
M — mineral – may be vitamin or mineral, naturally occurring or synthesized, or may be totally synthetic

		Animal	Vegetarian	Vegan	Mineral
Colours					
E100	Curcumin				M
E101	Riboflavin (Lactoflavin)		V	√	M
101(a)	Riboflavin-5'-phosphate				M
E102	Tartrazine				M
E104	Quinoline Yellow				M
107	Yellow 2G				
E110	Sunset Yellow FCF (Orange Yellow S)				M
E120	Cochineal (Carmine of Cochineal or Carminic acid)	A			
E122	Carmoisine (Azorubine)				M
E123	Amaranth				M
E124	Ponceau 4R (Cochineal Red A)				M
E127	Erythrosine BS				M
128	Red 2G				M
E131	Patent Blue V				M
E132	Indigo Carmine (Indigotine)				M

Table 2 – continued

		Animal	Vegetarian	Vegan	Mineral
133	Brilliant Blue FCF				M
E140	Chlorophyll		✓	✓	
E141	Copper complexes of chlorophyll and chlorophyllins		✓	✓	
E142	Green S (Acid Brilliant Green BS or Lissamine Green)				M
E150	Caramel		✓		M
E151	Black PN (Brilliant Black BN)				M
E153	Carbon Black (Vegetable Carbon)	A	✓	✓	M
154	Brown FK				M
155	Brown HT (Chocolate Brown HT)				M
E160(a)	Alpha-carotene, beta-carotene, gamma-carotene		✓	✓	M
E160(b)	Annato, bixin, norbixin		✓	✓	
E160(c)	Capsanthin (Capsorubin)		✓	✓	
E160(d)	Lycopene		✓	✓	
E160(e)	Beta-apo-8'-carotenal (C_{30})		✓	✓	M
E160(f)	Ethyl ester of beta-apo-8'-cartenoic acid (C_{30})		✓	✓	
E161(a)	Flavoxanthin		✓	✓	M
E161(b)	Lutein		✓	✓	
E161(c)	Cryptoxanthin		✓	✓	
E161(d)	Rubixanthin		✓	✓	
E161(e)	Violaxanthin		✓	✓	
E161(f)	Rhodoxanthin		✓	✓	
E161(g)	Canthaxanthin	A	✓	✓	

E162	Beetroot Red (Betanin)	✓	✓	
E163	Anthocyanins	✓	✓	
E170	Calcium carbonate			M
E171	Titanium dioxide			M
E172	Iron oxides, iron hydroxides			M
E173	Aluminium			M
E174	Silver			M
E175	Gold			M
E180	Pigment Rubine (Lithol Rubine BK)			M

Preservatives

E200	Sorbic acid	✓	✓	
E201	Sodium sorbate	✓	✓	
E202	Potassium sorbate			M
E203	Calcium sorbate	A		M

Table 2 – continued

		Animal	Vegetarian	Vegan	Mineral
E210	Benzoic acid				M
E211	Sodium benzoate				M
E212	Potassium benzoate				M
E213	Calcium benzoate	A			M
E214	Ethyl 4-hydroxybenzoate (Ethyl para-hydroxybenzoate)		⎫		M
E215	Ethyl 4-hydroxybenzoate, sodium salt (Sodium ethyl para-hydroxybenzoate)		⎪	Benzoic acid and its derivatives occur naturally in some fruits, but produced synthetically as a food additive	M
E216	Propyl 4-hydroxybenzoate (Propyl para-hydroxybenzoate)		⎬		M
E217	Propyl 4-hydroxybenzoate, sodium salt (Sodium propyl para-hydroxybenzoate)		⎪		M
E218	Methyl 4-hydroxybenzoate (Methyl para-hydroxybenzoate)		⎪		M
E219	Methyl 4-hydroxybenzoate, sodium salt (Sodium methyl para-hydroxybenzoate)		⎭		M
E220	Sulphur dioxide				M
E221	Sodium sulphite				M
E222	Sodium hydrogen sulphite (Sodium bisulphite)				M
E223	Sodium metabisulphite				M
E224	Potassium metabisulphite				M
E226	Calcium sulphite				M
E227	Calcium hydrogen sulphite (Calcium bisulphite)	A			M

E230	Biphenyl (Diphenyl)				M
E231	2-Hydroxybiphenyl (Orthophenylphenol)				M
E232	Sodium biphenyl-2-yl oxide (Sodium orthophenylphenate)				
E233	2-(Thiazol-4-yl) benzimidazole (Thiabendazole)				M
234	Nisin	A			M
E236	Formic acid ⎫ not permitted	A	√		M
E237	Sodium formate ⎬ in the UK	A	√	√	M
E238	Calcium formate ⎭	A	√	√	M
E239	Hexamine (Hexamethylenetetramine)				M
E249	Potassium nitrite				M
E250	Sodium nitrite				M
E251	Sodium nitrate				M
E252	Potassium nitrate				M
E260	Acetic acid				M
E261	Potassium acetate				M
E262	Sodium hydrogen diacetate				M
262	Sodium acetate				M
E263	Calcium acetate	A			M
E270	Lactic acid				M
E280	Propionic acid				M
E281	Sodium propionate				M
E282	Calcium propionate	A			M
E283	Potassium propionate				M
E290	Carbon dioxide		√		M
296	DL-malic acid, L-malic acid		√-L form	√-L form	M
297	Fumaric acid	A	√	√	√ DL form
					M

105

Table 2 – continued

	Animal	Vegetarian	Vegan	Mineral
Antioxidants				
E300 L-ascorbic acid			✓	M ⎫
E301 Sodium L-ascorbate				M ⎬ Vitamin C
E302 Calcium L-ascorbate	✓			M ⎭
E304 6-O-palmitoyl-L-ascorbic acid (Ascorbyl palmitate)	✓	✓		
E306 Extracts of natural origin rich in tocopherols		✓	✓	M ⎫
E307 Synthetic *alpha*-tocopherol				M ⎪
E308 Synthetic *gamma*-tocopherol				M ⎬ Vitamin E
E309 Synthetic *delta*-tocopherol				M ⎪
E310 Propyl gallate				M ⎪
E311 Octyl gallate				M ⎪
E312 Dodecyl gallate				M ⎭
E320 Butylated hydroxyanisole (BHA)				M
E321 Butylated hydroxytoluene (BHT)				M

Emulsifiers, stabilizers, thickeners				
E322 Lecithins	A			
E325 Sodium lactate	A	✓		
E326 Potassium lactate	A	✓		M
E327 Calcium lactate	A	✓		M
E330 Citric acid		✓	✓	

E331	Sodium dihydrogen citrate (monoSodium citrate), diSodium citrate, triSodium citrate				M
E332	Potassium dihydrogen citrate (monoPotassium citrate), triPotassium citrate				M
E333	monoCalcium citrate, diCalcium citrate, triCalcium citrate	A			M
E334	L-(+)-tartaric acid	A	>		
E335	monoSodium L-(+)-tartrate, diSodium L-(+)-tartrate		>	>	M
E336	monoPotassium L-(+)-tartrate (Cream of tartar), diPotassium L-(+)-tartrate		>	>	M
E337	Potassium sodium L-(+)-tartrate		>	>	M
E338	Orthophosphoric acid (Phosophoric acid)	A			M
E339	Sodium dihydrogen orthophosphate, diSodium hydrogen orthophosphate, triSodium orthophosphate				M
E340	Potassium dihydrogen orthophosphate, diPotassium hydrogen orthophosphate, triPotassium orthophosphate	A			M
E341	Calcium tetrahydrogen diorthophosphate, Calcium hydrogen orthophosphate, triCalcium diorthophosphate	A			M
350	Sodium malate, sodium hydrogen malate		>	>	M
351	Potassium malate		>	>	M
352	Calcium malate, calcium hydrogen malate	A			M
353	Metatartaric acid		>		M

107

Table 2 – continued

		Animal	Vegetarian	Vegan	Mineral
355	Adipic acid		✓	✓	M
363	Succinic acid		✓	✓	M
370	1,4-Heptonolactone				M
375	Nicotinic acid				
380	triAmmonium citrate				M
381	Ammonium ferric citrate				M
385	Calcium disodium ethylenediamine – NNN'N'-tetra-acetate (Calcium disodium EDTA)				
E400	Alginic acid		✓	✓	M
E401	Sodium alginate		✓	✓	M
E402	Potassium alginate		✓	✓	M
E403	Ammonium alginate		✓	✓	M
E404	Calcium alginate		✓	✓	
E405	Propane-1,2-diol alginate (Propylene glycol alginate)	A			
E406	Agar		✓	✓	
E407	Carrageenan		✓	✓	
E410	Locust bean gum (Carob gum)		✓	✓	
E412	Guar gum		✓	✓	
E413	Tragacanth		✓	✓	M
E414	Gum arabic (Acacia)		✓	✓	
E415	Xanthan gum		✓	✓	
416	Karaya gum		✓	✓	

Synthetic sweetners

E420	Sorbitol, sorbitol syrup			M
E421	Mannitol			M
E422	Glycerol			M
430	Polyoxyethylene (8) stearate	A	rarely	M
431	Polyoxyethylene (40) stearate	A		
432	Polyoxyethylene (20) sorbitan monolaurate (Polysorbate 20)	A		M
433	Polyoxyethylene (20) sorbitan mono-oleate (Polysorbate 80)	A		M
434	Polyoxyethylene (20) sorbitan monopalmitate (Polysorbate 40)	A		M
435	Polyoxyethylene (20) sorbitan monostearate (Polysorbate 60)	A		M
436	Polyoxyethylene (20) sorbitan tristearate (Polysorbate 65)	A		M

Emulsifiers, stabilizers, thickeners

E440(a)	Pectin		✓	
E440(b)	Amidated pectin		✓	
442	Ammonium phosphatides		✓	M
E450(a)	diSodium dihydrogen diphosphate, triSodium diphosphate, tetraSodium diphosphate, tetraPotassium diphosphate	A	✓	M
E450(b)	pentaSodium triphosphate, pentaPotassium triphosphate	A		M

109

Table 2 – continued

		Animal	Vegetarian	Vegan	Mineral
E450(c)	Sodium polyphosphates, Potassium polyphospates	A			
E460	Microcrystalline cellulose, alpha-cellulose (Powdered cellulose)				M
E461	Methylcellulose		✓	✓	M
E463	Hydroxypropylcellulose		✓	✓	M
E464	Hydroxypropylmethylcellulose		✓	✓	M
E465	Ethylmethylcellulose		✓	✓	M
E466	Carboxymethylcellulose, sodium salt (CMC)		✓	✓	M
E470	Sodium, potassium and calcium salts of fatty acids	A	✓	✓	M
E471	Mono- and di-glycerides of fatty acids	A	✓	✓	M
E472(a)	Acetic acid esters of mono- and di-glycerides of fatty acids	A	✓	✓	M
E472(b)	Lactic acid esters of mono- and di-glycerides of fatty acids (Lactoglycerides)	A	✓	✓	
E472(c)	Citric acid esters of mono- and di-glycerides of fatty acids (Citroglycerides)	A	✓	✓	M
E472(e)	Mono- and diacetyltartaric acid esters of mono- and di-glycerides of fatty acids	A	✓	✓	
E473	Sucrose esters of fatty acids	A	✓	✓	M
E474	Sucroglycerides	A	✓	✓	M
E475	Polyglycerol esters of fatty acids	A	✓	✓	M

476	Polyglycerol esters of polycondensed fatty acids of castor oil (Polyglycerol polyricinoleate)			
E477	Propane-1,2-diol esters of fatty acids	A	✓ ✓	M M
478	Lactylated fatty acid esters of glycerol and propane-1,2-diol			
E481	Sodium stearoyl-2-lactylate	A	✓	M
E482	Calcium stearoyl-2-lactylate	A	✓	M
E483	Stearyl tartrate	A	✓	M
491	Sorbitan monostearate	A	✓	M
492	Sorbitan tristearate	A	✓	M
493	Sorbitan monolaurate		✓	M
494	Sorbitan mono-oleate			M
495	Sorbitan monopalmitate			M
500	Sodium carbonate, Sodium hydrogen carbonate (Bicarbonate of soda), Sodium sesquicarbonate		✓ ✓	M

Acids, bases

501	Potassium carbonate, Potassium hydrogen carbonate	M
503	Ammonium carbonate, Ammonium hydrogen carbonate	M
504	Magnesium carbonate	M
507	Hydrochloric acid	M
508	Potassium chloride	M
509	Calcium chloride	M

Table 2 – continued

		Animal	Vegetarian	Vegan	Mineral
510	Ammonium chloride				M
513	Sulphuric acid				M
514	Sodium sulphate				M
515	Potassium sulphate				M
516	Calcium sulphate				M
518	Magnesium sulphate				M
524	Sodium hydroxide				M
525	Potassium hydroxide				M
526	Calcium hydroxide				M
527	Ammonium hydroxide				M
528	Magnesium hydroxide				M
529	Calcium oxide				M

Anti-caking agents

		Animal	Vegetarian	Vegan	Mineral
530	Magnesium oxide				M
535	Sodium ferrocyanide (Sodium hexacyanoferrate II)				
536	Potassium ferrocyanide (Potassium hexacyanoferrate II)				M
540	diCalcium diphosphate				M
541	Sodium aluminium phosphate				M
542	Edible bone phosphate	A			
544	Calcium polyphosphates				M
545	Ammonium polyphosphates				M

112

551	Silicon dioxide (Silica)			M
552	Calcium silicate			M
553(a)	Magnesium silicate synthetic, Magnesium trisilicate			M
553(b)	Talc			M
554	Aluminium sodium silicate			M
556	Aluminium calcium silicate			M
558	Bentonite			
559	Kaolin			
570	Stearic acid	A		M
572	Magnesium stearate	A	✓	M
575	D-glucono-1,5-lactone (Glucono delta-lactone)		✓	
576	Sodium gluconate			M
577	Potassium gluconate			M
578	Calcium gluconate			M

Flavour enhancers, sweeteners

620	L-glutamic acid			M
621	Sodium hydrogen L-glutamate (*monoSodium glutamate or MSG*)		✓	
622	Potassium hydrogen L-glutamate (*monoPotassium glutamate*)			M
623	Calcium dihydrogen di-L-glutamate (*Calcium glutamate*)			M
627	Guanosine 5'-(disodium phosphate) (*Sodium guanylate*)	A		

Table 2 – continued

		Animal	Vegetarian	Vegan	Mineral
631	Inosine 5′-(disodium phosphate) (Sodium inosinate)	A			
635	Sodium 5′-ribonucleotide		√		M
636	Maltol				M
637	Ethyl maltol				M

Glazing agents

900	Dimethylpolysiloxane				M
901	Beeswax	A			
903	Carnauba wax		√		
904	Shellac	A			
905	Mineral hydrocarbons				M
907	Refined microcrystalline wax				M

Improving and bleaching agents

920	L-cysteine hydrochloride	A			
924	Potassium bromate				M
925	Chlorine				M
926	Chlorine dioxide				M
927	Azodicarbonamide (Azoformamide)				M

No E numbers

Sweeteners

—	Saccharin		∑	
—	Saccharin calcium		∑	
—	Saccharin sodium		∑	
—	Aspartame	A	∑	
—	Acesulfame potassium		∑	
—	Thaumatin	✓		Vegetable source of amino acids
—	Hydrogenated glucose syrup	✓		
—	Isomalt		∑	mixture of proteins from W. African fruit
—	Xylitol	✓	✓	occurs widely in natural fruit and vegetables

Solvents

—	Ethyl alcohol	✓	✓	
—	Ethyl acetate	✓	✓	∑
—	Diethyl ether	✓	✓	∑
—	Glycerol monoacetate	✓	✓	∑
—	Glycerol triacetate	✓	✓	
—	Isopropyl alcohol	✓	✓	∑
—	Propylene glycol	✓		∑

Table 2 – continued

	Animal	Vegetarian	Vegan	Mineral
Miscellaneous				
Ethoxyquin				M
Dioctyl sodium sulphosuccinate				M
Extract of quillaia		✓		
Dichlorodifluoromethane				M
Calcium phytate		✓	✓	M
Glycine	A	✓	✓	
Sodium heptonate				M*
Calcium heptonate				M*
Hydrogen				M
Nitrogen				M
Nitrous oxide				M
Oxygen				M
Octadeyl ammonium acetate				M
Oxystearin	A			

* Or biologically derived.

Table 3
Additives Not Permitted in Food Specifically for Babies and Young Children

E310	Propyl gallate
E311	Octy gallate
E312	Dodecyl gallate
E320	Butylated hydroxyanisole (BHA)
E321	Butylated hydroxytoluene (BHT)
E420	Sorbitol
E421	Mannitol
E422	Glycerol
621	Sodium hydrogen L-glutamate (monosodium glutamate)
622	Potassium hydrogen L-glutamate
623	Calcium dihydrogen di-l-glutamate
627	Guanosine 5'-(disodium phosphate)
631	Inosine 5'-(disodium phosphate)
635	Sodium 5'-ribonecleotide

Table 4
Additives Recommended for Avoidance by Hyperactive Children

E102	Tartrazine
E104	Quinoline Yellow
E107	Yellow 2G
E110	Sunset Yellow
E120	Cochineal
E122	Carmoisine
E123	Amaranth
E124	Ponceau
E127	Erythrosine
E128	Red 2G
E131	Patent Blue V
E132	Indigo Carmine
E133	Brilliant Blue FCF
E150	Caramel
E151	Black PN
154	Brown FK
E155	Brown HT
E180	Pigment Rubine
E210	Benzoic acid

Table 4 – continued
Additives Recommended for Avoidance by Hyperactive Children

E211	Sodium benzoate
E212	Potassium benzoate
E213	Calcium benzoate
E214	Ethyl 4-hydroybenzoate
E215	Ethyl 4-hydroxybenzoate, sodium salt
E216	Propyl 4-hydroxybenzoate
E217	Propyl 4-hydroxybenzoate, sodium salt
E218	Methyl 4-hydroxybenzoate
E219	Sodium methyl hydroxybenzoate
E220	Sulphur dioxide
E250	Sodium nitrite
E251	Sodium nitrate (Chile saltpetre)
E310	Propyl gallate
E311	Octyl gallate
E312	Dodecyl gallate
E320	Butylated hydroxyanisole (BHA)
E321	Butylated hydroxytoluene (BHT)
E621	Sodium hydrogen L-glutamate (monosodium glutamate)
E622	Potassium hydrogen L-glutamate
E623	Calcium dihydrogen di-L-glutamate
E627	Guanosine 5'-(disodium phosphate)
E631	Inosine 5'-(disodium phosphate)
E635	Sodium 5'-ribonucleotide

Table 5
Sodium-containing Additives to be Avoided by Those on a Low-salt Diet

E201	Sodium sorbate
E211	Sodium benzoate
E215	Sodium ethyl para-hydroxybenzoate
E217	Sodium propyl para-hydroxybenzoate
E219	Sodium methyl para-hydroxybenzoate
E221	Sodium sulphite
E222	Sodium bisulphite
E223	Sodium metabisulphite
E232	Sodium orthophenylphenate
E250	Sodium nitrite

E251	Sodium nitrate
E262	Sodium hydrogen diacetate
262	sodium acetate
E281	Sodium propionate
E301	Sodium L-ascorbate
E325	Sodium lactate
E331	Mono sodium citrate (also di and tri)
E335	Mono sodium L-tartrate (also di)
E337	Potassium sodium L-tartrate
E339	Sodium dihydrogen orthophosphate (also di and tri)
E350	Sodium malate, sodium hydrogen malate
E401	Sodium alginate
E450	Disodium dihydrogen diphosphates (E450a-c)
E470	Sodium salts of fatty acids
E481	Sodium stearoyl-2-lactylate
E500	Bicarbonate of soda
E514	Sodium sulphate
E524	Sodium hydroxide
E535	Sodium hexacyanoferrate
E541	Sodium aluminium phosphate
E554	Aluminium sodium silicate
E576	Sodium gluconate
E621	Monosodium glutamate (MSG)
E627	Sodium guanylate
E631	Sodium inosinate
E635	Sodium 5'-ribonucleotide

No code
- Saccharin sodium
- Dioctyl sodium sulphosuccinate
- Disodium edetate
- Sodium heptonate

4. Cooking for Health

Cooking for health is just as important as shopping for health. Even if your basket is full of the freshest and best food, if you don't prepare it properly you will not get much advantage from the effort you have put into your shopping. Although enthusiasm and imagination are two excellent ingredients for a good cook, a little knowledge of food preparation is also a vital ingredient.

Keep it clean

This is not just a reference to the language in the kitchen when things get a bit too hot. It is also about going back to basics and reminding ourselves that one of the most important things in food preparation is hygiene.

When preparing food always

- Wash hands before and frequently during food handling.
- Keep raw and cooked meat separate, because food poisoning bacteria can easily be transferred from raw to cooked.
- Keep food refrigerated and chill cooked food as soon as possible; if it sits around at room temperature, bacteria will grow very quickly.
- Thaw frozen meat very thoroughly before cooking, especially poultry.

Store it well

Store food in a cool place or in the fridge. Keep meat and fish in the coldest part of the fridge. Unwrap meat and fish when you get them home and place on a plate. Lightly cover so the air can circulate around them.

Store fresh vegetables and salad in the salad compartment of the fridge and make a point of getting to the bottom of the crisper at least once a week to give it a clean.

Throw away all food with any mould on it. Moulds are the subject of toxicity investigations at the moment and it seems as though they are more harmful than we previously thought, as they penetrate far deeper than the surface areas on which they appear.

Don't *buy* mouldy food, either; always check beneath the cling-film wrapper to see if there is mould lurking.

Equipping your kitchen

Having the right tool for the job saves a lot of time and it saves your temper, too. It also means the food you are preparing has a better chance of turning out how you want it to be and not disappointing you.

Sharp **knives** are essential for making tasks easier and for minimizing vitamin loss – they do less damage to the food being cut than does hacking at it with a blunt knife. The cook is also less likely to be cut using a sharp knife because less force has to be used and things are less likely to slip. (It is also usual to take more care when the knives are known to be sharp!)

Stainless steel knives are best and, contrary to myth, they can be sharpened without ruining the blade. A kitchen steel is useful, or you can take knives to be sharpened at a local hardware or department store. Laser knives have stainless steel cutting edges cut by laser and are said to stay sharp for twenty-five years; I haven't had one for long enough to endorse the claim. Always keep knives in a knife block, plastic wallet, cloth wrap-around or cardboard sheaths. It is dangerous to go fumbling in drawers where upturned blades can cause nasty accidents. A carving knife, fruit and vegetable knife and palette knife are essential for the keen cook.

Choose stainless steel **saucepans** in preference to aluminium ones – stainless steel does not react with food. When some foods are cooked in aluminium pans the acids in them, particularly fruits and vinegary foods, react with the metal, making it shiny. Whether the aluminium absorbed in the food is harmful is debatable, but why risk it?

Good-quality (heavy) stainless steel pans may cost more than aluminium pans but they will last a lifetime. They also clean easily and look good after twenty years' wear if looked after properly. Many of the Scandinavian brands are good and they are also well designed (too handsome to hide in cupboards). Consider choosing pans that can also be used in the oven as casseroles and that are attractive enough for serving food in.

French cast-iron pans are also extremely useful. Because they are so heavy, with thick, well-constructed bases, they conduct the heat extremely well and can be used on the stove top on the minimum gas or electric setting. With a well-fitting lid it is possible to cook a casserole on top of the stove in these pans and to cut down on the amount of liquid added to food for cooking. The lids trap the steam and food cooks in its own moisture, preventing vitamins leaching out into water which may be thrown away.

It is easy to cook one-pot meals in these pans. Place a layer of sliced onion in the base of the pan with a little vegetable oil. Cover, and let it sweat (cook in its own moisture) for a few minutes. Add some unpeeled, sliced apple and potato seasoned with freshly ground black pepper and chopped sage, and place thin slices of liver on top. Top with sliced potato and cover. The meal will cook in its own steam without added liquid in about 20–25 minutes. Remove from the pan, add a little brown stock or vegetable stock (p. 385), boil vigorously and serve as gravy with the meal.

Lots of other meat, fish and vegetable dishes can be cooked in the same way using good-quality cast-iron pans that will cook over a very low heat without burning the food in them.

Cooking for Health

Non-stick pans have become more popular because they help cut down on the amount of fat and oil used in cooking. Foods like bacon can be fried without the addition of any oil. Vegetables may also be sweated in non-stick pans if they have a well-fitting lid.

A **wok** is also a handy piece of equipment because it minimizes the amount of fat needed for cooking. The food is cooked at a high temperature, cutting down on cooking time, and therefore on vitamin and mineral loss. Crunchier stir-fries are possible in a wok and a wok with a lid will keep the steam in to cook the veg even faster. A good-quality cooking oil is essential for this kind of cooking – although the oil has to be at a high temperature, it should not be smoking. Smoke means the oil is beginning to break down and it should not be used that hot. Oils such as corn, soya or sesame are good for this kind of cooking. Olive oil is also good, if you like the flavour.

A **double boiler** is another useful piece of equipment, but not essential, because it can be improvised using a heatproof basin stood on a metal trivet (or a small price of wood) inside a pan of boiling water. This piece of equipment is used for making sauces, custards or mixtures that must not boil (boiling would result in a curdled mixture). Put aside an old saucepan for this job because it will become furred by mineral deposits like the inside of a kettle. This pan can also be used for boiling eggs – eggs will spoil saucepans used for general cooking.

A **steamer** is another useful way of cooking food without it coming into contact with the fat or water in which it is being cooked – this cuts down on calories and on loss of nutrients. Collapsible stainless-steel steamers which sit inside a variety of saucepans are very handy and take up little storage space.

A pair of **scales** and a **measuring jug** are essential. There is no point in wasting expensive raw ingredients by not bothering to weigh them out. Sometimes guesswork will get you by, but correct weights and liquid measures are essential for recipes like choux pastry, soufflés and mousses. Check the pan on the scales – it may be clumsy to lift and difficult to pour from. It may also not come away from the scales very easily (check this on wall-mounted

Shopping for Health

scales). A transparent glass measuring jug that is also heatproof is very useful.

There are some very attractive **kettles** available which look more like ceramic coffee-pots. Before you buy, check the volume if you have any special needs (like an extra large/small family) and make sure it's stainless steel. When you use it, put in only the amount of water you need; don't boil a whole kettleful for one cup of tea – it wastes fuel and money. Fill fresh from the tap each time you want water; don't keep reboiling the same old water all day!

Mixing bowls are essential. Have a large one for jobs like bread-making and a small one for making cakes or whisking an egg white. If you have a large food-mixer, use that bowl for lots of jobs – don't clutter the cupboards with more than you need. Both transparent glass Pyrex bowls and the old-fashioned-Greens' brown mixing bowls can be used for whisking mixtures over a pan of hot water – it is a matter of personal taste which is chosen. When using the mixing bowl it is often helpful to place a damp cloth beneath it to prevent it slipping all over the work-surface.

Ceramic basins are useful, not only for cooking in, but also for storing leftovers or stock in the fridge. They do not absorb aromas and flavours like polythene fridge containers and they can be effectively covered, leaving a headspace above the material in them, with clingfilm.

Wooden **spoons** for beating and creaming mixtures and stirring food over heat are essential. It is useful to have one for savoury mixtures that might contain garlic and another for sweet use. A tablespoon, dessertspoon and teaspoon are needed for measuring (or a set of measuring spoons). A metal tablespoon is useful for folding egg whites into some dishes because it cuts through the mixture, losing less air than a thick wooden spoon would do. A large **fork** is handy for mixing drier mixtures or mashing, and a pliable **spatula** will enable every bit of mixture to be scraped from the sides of the bowl for economy and easier washing up.

Kitchen scissors are invaluable for cutting large quantities of herbs, which can be used as flavouring in place of salt. Scissors are also useful for dealing with gooseberries and currants, for cutting

Cooking for Health

paper to cook fish, etc., *en papillote* (which does not require fat) and for cutting paper to line baking tins.

A plain wooden **rolling pin** without fancy handles is the easiest to work with and to clean. A good **sieve** is essential for light baking when using wholemeal flour. Not for sieving out the bran and throwing it away (!) but for introducing air to wholemeal goods. The bran is put back into the mixture.

You will need a small hand **juicer** to squeeze juice from lemons with. (You can baste grilled foods with it rather than brushing them with oil.) A juicer with a strainer to catch the pips and pulp is the most useful type.

A good **tin-opener** is essential (not that you will be using that many tins) -- one that does not make jagged cuts which are dangerous and messy is the type to buy. A Magican one that takes off the whole lid so that you don't risk cut fingers is useful, or the butterfly-nut type.

A good **hand grater** is necessary for grating small amounts of fruit and veg, and for hard cheese and nutmeg. A **garlic press** will save you getting smelly fingers. Choose a rigid one that does not bend. Don't forget, either, a **colander** (a stainless steel one can double up as a steamer if necessary).

Oven gloves are essential if you don't want to ruin all your tea-towels. Gauntlet ones are best, as they prevent painful burns on the arms and they are easier to handle than those joined gloves.

A **perforated spoon** is handy for skimming stocks and a **skewer** for testing whether food is cooked. A **fish slice** is handy too. Not for frying, but for removing fish fillets whole from the grill pan.

If there is no **timer** on your cooker you will need to buy a separate one, especially if you are in the habit of wandering off and leaving things to cook.

If you like to do Indian or Malaysian cooking, a **pestle and mortar** is handy for grinding your own spices as you want them. You can then roast them immediately before you grind them for extra flavour (and you will need less salt). Also useful for making the Japanese condiment *gomasio*, which is toasted sesame seeds ground with a little salt (this makes the salt go further and gives it a more exciting taste).

Shopping for Health

Wire **cooling trays** will prevent worktops or wooden surfaces being burned or damaged by hot tins from the oven or hob. There is a great variety of **baking trays** and **tins** to chose from. Many are now available in stainless steel but those that are not can always be lined with greaseproof paper. To line a tin, first grease the inside of the tin and then the side of the paper that will be in contact with the food. Draw around the base of the tin to cut the lining for the bottom.

Loose-bottom tins are especially useful for cheesecakes and other soft-set mixtures; those with spring-form sides make the job of unmoulding much easier. The cake can be left on the metal base and placed on the serving dish if it is too fragile to remove from the base. Non-stick tins do not have to be greased and non-stick baking trays and bun tins are extremely easy to clean after use.

Glass or ceramic **flan dishes** and baking dishes often cut out the need for serving dishes because they are designed for use from oven to table (but they don't make crisp pastry!). A **soufflé dish** is another useful oven-to-table dish that can also be used for baked desserts or simply as a serving dish for vegetables, etc.

For roasting, choose a pan with a built-in rack so that meat and poultry can be roasted without added fats and the fats from the meat can drain away into the pan below and be discarded.

A reversible **chopping board** is a good idea. You can keep one side for vegetables such as onions and garlic which penetrate wood, and the other side for sweet ingredients. It is better to use a non-wood board for meat because this will prevent salmonella from being transferred to other foods should the board be cracked or the meat infected.

An **oil well** is extremely useful for keeping down the amount of oil used. It is a small plastic container with a well of oil into which a brush is depressed. As the brush is withdrawn, most of the oil is squeezed out of it, so far less oil ends up in the pan than it would do when pouring from a bottle.

Larger equipment

Larger pieces of kitchen equipment are only useful if you do a lot of cooking or prepare food for larger numbers of people.

Food processor

A food processor is probably the most versatile; a Kenwood Chef or Kenwood Chef Excel with its various attachments will give you a larger capacity than most. These are especially helpful if you are going to make a lot of salads, because they can slice and prepare food very quickly. They also are very sharp, thus cutting down on losses of nutrients. They will also mince meat for you at home, so you can buy lean meat and prepare it yourself – no more fatty or watery butchers' mince.

Home-made soups are made much more quickly and easily with the liquidizing and blending attachments, and breadcrumbs and nuts can be milled very quickly without a lot of fuss and mess. (A grinder/liquidizer will also make soup and grind breadcrumbs, nuts, etc.; it can be bought much more cheaply than a food processor.)

Pressure cooker

This will cut cooking time by about two thirds and so it will also cut vitamin and mineral losses. Pressure cooking also minimizes the amount of water used, so it cuts losses in that way, too. The high temperature of the cooker destroys the enzyme that destroys vitamin C in food, and food cooked in a pressure cooker can be tastier than that which is boiled, where a lot of the aroma is lost. Shape, colour and firmness are also better retained, making the food more appetizing as well as healthier.

A pressure cooker reduces the cooking time of beans and rice, encouraging you to make more use of these low-fat, high-fibre foods. (Microwaves do not speed up beans and other legumes.)

Shopping for Health

Microwave ovens

Britain is the largest market for microwave ovens outside America and Japan, no doubt due to our liking for convenience foods. You can also use a microwave oven for healthier cooking because it can

cook fruit and vegetables quickly with a minimum of, or no, water
reheat fresh chilled READY MEALS
thaw foods quickly
cook things like nut roasts and cutlets in far less time than a conventional oven
reduce the cooking time of brown rice and baked potatoes to make these valuable foods more convenient
make porridge very quickly to get you off to a good start in the morning
bake wholemeal loaves quickly, if you don't mind them looking a bit pale. (With a microwave oven which incorporates convection heating, this is, of course, no problem.)

Microwave ovens reheat food with less nutritional loss than other forms of reheating. (Although reheating is not to be encouraged!) They also result in more nutrients being retained in the vegetables cooked in them, especially if no water is used during the cooking.

They are also especially useful for making sauces in a hurry – a good sauce can be the basis of many nutritious dishes, from topping pasta and pizzas to making lasagne and moussaka.

Baked potatoes are, of course, an old favourite and they are a better bet nutritionally than popping out to the chip shop. Other vegetables can also be stuffed and baked quickly in a microwave.

Effect of Cooking Method on Energy and Fat Levels

	Energy (kcal per 100 g)	Fat (g per 100 g)
Potatoes		
boiled	80	0.1
roast	157	4.8

Cooking for Health

	Energy (kcal per 100 g)	Fat (g per 100 g)
chips (deep fat fried)	253	10.9
(frozen, deep fat fried)	264	13.8
(frozen, shallow fat fried)	291	18.9
(oven chips, oven cooked)	188	6.0
crisps	533	36
Beefburgers		
raw	338	29
grilled	277	19
fried	294	21
Fish-fingers		
raw	178	7.5
grilled	230	11.5
fried	259	15.7

Source: Eat Right, Eat Well, Co-op.

Cooking to keep the vitamins

To preserve the vitamins in fruit and vegetables prepare them for cooking when they are needed. Potatoes peeled and left all day soaking in cold water (in or out of the fridge) will lose much of their vitamin C and B vitamins, which will leach out into the water and be thrown away down the sink.

As well as leaching out into soaking or cooking water, vitamins are also lost through oxidation. When the surface of the vegetable is cut it exposes the vitamins to oxygen which destroys them. The smaller the pieces are cut the more surface is exposed to the air. In the case of salads, make up the salad dressing before washing and slicing the vegetables and then toss the vegetables in dressing as soon as they have been cut. The vegetable oil used in salad dressings will seal the surface against contact with the air and the vitamin E present in cold-pressed vegetable oils also helps prevent oxidation. (Heat-treated oils – all those *not* labelled cold-pressed

Shopping for Health

– will have had a certain amount of their vitamin content destroyed during processing.)

In the same way, vegetables for cooking should be put straight into the cooking medium. If they are to be boiled, have the water ready boiling, so that the oxygen in the water has been driven off; it will also help the vegetables cook more quickly, and quicker cooking means less time in contact with water and less vitamin and mineral (these also leach out into cooking water) loss. Plunging vegetables straight into boiling water also inactivates the enzyme in vegetable cells that destroys vitamin C (it is destroyed at 60°C). The enzyme is activated when cells are damaged by bruising or cutting, i.e. scrubbing, peeling and dicing.

Steaming vegetables is a better way of protecting their nutrients than boiling. Steam is a very efficient cooking medium and it keeps the vegetables out of the water.

Whether steaming or boiling, keep the water to a minimum. If boiling try to use the water in an accompanying sauce or save it for stock. (Water from cabbage, sprouts, broccoli and other vegetables of the cabbage family should not be kept, however – use it the same day.) Always use a well-fitting lid on the saucepan. This keeps heat in, speeds cooking and keeps oxygen out.

Having taken the trouble to prepare the vegetables just before cooking, don't ruin the good work by keeping the vegetables warm for a long time. Try to eat them as soon after they have been cooked as possible – keeping them warm encourages more vitamin loss.

Some green leafy vegetables do not need any added cooking water. Spinach, for instance, can be cooked in a saucepan with just the water it was washed in left on its leaves. Use a pan with a well-fitting lid and turn the spinach once or twice during about five to ten minutes cooking (depending on the amount). A pan full of mixed sliced vegetables, cut as for stir-fry, will cook in its own steam if a good-quality heavy-based pan with a well-fitting lid is used.

Fruit purées can also be cooked with the addition of just a couple of tablespoonfuls of water. Cook them in a good-quality stainless-steel pan placed over a low heat. The fruit will have to be

Cooking for Health

stirred to ensure even cooking if there is a lot in the pan.

Ideally fruit and vegetables should not be peeled if the skin is edible because in many instances the greatest concentration of vitamins is just below the skin. The skin also provides extra fibre. However, unless fruit and vegetables are organically grown there may be residues on the skin from chemical sprays applied as pesticides or even sprays to kill insects that might threaten the harvested crop. Thorough washing, or even peeling, is advisable if the origin of the fruit and vegetables is not known.

Incidentally, waxes are often used as preservatives on the rind of citrus fruits, so if you want to use the rind in cooking, it would be wise to look for the greener looking types, which may not have been sprayed. (Seville oranges should not have been sprayed, as they are used to make marmalade.)

Cooking for flavour

Vegetables

Most vegetables should be served while they still have some crispness left. *Al dente* is the term used when cooking pasta, meaning that it should be cooked but still offer some resistance to the teeth when bitten. The same should apply to well-cooked vegetables. The broccoli spear should not flop over completely in a water-sodden state; it should be almost able to remain turgidly supporting itself – though soft enough to bite into easily. Shorter cooking times help retain the flavour and appearance of food, as well as retaining the nutrients.

Keeping the colour of green vegetables has been an obsession of the British, who devised the disastrous practice of adding bicarbonate of soda to cooking water to retain the green colour. Bicarbonate of soda should never be added to cooking water because it destroys the vitamin C and the B vitamins. Shorter cooking times will help preserve colour, especially in French beans, which turn khaki when overcooked, because of chemical

Shopping for Health

reactions involving the naturally present acids in the bean. Some chefs suggest cooking French beans in copper pans to preserve their bright green colour, but copper pans encourage oxygenation and increase the loss of vitamin C. The younger the bean the less colour it will lose on cooking. Those straight from the garden keep their green colour well if cooked until just *al dente*.

Fish

The delicate flavours of fish are often destroyed by clumsy cooking. Coating in a heavy batter and frying is out. The batter adds unnecessary calories and interferes with the flavour of the fish – it acts as a sponge for the frying fat which becomes the predominant taste. (However, if you *must* fry, deep-fat frying is preferable to shallow frying because the food cooks quicker and stays in the fat for a shorter time. Do not re-use cooking oils and fats.)

Naturally oily fish like mackerel and herring (both much under-used and full of vitamins A, D and essential and protective marine fish oils) can be grilled without the addition of any fat. They can also be baked in the oven wrapped in greaseproof paper or vegetable leaves, or laid in a casserole, on a bed of finely diced onions, mushrooms and apples, which is then covered and cooked without any fat being added. For slightly less oily whole fish such as trout, the juice of a lemon may be used to baste them with under the grill. Place a sprig of fresh herbs in the gut cavity (parsley, thyme or fennel or fennel seeds) for a delicious aroma and flavour.

Herbs, spices and seasoning

Herbs and spices are very important in healthy cooking. Most diets contain too much added salt, which contributes to health problems such as high blood pressure. It also upsets the natural balance of mineral salts in the body, which is necessary for healthy functioning.

For most people there is more than enough salt naturally present in foods, and in the correct balance with potassium, its counter-balance in the body. So get out of the habit of adding salt during cooking and of using it at the table. The taste for salt in highly salted foods is acquired through habit and it can be lost in the same way. This will take some effort because the amount of salt in the diet is insidiously increased by food manufacturers in almost every product, in an attempt the seduce the palate into eating more. This fact is recognized by doctors, who have called on food manufacturers to use less salt.

Concentrate on bringing out the true taste of the food in cooking and make sauces from fresh vegetables or vegetable purées rather than using heavy cream-and-egg-based sauces or thick white sauces with high-calorie hard cheese.

Cooking for health summary

1. Remember the rules of hygiene.
2. Keep food refrigerated and cool cooked food quickly, especially meat.
3. Keep cooked and uncooked meat separate.
4. Don't fry (deep or shallow); add as little fat as possible in cooking.
5. Prepare as near to eating or serving as possible – don't soak food or keep it warm.
6. Keep the skins on and avoid peeling wherever possible. This gives fibre and saves nutrients.
7. Cook in the minimum of water and/or use the cooking water in the sauce. Plunge food into already boiling water or hot oil.
8. Don't overcook – keep it crunchy!
9. Use the right tools for the job to avoid accidents and cut down on nutrient losses.

The Shopping List

Writing your shopping list and going shopping

Before you go shopping here is a quick checklist of points you should remember and a few handy tips for getting it right. They may seem obvious, but they are the things we always forget to do . . .

- Check the fridge and food cupboard before you go – you may not have the item you thought was there.
- Write a list to sort out your ideas about what you are going to buy and cook.
- Even though you have a list, try to remain flexible so you can take advantage of any bargains you see while you are shopping.
- Don't be taken in by the 'reduced' labels on perishable foods like fruit, veg and dairy produce; it is not a real saving if they are nutritionally poor.
- Check the sell-by date.
- Get to know the delivery days for fresh foods in your local shops and buy on those days.
- Don't shop when you are hungry – you will buy more than you need and you will be tempted when you are standing by the sweets at the checkout or at the cake counter.
- Use a basket rather than a trolley, if possible; if you have to carry it you will think twice about putting in unnecessary items.
- Read the labels even if the picture on the packet looks like 'real' food.

The Shopping List

- Don't buy battered cans or boxes.
- Don't be afraid to buy as small an amount as you want – be ready with a smart reply for the assistant who calls you the 'last of the big spenders' if you want only 2 oz of cheese or 4 oz of meat.
- If you don't see what you want, ask for it – stating a preference is the only way to get things stocked.
- Always take back items that are off, bad, going bad or damaged when you open them.

Taking avoiding action

If you want to avoid a particular food additive or ingredient, keep a piece of paper or card in your purse or wallet with the E number and common name of the additive(s) you want to avoid so you can do a quick double-check before buying. Keep a copy of the list at home, on a notice board or somewhere central, so that when another person does the shopping for you they have the information to hand. It is useful also to keep a note on the same paper of foods that any one in the family is allergic to.

```
SHOPPING REMINDER


E Number   212        Name    Potassium benzoate
           250                Sodium nitrite

Name       Adam       Item    Tomatoes
           Jane               Cow's milk
                              (lactose, whey, etc.)
```

'My choice'

Throughout this section I have highlighted my personal choice of best product, or products, in each category. These are entered under the heading 'My Choice'. The criteria here were nutritional value,* taste and general acceptance, but of course some element of subjectivity is bound to enter such a selection – my likes and dislikes will be different from yours. These 'choices' may lead you at once to a product you like, but don't let them put you off trying the many other excellent items listed in the Shopping List.

While every effort has been made to ensure that all entries are completely up to date, some manufacturers may have changed their recipes/formulas since this book was produced.

BABY FOOD

Breast is best, as the old saying goes, and this is still true today. Babies benefit from being breastfed for as long as practicable and certainly for at least three months. Between three and six months the baby may be introduced to its first solid foods. There is no reason why special foods should be bought for a baby – healthy adult food is healthy baby food, so long as it is puréed or strained, is free from added salt and sugar, and is not highly spiced or seasoned. After all, until comparatively recently, there were no canned baby foods, baby meals in jars or dried packet foods.

Formula feeds

Formula feeds, substitutes for breast-milk, are made from specially modified cow's milk. A baby's kidneys cannot cope with the amounts of protein and sodium contained in cow's milk or dried cow's milk, and this should never be given to a baby under six months old. (This is why tins of dried milk powder are labelled 'not suitable for babies'.) Goat's milk may be used for toddlers

---

* By nutritional value, I mean foods that are as near to their natural state as possible and as free from additives as possible. This results in a choice of foods with high nutrient value and lower calorific value – a diet high in fibre and low in fat, sugar and salt.

Baby Food

with an allergy to cow's milk, but is as unsuitable for small babies as cow's milk.

Non-dairy soya-based milks are available for babies who cannot tolerate cow's milk or whose parents prefer them to have a vegetarian (non-animal) product. Special formulas are also available for the very few babies who have problems such as phenylketonuria, histidinaemia, fat malabsorption and other conditions needing professional care and advice.

Weaning

The age at which a baby is weaned from breast or bottle depends on personal development, but today weaning generally starts when a baby is from four to six months old. Too early an introduction to cow's milk or cereals, especially wheat protein, can lead to allergies. As a general rule avoid baby foods with added sugars, added salt and additives. There are some additives which manufacturers are not allowed to put in baby food (see Table 4). The 1984 Labelling Regulations banned the use of any claims that formula milks are better than or even as good as the milk of a healthy mother.

Food claiming to be specially for babies or young children must fulfil all the claims made for it; it must be prepacked and completely enclosed to ensure it is totally hygienic. Special instructions for use also have to accompany baby foods, together with a nutritional statement about the energy (calories/kilojoules) it will provide, to protect babies from undernourishment or overnourishment (which could lead to obesity).

Salt and sugar

Salt and sugar may legally be added to commercial baby foods, but are better avoided. Salt is not recommended for babies because their sodium needs are met from the naturally present levels of sodium in milk and solid foods and infant kidneys cannot cope with an excess. Salt added to infant food (and to adult food)

Baby Food

has no nutritional function, and it is better not to encourage the development of the taste for salty foods.

Remember that sugar in baby and children's foods goes under many names other than sugar, including sucrose, glucose, fructose and dextrose. (See SUGAR.)

Most baby-food manufacturers are responding to demands from parents for more 'natural' baby foods and you will see 'low sugar' or 'reduced sugar' claims on many ranges, but even these are not always as low in sugar as you might think. Manufacturers have responded to later weaning by making larger jars or packets of their products – which goes to show that shoppers should make their needs known.

Hyperactivity

Many manufacturers supply tables and lists of products that are suitable for babies on special diets: vegetarian, vegan, gluten-free, milk/lactose/galactose-free, egg-free, etc. Heinz even list their tomato-free products, which might be useful for hyperactive children, because tomatoes contain salicylates, which have been implicated in hyperactivity. The other fruits and vegetables containing salicylates are: apples, apricots, blackberries, cherries, cucumbers, currants, gooseberries, grapes, peaches, plums, prunes, oranges, raisins, raspberries and tangerines.

Organic foods

It is now possible to buy convenience baby products made from organically grown produce (see ORGANIC FOODS) by Johannus and Holle. Milupa also analyse their raw ingredients for pesticide residues in cereals, fruit and vegetables, and the meat used in their products is analysed for hormones and antibiotics.

Most baby-food manufacturers have two ranges of baby foods. One is for the baby's first introduction to solids and the second for older babies. They usually offer ranges of main meals, either meat or vegetable based, and desserts. There is one 'tea-time' range, from Milupa. Special cereal feeds for smaller babies should never

Baby Food

be put into the baby's bottle to 'boost' its food or get it off to sleep – they should be given with a spoon to encourage chewing. Cereals should never be introduced earlier than three months, and many specialists recommend four months. Special baby mueslis are available.

Sweet tooth

Rusks are also popular for babies. They don't really help the teeth come through but they keep babies quiet and give them something to do! Rusks for babies over six months can be easily made at home from oven-dried fingers of wholemeal bread or egg-soaked dried bread. If you are buying them watch out, again, for added sugar. There are some sugar-free and some low-sugar versions, but the low-sugar ones are usually very similar to the normal ranges. If you don't use sugar-free versions you will be giving 'teeth-rotting' rusks rather than teething rusks. Some manufacturers have introduced wholemeal rusks made with specially finely ground wholemeal flour or a mix of white and wholemeal. The flour needs to be very fine to prevent choking.

Special drinks can also encourage a sweet tooth. Generally 'juices' are better than 'drinks', because the latter may have added ingredients like sugar, colour, etc. If buying baby juices and drinks, check the ingredients panel. (Similarly, beware of teething gels – they often contain sugar.) Avoiding sugary foods early on saves a lot of trouble later. Although a young baby has no teeth for the sugar to cause decay, a 'sweet tooth' can easily develop.

Home-prepared baby foods are certainly a lot cheaper than bought baby foods, but the ready-prepared meals are convenient at times. When you are evaluating commercial baby foods, ask yourself:

- Are they sugar-free and salt-free?
- Are they low in saturated fats?
- Are they free from additives?
- Are they made from 'whole' grains such as wholemeal flour and pasta, where appropriate?
- Will they encourage a sweet tooth?

Baby Food

Remember, baby foods may seem bland to our over-stimulated adult palates, but they don't need jazzing up for a baby. So don't be tempted to add a little sugar or salt – it would be harmful. Avoid 'chocolate' and 'caramel' flavoured baby foods; they will develop a taste for these flavours too soon.

See CANNED FOOD for general notes on buying food in cans.

Infant formula foods

Cow & Gate Formula S is a soya-food dried formula which is free from cow's milk and is suitable for vegetarian babies and those intolerant of cow's milk. Vegan mums might like to know that the vitamin D is derived from sheep's wool lanolin. It is free from sugar, but contains glucose syrup.

Wysoy soy protein baby formula is another milk-free formula, from the makers of SMA baby food.

NB. There are many regular formula feeds based on modified cow's milk which do not contain added sugar; the above are mentioned because they are of interest to those with special requirements.

All special baby problems should of course be tackled with the help of a qualified practitioner.

Cereals

Familia Swiss Baby Food and Familia Swiss Baby Cereal – No Added Sugar are mueslis made from natural ingredients without any additives. They are imported, you will have noted, from the home of the original muesli!

Robinson's Baby Rice is based on rice flour and, as well as being free from additives, sugar and salt, is also gluten-free and lactose free. A very versatile introduction to solids.

Robinson's Breakfast Cereals are mixed-grain and skimmed-milk cereals which are sucrose free.

Baby Food

Cow & Gate Muesli Breakfast with Vitamin C is free from additives, sugar and salt, and is based on fruit and low-fat yoghurt.

Boots Breakfast Porridge Oats, Mixed Cereal Breakfast, Protein Baby Cereal and Baby Rice are flaked baby cereals which are all free from added sugar and salt. The Baby Rice is gluten-free and is suitable for vegan babies; the others have some milk products, but are suitable for vegetarian babies. Boots granulated breakfast cereals are free from added salt and 'low in sugar'.

Farley's Farex Weaning Food is a rice-based cereal which is free from sugar, salt, milk, milk products and egg, making it suitable for vegetarians and vegans, and babies on a gluten-free diet.

Milupa do a range of breakfast cereals which are all suitable for vegetarian babies and free from artificial additives, but they contain cow's milk protein and lactose, which rules them out for vegans. They also contain some sugar. However, all Milupa raw ingredients are analysed to ensure they are free from pesticides and other chemical contamination. They are also screened for heavy metals, such as lead, which can enter fruit and vegetables, in particular from car-exhaust fumes. Pure Rice Cereal is Milupa's weaning cereal and there is also a Junior Muesli.

> **My choice**
>
> Milupa, or Familia Swiss Baby Cereal – No Added Sugar.

Rusks

These can be used as a 'teething aid' or as a meal, topped with mashed banana, for example, or scrambled egg. The listed rusks are all free from additives and from added salt.

Bickiepegs is the one brand of rusks that is completely sugar- and salt-free; they contain only flour, wheatgerm and water.

Farley's Low Sugar Rusks have a sucrose level of 15 per cent (their ordinary Osterusks contain 18 per cent from sucrose and glucose syrup), but when other sugars in the low-sugar rusk are included the total sugars are 28 per cent. They are suitable for vegetarian babies because they are egg-free, but contain whey. Farley's Rusks with Wholemeal contain 48 per cent finely ground wholemeal flour, but they also contain 23.5 per cent sugar, including 17 per cent sucrose. Farley's state the rusks are free from 'animal tissue' and so are suitable for vegetarians. They are egg-free, but they do contain whey (from milk) and are not suitable for vegans.

> **What Baby Needs**
>
> Remember baby's needs are not the same as yours. Babies do not need added salt and sugar, no matter how bland their food tastes to you. Neither do they need high-fibre, low-fat foods. A Cow & Gate survey showed that mothers thought their babies might need added fibre, or low-fat milk, but this is not so, as they need lots of calories, which are provided by fat. If they didn't have the concentrated calories of fat from breast milk or bottle milk they would have to drink far larger quantities than they could manage. For toddlers and the under-fives it's not quite so simple. If they get enough calories from elsewhere it should not be necessary to give them whole milk, which adds a lot of saturated fat to the diet; they may get their calcium and dairy vitamins from yoghurt and other foods. However, the official line is still to give full fat milk to the under-fives.

Boots rusks are available in a Low Sugar version and a Low Sugar Apricot Flavour. They are egg-free and suitable for vegetarians. The Low Sugar rusks contain 13.5 per cent added sugar and 5.2 per cent glucose syrup – a total of 18.3 per cent sugars. The Low Sugar Apricot Flavour rusks contain 13.5 per cent sucrose and 5.4 per cent glucose syrup – a total of 18.5 per cent sugars. (The apparent discrepancy in the figures arises because glucose syrup is partly water and so its contribution to the total percentage is less than the proportion of the ingredient would indicate. Some of the water is lost during cooking.) Boots's regular rusks and Ruskmen have a total of around 30 per cent sugars.

Baby Food

Holle rusks are imported from Switzerland and are part of the *Johannus* range of baby foods. They have the German Demeter trademark, which indicates that they are grown to biodynamic standards. (This means that the ingredients are organically grown, taking into consideration also the effects of the moon and the conjunctions of the planets on planting and growing time.) They are salt-free and are made from wholemeal flour and honey. They are stocked by some wholefood and health-food shops; they are imported by the Infinity Foods Cooperative, in Brighton (see ORGANIC FOODS).

Milupa claim that their rusks have the lowest total sugars of the most widely available rusks. They say that although some competitors' quoted sugar levels may appear lower, this is because they are quoting added sucrose only, and not including other forms of added sugar. Milupa Fruit Rusks contain 19.5 per cent total sugars, their Muesli Rusks contain 17.5 per cent total sugars and their Granulated Rusks not more than 10 per cent sugars. The rusks are all free from additives and suitable for vegetarian babies.

> **My choice**
> Bickiepegs – they are the only *really* sugar-free rusks.

Baby meals – main courses and desserts

Main courses are available in cans, glass jars or dehydrated in packets. Ingredients panels may reveal unexpected items in savoury dinners such as the ubiquitous sugar, as well as modified starches and cornflours. The government's Food Additives Committee has recommended limiting the amount of modified starches in baby foods, as these are considered a 'suspect' food additive (see Table 1). Dried skimmed milk powders are also found in savoury dishes. (Most manufacturers provide lists of milk-free products.)

Although most baby foods are free from additives, the majority

Baby Food

of main courses rely on meat – few are solely vegetable products and virtually none offers a balanced form of vegetarian protein. Little use is made of fish, or vegetable proteins like lentils and other pulses.

> **Babyfood Key**
>
> Meat-based meals form the majority of most manufacturers' ranges; listed here are the ones that can be used by vegetarians or vegans. I have also tried to give a brief taste of each company's approach to baby foods. Only one makes a fish dish and that is Cow & Gate.
> All the foods listed are gluten free, unless stated otherwise; an * indicates sugar-free dishes.

Beech-nut stages

Beech-Nut is an American range of baby foods available in health-food shops and chemists in London, Manchester and Leeds. Most are sugar free and low in, or free from, fillers such as starches. They offer fruits and vegetables not otherwise available. There are three 'stages': one for weaning which consists of single ingredients because paediatricians say they are easier for a baby's immature digestive system, and also because it's easier to identify baby's likes and dislikes; stage two has mini-bite pieces of food; other manufacturers offer strained foods for the first stage and textured for the second.

Stage 1 (4.5 oz/127.6 g)
Vegan – *Golden Delicious Applesauce, *Chiquita Bananas, *Sweet Potatoes, *Bartlett Pears, *Yellow Cling Peaches, *Squash, *Royal Imperial Carrots, *Green Beans, *Peas.
Stage 2 (4.5 oz/127.6 g)
Vegetarian – Banana Custard Pudding, *Creamed Corn, *Dutch Apple Dessert, *Mixed Fruit and Yoghurt.
Vegan – *Oatmeal with Applesauce (not gluten free), *Plums with Rice, *Applesauce and Cherries, *Bartlett Pears and Pineapple, *Garden Vegetables, *Fruit Dessert, *Mixed Vegetables, *Apricots with Pears and Applesauce, *Applesauce and Banana, *Mixed Cereal with Applesauce and Banana (not gluten free),

Baby Food

*Pears and Carrots, *Prunes with Pears, *Pears and Applesauce, *Banana with Pears and Applesauce.
Stage 3 (7.5 oz/212.6 g)
Vegan – *Sweet Potato, Applesauce and Banana, *Banana with Pears and Applesauce, *Apricots with Pears and Applesauce.

Boots

One of the most widely available ranges. Based mainly on meat but the products listed below are suitable for vegan or vegetarian babies. Boots Instant Baby Food and Granulated are dried and have to be mixed with warm, previously boiled water. Boots baby food in jars is ready to eat. The range is free from preservatives and added salt, but the majority of the Stage 2 instant dried savouries contain sugar.

Instant babyfood Stage 1 (43 g)
Vegetarian – *Cheese and Tomato Savoury, *Cauliflower Cheese, *Scrambled Egg Breakfast, Pineapple and Banana Dessert, Strawberry and Orange Yoghurt Dessert, Rice Pudding with Rosehips, Egg Custard.
Vegan – *Savoury Mixed Vegetables.

Instant Babyfood, Stage 2 (105 g)
Vegetarian – *Egg and Cheese Savoury, Rosehip and Raspberry Yoghurt Dessert, Apple and Sultana Dessert, Tropical Fruit Treat, Banana Hazelnut Treat.
Vegan – Country Vegetable Bake.

Boots Babyfood in jars Stage 1 (100 g)
Vegetarian – *Cheese Savoury, Pear Dessert, Mixed Fruit Dessert, Apple Dessert.
Vegan – *Mixed Vegetable Savoury Variety

Boots Babyfood in jars, Stage 2 (120 g)
Vegetarian – *Cheese Supper, Pear Treat Dessert.
Vegan – *Savoury Vegetable Casserole, Mixed Fruit Salad, Orchard Apple Pudding.

Granulated Infant Food (140 g)
Vegetarian – Strawberry Rice Dessert, Apple and Blackberry Treat, Orange and Banana Dessert.

Baby Food

Vegan – *Garden Vegetable Casserole, *Garden Vegetable Hot-pot.

Cow & Gate

After doing market research to find out what mothers wanted, Cow & Gate changed the sizes of their baby foods because more babies are still on Stage 1 at six to seven months, as a result of later weaning, which means that they have larger appetites. Stage 2 is still eaten by some babies of ten months and over. These foods are in jars and are ready to eat. No sugar is added to the savoury meals, and all are free from additives and added salt.

Trial size (80 g)
Vegetarian – Fruit Delight Dessert, Peach Melba, Strawberry Yoghurt Dessert.
Vegan – Vegetable and Rice Casserole.

Stage 1 (110 g)
Vegetarian – Cheese and Tomato Savoury.
Vegan – *Apple Dessert, *Apple and Banana Dessert, *Apple and Orange Dessert, Cherry Treat Dessert, *Fruit Delight Dessert.

Stage 2 (150 g)
Vegetarian – Cheese and Tomato Savoury (not gluten-free)
Vegan – Vegetable Casserole with Pasta (not gluten-free, but contains wholemeal pasta).
The same desserts as Stage 1 are available in Stage 2 sizes, plus one additional vegan dessert, *Pineapple Dessert.

Heinz

Heinz have been gradually reducing the sugar in their baby foods from a maximum of 10 per cent in 1982 to 5 per cent in 1986. They also have foods which are free from added sugar and they carry a flash 'no added sugar' on the jars or cans. Heinz baby foods are all in one size – 128 g – packed either in cans or jars. For weaning there is Strained Food and for older babies Junior Cans. Both ranges free from salt and artificial additives.

Strained cans
Vegetarian – Apples with Vitamin C, Apricot Custard, Creamed

Baby Food

Caramel Dessert, Creamed Rice Pudding, Egg Custard with Rice, *Pear Dessert and two Savoury Specials: Cauliflower Cheese, Macaroni Cheese.
Vegan – Banana Dessert with Vitamin C, Fruit Salad.

Strained jars
No vegetarian or vegan meals available.

Dessert jars
Vegetarian – Egg Custard with Rice, Orange Dessert with Vitamin C, *Pineapple Dessert with Vitamin C.
Vegan – Fruity Juice Desserts: *Apple, *Apple and Banana, *Apple and Blackcurrant, *Apple and Orange, *Fruit Salad, *Pear and Cherry.

Baby Yoghurt Dessert jars
Vegetarian – Apple, Apricot, Banana, Orange, Pear, Strawberry.

Pure Fruit cans
Vegan – *Apple and Apricot, *Apple and Banana, *Apple and Orange, *Apple and Pear, *Just Apple, *Mixed Fruit.

Vegetable Meals cans
Vegan – *Carrot and Tomato, *Golden Vegetable, *Mixed Vegetable, *Spring Vegetable, *Winter Vegetable.

Junior cans
Vegetarian – *Apple Dessert, Apricot Dessert with Rice, *Banana Rice with Rose Hip Dessert, Creamed Rice Pudding, Egg Custard with Tapioca, *Fruit Dessert with Tapioca.

Milupa

The ingredients used in Milupa foods are checked for herbicide and pesticide contamination, say the manufacturers, and contamination such as lead and other heavy metals is also checked. They are packed in plastic-lined foil bags inside cartons and, being dried foods, they need to be mixed with warm, previously boiled water.

Infant Foods, Dinner Time Savouries (120 g)
Vegetarian – *Carrot and Tomato, *Summer Salad Variety.

Baby Food

Dinner Time Desserts – (150 g)
Vegetarian – Autumn Fruit Harvest, Caribbean Fruit Dessert, Rice Dessert, Semolina and Honey.

Fruit (150 g)
Vegetarian – Apple and Rosehip Delight, Banana, Mixed Fruit, Pear and Orange.

Yoghurts (150 g)
Banana and Apple, Orange and Mandarin, Soft Fruit, Summer Fruits.

Junior Foods
There are no vegetarian or vegan meals in the junior range.

Robinson's

Robinson's claim a lower total sugar content than other baby food manufacturers, but not all are sugar-free. They are dried foods and need to be mixed with warm, previously boiled water.

Infant Meals (100 g)
Vegetarian – *Egg and Cheese Savoury, *Cauliflower Cheese.
Vegan – *Mixed Vegetable Dinner (45 g), Country Vegetable Casserole (100 g).

Junior Meals (80 g)
*Tomato, Cheese and Egg Noodles (not gluten-free)
Vegan – Vegetable Hot Pot (80 g) (not gluten-free)

Desserts (55 g)
All contain skimmed milk and sugar.
Vegetarian – Egg Custard, Banana Yoghurt Dessert, Apple and Banana Pudding with Vitamin C, Apple Dessert with Vitamin C.
Larger packs (125 g) – Creamed Rice Pudding, Summer Fruit Salad with Vitamin C, Strawberry Surprise, Banana and Pineapple Treat with Vitamin C.

Baby Food

> **My choice**
>
> If they were available, I would choose Johannus and Holle organic baby foods, but since the Chernobyl disaster most have been bought up in Germany and Switzerland where they are made, so supplies to Britain are short – because of the radioactive fallout, none may be made during 1986.
>
> Beech-nut would be my first choice of the non-organic foods, followed by the varieties free from added sugar (marked with an *), preferably ready to eat. Of the dried foods, I think Milupa are my first choice.

Juices
Robinson's Baby Juices are free from sugar, other sweetners and additives, and have added vitamin C. They are ready-diluted.

Cow & Gate Pure Juices are pure fruit combinations with added vitamin C. They are free from sugar, additives and other sweeteners. Pure Concentrate Juice has added vitamin C and is free from added sugar and additives. The juice has to be diluted with previously boiled cool water and comes in four flavours. It must be stored in a fridge after opening because it does not contain preservatives or sugar.

Holle also have a range of sugar-free baby juices under the Johannus brand label. From the Infinity Foods Cooperative (see ORGANIC FOODS).

BAKED BEANS
See also under PULSES.

Baked beans originated from a dish called Boston baked beans, which was a staple American food, just like the peas pottage of medieval and Tudor England. According to Heinz, who still can a million cans a day, the first canned beans appeared in 1875 made by a company named Burnham and Morrill, who supplied the crews of their fishing fleets with this food. The traditional New

Baked Beans

England recipe included mustard, salt pork, and blackstrap molasses.

The small round white beans are actually a type of haricot bean called the 'navy' bean or pea bean; they are grown mainly in the US around the Great Lakes. Britain imports 800,000 tons of these beans each year to make baked beans and one firm, Whole Earth, which makes no-added-sugar beans, has even succeeded in exporting them back to the States where, when the rate of exchange is favourable, they can compete on price terms with American canned beans.

The second main ingredient of baked beans is tomatoes, used in the form of a concentrated purée; this sauce is usually thickened with modified starch and flavoured with sugar, salt, vinegar and spices.

Nutritionally, beans are a cheap source of protein, very low in fat and high in fibre but, like many sources of vegetable protein, beans are low in one of the amino acids needed by the body to make its own protein – in the case of beans, methionine. By combining beans with other vegetables that have higher levels of methionine (and probably lower levels of other amino acids that beans are high in) we can give the body a good source of vegetarian protein. Fortunately cereals are higher in methionine, so baked beans on toast are a good source of vegetable protein.

Two types of fibre

Beans are high in fibre. Most of our fibre is the insoluble fibre and bran which comes from cereals like wheat (made into bread and pasta) or from rice (brown rice and wild rice are highest in fibre). This insoluble fibre helps to make food more bulky, so getting toxins and waste out of the system quickly and preventing constipation. Beans, however, are also a good source of soluble fibre (as are oats), which helps regulate blood fat levels and so reduces the risk of heart disease.

Baked beans are about 60 per cent carbohydrate, so they are also a good, unrefined source of slow-release energy. But as well as these beneficial starches there are also the sugars that virtually

Baked Beans

every baked-bean manufacturer adds. In fact there is very little difference between one brand of baked beans and another, in this respect: on average Heinz and Crosse & Blackwell contain around 5 per cent, Safeway 4.8 per cent, International and Waitrose 4.5 per cent, and Sainsbury's and Tesco 4.3 per cent. That means there is 5 g of sugar per 100 g of baked beans on average, compared with just under 1 g per 100 g in plain, boiled haricot beans. The total sugars will be higher than this, because there are also natural sugars in the tomatoes and beans themselves.

Added salt is around 1.2 per cent in Crosse & Blackwell and Safeway baked beans, 1.3 per cent in Heinz, 1–1.25 per cent in Waitrose and 0.7 per cent in International and Sainsbury's.

As a convenience food baked beans are one of the healthiest around because they are usually free from additives and (to recap) relatively low in salt and sugar and high in fibre.

Proteins and baked beans

Combining baked beans with grains at a meal will increase the usable protein by about one third. There is lots more about making the most of vegetable proteins in *Diet for a Small Planet* by Frances Moore Lappe (Ballantine Books, New York), sold in health-food shops.

	Protein	Available carbohydrate	Fibre
5 oz (140 g) baked beans	6.4 g	18.6 g	10.3 g
5 oz (140 g) baked beans, with 1½ oz (45 g) wholemeal toast and ½ oz (15 g) butter	9.6 g	33.2 g	13.3 g

Source: Heinz.

Buying cans
See CANNED FOOD.

Low-sugar/low-salt baked beans

Crosse & Blackwell have a range of baked beans called *Healthy Balance*. The beans have 2 g sugar added to every 100 g compared with 4 g in their standard beans and 0.8 g of salt compared with 1 g. However, for those wishing to avoid additives the ingredients are: beans, tomatoes, water, sugar, modified starch, salt, onion, spices, artificial sweetener – saccharin.

HP have reduced the sugar in their baked beans by half, to 2.4 g per 100 g and the amount of salt by a quarter, to 0.9 g per 100 g. These beans are also free from artificial colours and preservatives.

Sainsbury's do reduced salt and sugar Beans in Tomato Sauce, containing 2 g sugar and 0.8 g salt compared with 4.4 and 1.1 g respectively in the standard product.

No-added-sugar baked beans

Whole Earth Campfire Style Baked Beans are sweetened with apple juice and contain a wider range of flavourings (natural).

TYPICAL BAKED BEAN	WHOLE EARTH CAMPFIRE STYLE BAKED BEANS
Beans, water, tomatoes, sugar, salt, modified starch, spirit vinegar, spices	Haricot beans, apple juice, tomato purée, sea salt, barley malt vinegar, guar gum, onion powder, kelp, cinnamon, dill herb, ground nutmeg, cayenne, cloves

There is no added sugar in Whole Earth baked beans; the apple juice content is 7.5 per cent and added salt is 0.9 per cent. They have a spicier flavour and are more savoury than the regular baked beans. The can is lined with a special white, non-migratory plastic that stops the food coming into contact with the can (some leaching of metals into food may occur in canned foods); it has a lead-free seam for the same reason.

Waitrose No Added Sugar Baked Beans in Tomato Sauce have no added sugar or starch. The tomato sauce is made with apple juice

Baked Beans

instead of sugar, and guar gum replaces modified starch as a thickener. Salt, spices and soya sauce are the other ingredients in this additive-free product.

Heinz Weight Watchers range includes a no-added-sugar baked bean, but this is still sweetened with artificial sweeteners.

> **My choice**
>
> Whole Earth Campfire Style Baked Beans, or Waitrose baked beans for a more regular taste.

Other canned beans

Canned versions of the less commonly used beans are also available. These are ready cooked and canned in water rather than sauce. They are convenient if you do not have the time to soak or boil red kidney beans, borlotti beans, cannellini beans, butter beans, chick peas or haricots, but they are an expensive way to buy these relatively cheap foods. A pressure cooker cuts down cooking time and fuel costs by about two thirds and cooked beans will freeze if you want to cook them in batches. All these beans are canned in salted water and they usually also have some sugar added, plus calcium chloride, a mineral used as a sequestrant to bind with the trace metals in the can to prevent them encouraging oxidation of the product (which would be detrimental to the food). Supermarket own brands and *Boots the Chemist* have good ranges of canned cooked beans. *Cirio*, the Italian brand leaders, also sell canned beans in British supermarkets and groceries. *Batchelors* Bean Cuisine range includes tasty Calypso Beans, Chili Beans and Cassoulet Beans.

Granose include a handy Mixed Bean Salad in their *Itona* brand; it contains kidney beans, navy beans, black beans and chick peas with sweetcorn and green and red peppers.

BEER
See under WINE.

BISCUITS
See also CEREAL BARS and CRISPBREAD AND CRACKERS.

If you have read the book this far, you will have realized that as a nation we are eating more fat and sugar than is good for us. You will also have noticed that in Britain we love biscuits (and cakes) and eat about £900 m worth of biscuits each year. These two facts have a lot to do with each other.

Hidden fat and sugar

The main link is that most of the fat used to make biscuits is saturated fat and, as we have seen, saturated fat is implicated strongly in the British epidemic of heart disease. Of course this cannot all be 'blamed' on biscuits, but biscuits are one of the major sources of 'hidden' fat in our diet. The latest figures from the National Food Survey (1984) show that 6.4 per cent of the fats in our diet come from biscuits, cakes and pastries and 7.3 per cent of the saturated fat in our food is from the same source. Sugars are present in biscuits in roughly the same proportion as fat.

The reason most biscuit manufacturers do not use 'healthier' polyunsaturated fats in biscuits is that these fats are not as stable as saturated fats. They have unsaturated double bonds in their make-up and can be oxidized by the oxygen in the air which makes them go rancid. That is why most of the fats used in baked goods are hydrogenated – hydrogen is added chemically to the double bonds, saturating them so that the fats can't go off. Hence many biscuit ingredients' panels state 'hydrogenated' vegetable oil. Unfortunately, it is this kind of fat in our food that adds to the risk of heart disease. Hydrogenation turns beneficial polyunsaturated cis fatty acids into trans fatty acids, which behave in the body in the same way as saturated fats.

Biscuits
Natural choices

Many biscuit manufacturers are now entering the 'health-food' biscuit market and using polyunsaturated fats in their products, despite the fact that they are more expensive because of their shorter shelf-life. For example, *McVities* have launched a *Natural Choice* range, which they expect to make £10 m profit after the first year. *Cadbury* have announced that all their biscuits are now made solely with vegetable fats. The chocolate biscuits now have vegetable fat in the biscuit and dairy and vegetable fat in the chocolate. *Burton's* have made their rich tea biscuits, digestives and ginger nuts free of animal fats.

Biscuits are high in sugar and the sugar may appear in many different forms: plain sugar, glucose, glucose syrup, brown sugar, raw cane sugar, honey, dextrose, malts, maltose syrup, invert sugar, caramel, fructose, fructose syrup. The chocolate coating on biscuits and in 'cream' and 'sandwich' biscuits is also high in fat and sugar.

Most biscuits, especially the cheaper ones, also contain a fair number of additives to give them colour and flavour (processed fats and sugars and refined white flour and starches are not only devoid of nutrients, but they are also devoid of flavour) and keep them stuck together, crunchy and crisp. Most classes of additive are allowed in biscuits including: colouring, flavouring, antioxidants, preservatives, emulsifiers, stabilizers, sweeteners and various miscellaneous additives. (*Burton's Bakers* have removed all synthetic colourings from their *Baker's Selection* biscuits.)

The biscuit habit

We all know, then, that biscuits are 'bad' for us, yet we persist in eating them for many reasons. They are associated with reward in childhood, they are associated with the British cuppa, they are part of social hospitality, and sadly they are one of the cheap foods used as 'fillers' by those who cannot afford fresher foods. We can do our children a great favour by not getting them hooked on the biscuit habit and giving them, instead, a sandwich or dried or

Biscuits

fresh fruit. We can make biscuits 'treats only' and the easiest way to do this is get out of the habit of buying them, so that we limit our intake. We can also make them at home using unrefined wholemeal flour and soft vegetable margarines that are high in polyunsaturated fats, sweetening them with dried fruits, spices and concentrated fruit juices; if we do use sugar, we can use a high-quality unrefined sugar.

No doubt we are a long way from giving up biscuits, so here are a few pointers to look for when buying them:

- Aim for biscuits made from wholemeal flour or wholegrain cereals because these will be high in fibre.
- Try to choose varieties that are less sweet or semi-sweet, such as digestives.
- Prefer varieties made with vegetable oils and margarines.
- Look for brands that are lower in salt or free from added salt (baking powder is sodium based and sodium additives also add 'salt').
- Look for the brands that are free from additives; invariably the cheaper biscuits use cheap ingredients that need additives, so buy the more expensive brands (this will be an added incentive to eat fewer of them!).
- Remember that 'chocolate' biscuits means added-fat-and-sugar biscuits. Chocolate is also a stimulant and 'addictive' so try a carob biscuit instead. Carob is a caffeine-free alternative to chocolate that is also less sugary and fatty.

   Applying these criteria to biscuits often means shopping in a health-food store, but some supermarket own-brands and some of the larger manufacturers are now supplying the demand for a more 'nutritious' biscuit.
- Even if it claims to be a 'healthy' biscuit or 'high in fibre', you should still read the ingredients panel . . .

Biscuits

Better buys

Here is a selection of some of the better biscuits and where you can buy them (Ch = chemists, HF = health-food or wholefood shops, G = grocers, S = supermarkets):

Allinson's, from the producers of Allinson's wholemeal flour and breads. A range of thirteen biscuits, plus three carob-coated biscuits. All are additive free and made from unrefined sugar and vegetable fat – some are made with wheatmeal flour. Their Carob Bites are especially good. These are carob coated mini biscuits available in lemon or orange flavour. Allinson's also produce a wholemeal shortbread – as do other companies in the health-food trade. (HF)

Prewett's are also producers of wholemeal flour; their six varieties of biscuits are made from 100 per cent wholemeal flour, raw cane sugar and vegetable margarine. They are free from additives (HF).

Country Basket biscuits are made by Newform Foods. This is a range of wheatmeal biscuits, free from additives; they use raw cane sugar and vegetable fats; generally a high-fibre, lower-calorie biscuit. (HF, Ch)

The *Holly Mill* range of additive-free wholemeal biscuits uses brown sugar and vegetable fat. Some are sweetened with fructose and are described as suitable for diabetics. Eggs are used in their Orange Biscuits and Farmhouse Biscuits, making them unsuitable for vegans. (HF)

Braycott have three styles of biscuit, all made from natural ingredients with no additives. The *Oat Crunch* range is based on oats with raw sugar and molasses, plus vegetable oil or shortening. *Wholefood Cookies* use 100 per cent wholemeal flour and oats, and are free from raising agents like baking powder (making them lower in salt). There are also two carob-coated biscuits. (HF, G)

Cheshire Cookies, manufactured by *Healthy Life,* use wheat flour, brown sugar and vegetable oil. They are not 100 per cent

Biscuits

wholemeal but are additive free. They also produce *Mitchelhill Digestives* made with honey and wheatmeal, one of the few digestives suitable for vegetarians. (HF)

Doves Farm wholemeal digestives are baked with organic flour; they are also available as half-coated digestives with sugar-free carob (just like conventional chocolate biscuits, but better!).

Infinity Foods (see ORGANIC FOODS) import a range of organic and sugar-free biscuits. (HF)

Moorlands hand-baked biscuits from J. H. H. Kippax are made from wholemeal flour, vegetable fat and brown sugar. Also Moorlands *High Fibre* range; all of these, except Honey Bran, are suitable for vegans. (HF, G)

Fox's Biscuits produce some biscuits that are free from additives. These include: Bran Crunch, made from wholemeal flour, brown sugar and vegetable fat, but also contain sugar syrup. A Wholemeal Honey Sandwich is made from wholemeal flour but contains hydrogenated vegetable fat and three types of sugars as well as honey. Muesli Biscuits are free from hydrogenated vegetable oil and made with wholemeal flour and oats, plus brown sugar. These are suitable for vegetarians, but vegans should avoid the Honey Sandwich and Muesli biscuits. Other biscuits from Fox's are suitable for vegetarians and some for vegans – they do not contain 'wholefood' ingredients, although many are free from hydrogenated fats. (S, G)

McVitie's (United Biscuits) produces the *Natural Choice* sub-brand – five varieties of additive-free wholemeal biscuits made with vegetable oils and hydrogenated vegetable oils. The range, which is widely available, includes: Yoghurt Creams, Blackcurrant Yoghurt Creams (both suitable for vegetarians) and Muesli, Fruit and Nut Crunch and Wholemeal (which are also suitable for vegans). (S, G)

Biscuits

> **My choice**
>
> We shouldn't really . . . but, if we must, digestives are usually lower in fat and sugar and some, such as Doves Farm, are also organic and wholemeal! Otherwise I prefer Allinson's, Country Basket and Infinity Foods biscuits.

BREAD

See also CRISPBREAD AND CRACKERS.

Bread is a good source of nutrients, and the old myth that bread is fattening has long been disproved – it is what you put on the bread that makes it fattening. Butter or marge are both high in calories and jam and marmalade are high in sugar. So be mean with the spread and cut the bread into thicker slices. Toast it under the grill, if necessary, because most toasters seem designed to cope only with ready-sliced, puny-sized pieces of bread.

Although in Britain we eat 10 million large loaves a day, the COMA report on bread (1983) says we should be eating more bread. Bread is nutritious, filling, very low in fat and, if wholemeal, very high in naturally occurring fibre. Although we are eating less bread, there is an increase in the amount of wholemeal bread being eaten. Compare our 1957 average of 48 oz a week, of which 85 per cent was white bread and 8 per cent brown, with the 1983 figure of 68 per cent white and 19 per cent brown and wholemeal (National Food Survey, reported in *Which?*).

There are three main types of bread

wholemeal
brown
white

and the difference is that each is made from a different flour.

Wholemeal bread

This is made from wholemeal flour – the flour is milled from the whole wheat grain and all of it goes into the flour. Traditionally it was made by crushing the grain between two millstones, giving equal distribution of the particles and all the contents such as the wheatgerm and the oils of the germ, which would be evenly spread throughout the flour. This type of flour can still be bought and is labelled 'stoneground' on the bag. Loaves made from stoneground flour are identified in the same way. The texture of these loaves (and the flour) is slightly coarser than flour produced by a roller mill where the metal rollers shear off the outer layers (the bran) and then crush the central endosperm. The oils in this type of flour remain in the starchy central part of the flour and are not so evenly distributed. This method of milling generates heat, which destroys a small amount of the heat-sensitive B vitamins; the very fast modern mills cause still greater losses.

Additives

Fewer additives are allowed in wholemeal bread than in brown or white and many wholemeal breads are entirely free from additives, although it is difficult to find wrapped supermarket wholemeal loaves free from additives. Yet as shoppers we are tending to reject additives.

Proposals in the 1983 COMA report included allowing three *additional* additives for wholemeal bread: ascorbic acid (vitamin C), L-cysteine hydrochloride and azodicarbonamide. The proposed regulations would also allow chlorine dioxide, chlorine and benzoyl peroxide, and all bleaching agents in bread; it is unlikely that these would be used in wholemeal bread, however. (Yeast-stimulating preparations, 'rope inhibitors', preservatives, emulsifiers and stabilizers are already permitted in wholemeal bread, although not all bakers use them.) It was requests from major bakeries to use additives to cut the costs of producing wholemeal bread, and to make wholemeal bread 'more like white bread' in texture, that led to the proposed change in the law. It met with strong opposition from the health food lobby and from members

Bread

of the Association of Master Bakers, however, and has so far been defeated.

Phytic acid

Critics of wholemeal bread have often said the phytic acid it contains will prevent minerals such as calcium and zinc from being used by the body, but research suggests that an enzyme breaks down the phytic acid during the proving of wholemeal bread, and cooking also destroys some of the phytates. It seems, too, that when wholemeal bread is eaten regularly, an enzyme is produced by the body to cope with the phytic acid. The idea that people are at risk of mineral deficiencies through eating wholemeal bread is rather a myth. The ones really at risk are those who use large quantities of raw bran on their food.

Brown bread

Brown bread is made from flour which has had some of its fibre removed so it does not contain 100 per cent of the grain like wholemeal. Until recently this included the 'wheatmeal' loaf, but the name was banned by the 1984 Bread and Flour Regulations from July 1986 because it is too similar to 'wholemeal' and therefore confusing to the shopper.

The 1984 Regulations say that brown bread must have a fibre content of not less than 0.6 per cent; otherwise, brown bread is often very similar to white bread – all the additives used in wholemeal, plus some others (see the table on pp. 174–5), are allowed in brown breads.

White bread

This is baked from white flour made from the starchy endosperm of the grain after the bran and wheatgerm have been removed; the resulting grey/yellow starchy flour is bleached to make it white. White breads usually have the highest number of additives, so pay particular attention to the labels when buying them.

Because most of the nutrients have been removed during milling

Bread

of white flour, any flour of less than 80 per cent extraction must, by law, be fortified with calcium carbonate (chalk), which is a form of calcium, iron, thiamin (vitamin B_1) and nicotinic acid (vitamin B_3) – this dates from the Government Flour Order of 1953, which was introduced in order to bring bread up to the nutritional standard of the wartime National Loaf (which was made from flour of about 85 per cent extraction rate and contained added calcium carbonate on nutritional grounds). Despite recent efforts to discontinue the practice following a 1983 COMA report on bread, it has been maintained in the 1984 Regulations, partly because of refutations of the COMA claim that it was no longer necessary to add these nutrients.

Although wholemeal bread is the best nutritional value, if you don't like it, you should continue to eat white bread, because it still has fibre and nutritional value – but try to find an additive-free white bread. Everybody enjoys a nice crusty white French stick at some time . . .

Buying bread

Most bread is baked and sold the same day so date-stamps and sell-by dates are not usually necessary, although wrapped bread is date-stamped. It will keep at home for a couple of days longer than unwrapped bread.

Finding a good traditional baker who does not use additives is the first step towards eating better bread; some specialist wrapped breads are free from additives and are made from whole grains (see below).

There is a great variety of bread and it is enjoyable to switch around and try several varieties, especially the wholemeal ones.

The Health Education Council has come up with a symbol which is a 'stamp of approval' for foods that are good sources of fibre. It has been adopted for Allinson wholemeal sliced breads, and VitBe and HiBran loaves. Remember, however, that it does not guarantee that these products are free from additives – label-checking is still necessary.

Bread

Know your breads

We have already looked at the main categories of bread: wholemeal, brown and white. The following is a guide to the varieties of bread within the main categories. See also the table of additives on pp. 174–5.

Wheatgerm

This has 10 per cent or more added wheatgerm. It can be made from brown and/or white flours. Hovis and Vitbe are examples. Many people buy these because they think the wheatgerm will give them extra B vitamins and vitamin E. In fact, there is no vitamin E in them because the stabilization or baking process destroys it; there are also far fewer B vitamins, except for thiamin, than there are in wholemeal bread. The real advantages are in taste and texture.

Rye

Rye bread is made from rye flour, which can be either dark (nearer wholemeal) or light. It tends to be denser than bread made from wheat flours and is traditionally made using a sour-dough method of fermentation rather than yeast, but yeast may be used in modern lighter rye breads.

Hi-fibre white bread

This is made from white flour with added fibre, not necessarily bran; sometimes the fibre is from peas or other sources. Some white bread claims to be as high in fibre as wholemeal or brown bread, but it is commonly of a cotton-wool texture, being sliced and steam baked. It may be popular with people who do not like wholemeal or brown bread, but it is often better to take fibre where it occurs naturally, rather than as an 'additive' in refined foods. (See Chapter 1.)

Malted bread

Malted bread is made from malted brown flour with cracked and malted wheat grains. 'Malted' means that the grains have been

Bread

moistened and germinated and then roasted. 'Granary' is a registered trade-name of a type of malted wheat-grain bread. (This is not to be confused with fruit malt loaf, recipes for which often contain additives. See CAKES.)

Bran bread
This is made from any type of flour enriched with added bran.

Soda bread
Soda bread is usually made from white flour; bicarbonate of soda must be used as an ingredient; it replaces yeast as a raising agent.

Milk bread
This must contain a minimum of 6 per cent milk solids.

Skimmed-milk bread
This must contain a minimum of 6 per cent skimmed milk solids; it may also be called lactein bread.

Butter bread
This must contain a minimum of 6 per cent milk fat.

Protein or high-protein bread
This must have a minimum of 22 per cent protein.

Cheese bread
This must be 'cheesy' but it does not have a specified cheese content.

Gluten bread
This must contain a minimum of 16 per cent protein.

Oat bread/muesli bread
These are examples of speciality breads; speciality breads can be called after any ingredient that is present in sufficient quantity to give the bread the 'characteristic' of that ingredient – oats and muesli in the example quoted.

Bread

Pitta bread
This Middle Eastern bread is available in wholemeal and white versions, often without added fat and additives. It is made by various bakeries in London and the regions, where it may go under different names. For example, *London Mediterranean Bakery* has a round pitta bread (most are oval) called 'khoubz', which is free from additives and added fat, and is made with wholemeal flour.

Gluten-free bread
For coeliacs who cannot tolerate gluten (the protein in wheat, rye barley and oats) gluten-free breads are a welcome addition to the diet. The *Juvela* Gluten Free Fibre loaf is especially useful because it contains dietary fibre from sugar beet, giving a 7 per cent fibre content. Juvela loaves are made in the Gluten Free Bakery of *GF Dietary Specialities* – other gluten-free products are also baked there. Available from Boots and other chemists and some health-food shops.

German breads
Pumpernickel and Vollkornbrot (rye breads), and also Leinsamenbrot (linseed bread), offer a good variety of tastes and make excellent open sandwiches. One additive-free brand is *Mestermacher*, which is low in salt and has no added fat.

Special breads

Whole Earth Bread
Made from 100 per cent wholemeal flour, filtered water, malted wheat grains, 100 per cent soya flour, sunflower seeds, sesame seeds, yeast, sea salt, linseed, carrots, alfafa and Norwegian kelp. This is bread for the shopper who likes every ingredient to count nutritionally; it is free from added sugar and additives, which goes without saying, really! Unique flavour – it is also high in fibre, worth trying. Available from health-food shops.

Bread

> **Additives Out – the Best Thing Since Sliced Bread . . .**
>
> The major bakeries have responded to the move away from food additives among their customers by removing the preservatives in loaves.
>
> *Allied Bakeries* was the first with the removal of preservatives from their Allinson's Wholemeal Bread in January 1986, but they left in some emulsifiers, added sugar and vegetable fat. Allied is also gradually reducing the amount of salt in its bread in line with Health Education Council suggestions. In February 1986 Allied also removed the preservatives from Vitbe bread and rolls.
>
> *British Bakeries* in April 1986 removed the preservatives from *Hovis, Windmill Bakery, Mother's Pride, Country Pride* and *Nimble* wrapped breads, rolls and baps. They are also gradually reducing the amount of salt and changing to unbleached white flour in white breads and rolls. Two emulsifiers and flour improvers are still used. A natural ingredient – white vinegar – is being added during warm weather to help prevent spoilage, a problem in polythene-wrapped breads.

Vogel Bread
A Swiss-style mixed-grain bread baked to a Swiss recipe devised by the nutritionist Alfred Vogel. It is free from additives and added fat. The ingredients are wheat flour, water, rye grains, wheat grains, dried whey, dried wheat protein, yeast, bran, rye flour and salt. A delicious loaf with a unique texture and chewy grains; baked regionally to the original recipe.

Boots
Boots the Chemists have brought out a range of wholemeal breads (and cakes) made from Prewett's stoneground 100 per cent wholemeal flour; they are free from additives, except for the 'safe' flour improver l-ascorbic acid, E300. Boots also produce mixed-grain rolls.

Doves Farm Organic
This bread is made with Doves Farm organically grown flour (which they also use for their digestives – see BISCUITS); this is an

Bread

additive-free wholemeal loaf with a pesticide- and herbicide-free guarantee as well.

Heart of Gold Low Salt Bread
Independent family bakers Starbake of Newport, Gwent, produce a low-salt bread in medium-sliced wholemeal and stoneground medium-sliced wholemeal. The sodium content is 288 parts per million, compared with the 9,800 p.p.m. of the average loaf. The bread is free from artificial additives and is sweetened with honey and orange juice. The small amount of salt used is sea salt.

Spring Hill Bread
The Spring Hill bakery produces a wide range of wholemeal breads made from organically produced flour and free from additives. The breads are made with vegetable oils and also contain sprouted grains. Their slogan says it all 'We grow the grain. We mill the flour. We bake the bread' – testament to their ethical no-additives approach. In texture the loaves are denser than British breads and are more like pumpernickel-style breads. Strong on flavour; long shelf life.

Granary
Granary bread is a registered trade-name of Rank Hovis. The ingredients are Granary malted flour (wheat flour, malted wheat grains), water, yeast, wheat protein, hydrogenated vegetable oil, preservatives E280, E281, soya flour.

Hovis Wheatgerm Bread
This is *not* a wholemeal bread. The ingredients are wheat flour, water, cooked wheatgerm, yeast, salt, wheat protein, hydrogenated vegetable oil, dried glucose syrup, emulsifier E472(e), soya flour.

Vitbe Wheatgerm
This is similar to Hovis, but with a slightly different ingredients listing: flour, water, cooked wheatgerm, yeast, vegetable fat, wheat protein, salt, malt flour, dextrose, permitted emulsifier E472(e) – of vegetable origin, soya flour.

Bread

Vitbe Hi-Bran
This has similar ingredients to its wheatgerm stable mate: flour, water, cooked wheatgerm, yeast, vegetable fat, wheat protein, salt, malt flour, dextrose, soya flour, emulsifier E472(e) – of vegetable origin, flour improver, ascorbic acid.

Allinson's
This is wholemeal bread made with Allinson's wholemeal flour by Allied Bakeries. It was the first of the larger ranges to go preservative-free, but still contains emulsifiers and some added sugar and vegetable fat. Both stoneground and ordinary wholemeal available, plus extra-thick sliced bread for toasting – good to see. Allied Bakeries are also reducing the salt in this bread by 20 per cent a year until they meet 'customer resistance'. At present the salt is at 1.1 per cent, down from 1.5 per cent.

Warburton's/Goswell
These are two specialist bakers, in Bolton and London respectively, who produce ranges of speciality breads which use a lot of wholemeal flours and wholegrain flours. Goswell's range is more additive-free than Warburton's, but both offer a large range of different breads to meet many healthy tastes!

Co-op
Co-op brand bread, produced by British Bakeries, is preservative free (white, brown and wholemeal).

Marks & Spencer
All their breads are now preservative-free, but none is completely additive-free.

White sliced
If you like white sliced, you might like to note that Allied Bakeries have removed the preservatives and bleaching agents (which artificially age the flour) from their *Sunblest* and *Danish* range.

Bread

> **My choice**
>
> Additive-free wholemeal bread from my local baker (Koblers of St Margaret's, Twickenham, to be found in the *Good Food Guide*) or sprouted grain bread from Spring Hill. Of nationally available bread I use Doves Farm and Vogel and Granary loaves to ring the changes.

Breadcrumbs

Most packets of purchased breadcrumbs are lurid yellow in colour; they are usually dyed with tartrazine. Two manufacturers offer a simple pack of wholemeal breadcrumbs without any artificial additives or any other ingredient. The first was Mr Harvey's Original Wholemeal Breadcrumbs, available in 250 g packs from health-food shops and Sainsbury's, made by *Just Naturally Foods*; second on the scene was *Supercook*'s brand in a 200 g shaker drum.

Summary

A quick round-up of the main points to remember when buying bread:

- Wholemeal (100 per cent) is best for health and is less likely to contain additives, but check the wrapper or ask the baker what is used to make the bread.
- If fat is used in the bread, choose a variety that uses unsaturated fats wherever possible.

Footnote: buying a toaster?

Choose one that can accommodate thick slices – that way you get more bread and less spread or sugary jam or honey. Alternatively, toast bread under the grill – then you can have the bread as thick as you like.

How nutritious is Britain's bread?

The most recent survey of the nutrient content of Britain's breads was made in 1983 by a team headed by Robert Wenlock of the Ministry of Agriculture, Fisheries and Foods. It took samples of thirteen different types of bread and rolls from seven regional centres in Britain and compared their nutritional status. 'Considerable differences were encountered in all regions in identifying wholemeal products,' says the report, published in the *Journal of Science of Food and Agriculture*.

Each type of bread was analysed for moisture, protein, fat, sugar, starch, dietary fibre, sodium, calcium, nitrogen, phosphorus, iron, calcium, zinc, manganese, chloride, thiamin, riboflavin, nicotinic acid, vitamin B_6 and folic acid. Here is a summary of the main findings:

- In England added salt showed no regional difference; bread was saltiest in Scotland.
- Unsliced and unwrapped wholemeal and brown loaves contained less moisture than sliced.
- The unsliced and unwrapped loaves also contained higher levels of nutrients than the sliced, wrapped versions.
- New analysis methods showed fibre was higher in white bread than had previously been thought (but it is still far less than in wholemeal or brown).
- The new analysis methods also concluded that calories, protein, fat, available carbohydrate, iron and thiamin levels were lower than had previously been shown in analytical figures.
- Plant-baked white loaves had less protein than unsliced white; they also had fewer nutrients and contained more water.
- The highest level of thiamin was in Hovis, where the added wheatgerm contributed that particular vitamin.
- Folic acid was higher in wholemeal, wheatgerm and malted breads, but low in white breads. This is another reason for switching to wholemeal bread, because folic acid is often low in the British diet and is essential for healthy nerves and reproduction. Bread is the major source of folic acid in our diet.

Additives Allowed in Bread

		Beware	Safe	Suspect	
	Allowed in all bread, including wholemeal				
E150	Caramel			✓	
E170	Calcium carbonate			✓	
E260	Acetic acid			✓	
E262	Sodium hydrogen diacetate			✓	
E270	Lactic acid			✓	except for v. young
E280	Propionic acid			✓	
E281	Sodium propionate			✓	except migraines
E290	Carbon dioxide (in aerated prepacked bread only)			✓	
E300	L-ascorbic acid			✓	
E322	Lecithins			✓	
E336	Mono potassium L-(+)-tartrate			✓	
E341	Calcium diorthophosphate	!			
E450(a)	Disodium dihydrogen diphosphate		?		
E471	Mono and diglycerides of fatty acids		?		
E472(b)	Lactic acid esters of E471		?		
E472(e)	Citric acid esters of E471		?		
	Mono and diacetyltartaric acid esters of E471		?		
E481	Sodium stearoyl-2-lactylate		?		
E482	Calcium stearoyl-2-lactylate		?		
E483	Stearyl tartrate		?		
E510	Ammonium chloride		?		
516	Calcium sulphate		?		
	Chlorine	!			
	Ammonium dihydrogen orthophosphate		?		
925	Diammonium dihydrogen orthophosphate		?		

Ammonium sulphate
Alpha-amylases proteinases

Allowed in all bread except wholemeal
920 L-cysteine hydrochloride
924 Potassium bromate
925 Chlorine
927 Azodicarbonamide
Benzoyl peroxide

Special uses
E150 Caramel — wholemeal, brown, malt.
E330 Citric acid
E333 Tricalcium citrate — rye
E460 Alpha-cellulose ⎫
E466 Carboxymethylcellulose, sodium salt ⎬ slimming breads
E500 Sodium hydrogen carbonate ⎫
E541 Sodium aluminium phosphate, acidic ⎬ soda bread
575 D-glucono-L, 5-lactone ⎭

Bread

- Wholemeal and wheatgerm breads were also good sources of polyunsaturated fats.

Fibre and Calorie Content of Common Breads

	Fibre g per 100g	Calories
Wholemeal	8.5	215
Hovis	5.8	211
VitBe	6.4	252
Small white	4	242
Scottish batch	4.3	232
French	5.6	270
Vienna	4.6	263
Slimming	4.3	247
Granary	7.3	235
Rye bread	6.4	220
Malt bread	7	260
Currant loaf	4.2	289
White rolls		
crusty	4.7	280
soft	4.2	268
Brown rolls		
crusty	7.8	255
soft	7	268
Wholemeal rolls	9.7	243
Morning rolls	4.5	269
Hamburger buns	4.4	264

Source: *Nutritional Composition of British Bread.* R. W. Wenlock and others, 1983. In the original figures, large loaves, small wrapped and small unwrapped were analysed; averages have been used in this table to give a general idea of the fibre and calorie content of each type of bread.

Selenium shock

New evidence from research by the West of Scotland Agriculture College has discovered that our bread (and flour) contains only a quarter of the selenium that published figures claim is present and this may have serious implications for health because low selenium levels are consistently being linked with heart disease and cancers as well as less serious arthritis.

Dr Ivy Barclay has been monitoring levels for two years and has found that since more British wheats have been used to make our bread the selenium levels have dropped. Previously bread was made from imported Canadian wheat and Canadian soils are high in selenium. More than half the selenium intake in the average diet is from bread.

BREAKFAST CEREALS

Cooked breakfasts are a thing of the past in most households. They have become a weekend treat or something eaten only on business trips or holidays. Replacing the slowly cooked traditional porridge, the middle-class kippers and the kidneys of the twenties and thirties, or the bacon, egg and sausage that came later, has come the bowl of breakfast cereal. Just shake the packet and pour on milk and you have one of the most popular convenience foods of the last thirty years.

Compare the 1950s, when 90 per cent of people ate breakfast, 50 per cent had a cooked breakfast and less than 25 per cent ate breakfast cereals, with a Kellogg's survey in the 1970s which revealed that 40 per cent ate cereals for breakfast, 25 per cent ate only bread or toast, 18 per cent had a cooked breakfast and 17 per cent ate nothing at all.

But manufactured breakfast cereals go back further than the fifties. Force Wheat Flakes claim to be the first breakfast cereal introduced to Britain in 1902, closely followed by Shredded Wheat in 1908; most of our breakfast cereals have been around since the Second World War. In the last decade the high-fibre breakfast-cereal market has been developed in response to the new popularity of fibre. In 1983 bran-based breakfast cereals boomed by 40 per cent and sales of muesli rose by 23 per cent, even though during that year overall growth was only 7 per cent. In the last few years crunchy Granola-type cereals have really

Breakfast Cereals

taken off, now claiming 25 per cent of the total muesli market, which was worth £52 m in 1984.

Fibre for breakfast

All this sounds very healthy for the bank balances of breakfast-cereal manufacturers, and it may sound good for our health too, but, unfortunately, just switching to a bran-based high-fibre cereal or sprinkling bran over your breakfast is not quite the answer (see Chapter 1), for several reasons.

First, to make the bran palatable, many recipes include a lot of fat and sugar to stick it together, making it less dry and easier to eat. Recipes that are high in fibre are good, but only if they are also low in fat and sugar – otherwise they are not contributing to healthy eating.

Second, especially with raw (uncooked/untoasted) bran, a substance called phytic acid might cause problems by binding with minerals such as zinc and calcium and making them unavailable for the body. So using large amounts of raw bran at breakfast is not a good idea (nor is it very tasty).

Third, taking bran from the whole grain and then adding it to refined breakfast cereal ingredients is not the best way to improve the diet. A better way to increase fibre intake is to eat fibre where it occurs naturally – and this applies to breakfast cereals as much as to other foods.

So, the criteria for a good breakfast cereal are

- Make sure it's a whole-grain cereal, not a refined product with lots of sugar and fat.
- Watch the amount of salt added – aim to buy salt-free or no-added-salt cereals.

Milk and sugar

Switching to skimmed or semi-skimmed milk with your breakfast cereal, and during the rest of the day, will cut down your fat intake considerably over the years.

Breakfast Cereals

Do you also put sugar on your breakfast cereal? Reading the ingredients panel of most cereals will reveal that there is already sugar in the cereal, so should you really be adding more? There is, for example, already 21 per cent added sugar (and a total of 31 per cent sugars) in *Weetabix Honey and Nut Farmhouse Bran* and 14 per cent (22 per cent total) in *Weetabix Toasted Farmhouse Bran* and 11 per cent (22 per cent total) in *Weetabix Apple Farmhouse Bran*. Not all breakfast cereals contain that amount of sugar and many contain much more; take a look at the table at the end of this section (p. 183) and compare the different Weetabix products. Nevertheless, most breakfast cereals do contain some sugar already.

Sugar and salt in breakfast cereals

Most cereal manufacturers do not disclose how much salt or sugar is added to their products because they say it is part of their secret recipe. Labelling laws require only that ingredients are listed in descending order by weight, so we are often none the wiser about the true content. However, many supermarkets' nutritional labelling now shows the amount of added sugar and salt in their own-label products; health-food products have for a long time given this sort of information.

For years breakfast-cereal manufacturers have proclaimed the added vitamins and minerals in their products, giving the percentage of the recommended daily intake of these that their products contribute – so why not go the whole hog and tell us all?

Sugar- and salt-free breakfast cereals

Shredded Wheat and Cubs
Quaker Puffed Wheat
Sainsbury's Miniwheats
Sainsbury's Puffed Wheat
Holly Mill Toasted Wheatflakes (sucrose free)
And, of course, porridge.

Breakfast Cereals

Sugar-free breakfast cereal
Kellogg's Nutri-Grain
This range offers Wholewheat with Raisins, Rye and Oats with Hazelnuts, and Brown Rice and Rye with Raisins. They all taste good and are so 'normal' you could fool any sugar addict into liking them!

Oat fibre

One of the traditional breakfast cereals – porridge – is completely free from added salt and sugar. The oats are 'stabilized' during the milling (which adds nothing and removes nothing) to prevent the naturally present oils from going rancid (at one time you had to keep oats in an airtight tin and they did not last very long). The stabilization process is a secret guarded by the manufacturers, but it is basically a steaming technique which does not involve chemicals.

Oats have recently been found to contain a valuable type of bran called soluble fibre, which is different from wheat bran. Soluble fibre helps to control our blood fat levels, especially the levels of the harmful types of cholesterol, and slows down the release of energy (sugars) to the bloodstream. This is less disruptive to our blood sugar levels and makes oats a particularly good food for diabetics, although we can all benefit from this type of fibre.

Porridge

Porridge can be made with water or skimmed milk and it is equally 'creamy' in texture whichever it is made from. Sweetness can be added by stirring in some sultanas or raisins or other chopped dried fruit rather than using sugar. Or a little honey or molasses may be stirred in. If adding salt, keep it a minimum – or better still wean yourself off salty porridge.

Breakfast Cereals

Porridge oats

Scotts Porage Oats
Scotts Piper Oats
Mornflake Jumbo Oats, Porridge Oats, Oatmeal (fine, medium, coarse)
Hofels Breakfast Oatflakes, Jumbo Oatflakes, Oatbran Porridge
Prewett's Scotch Breakfast Oats, Jumbo Oats, Oatbran and Oatgerm*

Instant porridges

Ready Brek
Quaker Warm Start (sweetened only with a little malt – it is 1 per cent of the total sugar)
Sainsbury's Instant Hot Oat Cereal
Waitrose Instant Porridge
Quaker Instant Hot Bran (sweetened with brown sugar and malt, total 0.5 per cent sugars)
Mornflake Superfast Oats

Muesli

Muesli was invented by Dr Bircher Benner, who made it a basis of his naturopathic (nature-cure) health hydro in Switzerland. It originally contained more fresh fruit and nuts than cereal and was soaked overnight to swell the grains and allow their sweetness to come through. Today's habit of pouring the milk on to muesli and eating it virtually dry does not let the grains swell and soften, which is why it seems dry and unpalatable to many people.

It is easier to chew and digest muesli after it has been soaked, and adding dried fruit to the oats, or freshly chopped fresh fruit or grated apple just before eating, will make it more delicious. It can be soaked overnight or for a few minutes while you shower before breakfast. You can soak it in apple juice or mineral water or skimmed milk. You will also find this makes the muesli go further because a small amount swells quite a lot – which can cause some

---

* Oat bran is similar to wheat bran; it is the product of milling oats, and it contains a substantial part of the germ. It can be used in the same way as standard wheat bran.

Breakfast Cereals

people to experience abdominal discomfort after eating muesli that has not been soaked.

As it is based largely on oats, muesli is an excellent source of fibre – see 'Oat Fibre' above.

No-added-sugar mueslis

Cheshire Wholefoods Muesli; Fruit and Nut Muesli
Just Naturally Sugar Free Muesli
Familia Swiss Birchermuesli
Waitrose Fruit and Nut
Sainsbury's Deluxe Muesli
Boots Second Nature No Added Sugar Muesli Cereal
Tesco Wholewheat Muesli
Kellogg's Summer Orchard
Sunwheel Muesli, De Luxe and Tropical Mix
Holly Mill Muesli; Paradise Muesli
Jordans Special Recipe Muesli (made with Conservation Grade* cereals)
Doves Farm Muesli
Bejam Fruit and Nut, Bran
Infinity Foods Organic Muesli
Fruitfort (Swiss sugar-free muesli)
Fine Fare Wholefood

There are many other smaller health-food companies and shops producing sugar-free mueslis and muesli bases to which you can add your own fruit and nuts – shop around your area.

Granola cereals

Whole Earth Orange Crunch and Almond Crunch and *Community Foods* Hazel Malt Crunch are all free from added sugar and salt; *Jordans* Original Crunchy, Natural, is free from added sugar and salt, but contains honey.

---

* Conservation grade is a standard of cultivation devised by Jordans – it is a half-way house between organic and standard chemical cultivation designed to exclude the most noxious of chemicals, but allow some of the least harmful. (See also ORGANIC FOODS p. 328.

Weetabix Products
(all figures are percentages)

	Weetabix	Weetaflake	Weetaflake 'n' Raisin	Alpen	Toasted Farmhouse Bran	Banana & Apple Farmhouse Bran	Honey & Nut Farmhouse Bran	Bran Fare
Added sugar	2.8	2.8	5	8	14	11	21	no
Total sugar	6	6	25	21	22	22	31	no
Salt	0.8	0.8	0.5	0.2	1.9	1.6	1.4	no
Oil	2	2	0.6	5	1.5	5.5	4	3
Wheat	93	93	70	34	78	64	59	100
Fibre	13	13	8	8.5	20	17.5	15	38
Antioxidants	no	no	no	no	no	no	no	no
Preservatives	no	no	yes*	yes*	no	yes*	no	no
Colouring	no	no	no	no	caramel	caramel	caramel	no
Suitable for lacto-vegetarians	yes	yes	yes	yes	yes	yes	yes	yes
Suitable for vegans	yes	yes	yes	no	yes	yes	yes	yes

* Very occasionally low levels of sulphur dioxide are found on the fruit.

Breakfast Cereals

Other cereals

These can be bought in health-food shops and used to make the base of your own muesli or breakfast cereal.

Brown's barley flakes, wheat flakes, maize flakes, millet flakes, rye flakes

Zwicky millet flakes

Hofels toasted rye flakes, barley flakes, toasted wheat flakes, rye flakes

Norfolk Village barley flakes, millet flakes, rye flakes, wheat flakes, oat flakes.

> **My choice**
>
> Shredded Wheat, Kellogg's Nutri-Grain and porridge; also the occasional Weetabix and Force Wheat Flakes for 'added-sugar' occasions! Of the mueslis, I prefer Hunza Wholefoods' (Syon Park, Middlesex) DeLuxe Muesli, or the nationally available Fruitfort and Jordans Special Recipe.

BURGERS

If you buy the usual frozen or butchers' burgers they will be high in fat, low in fibre and probably contain additives such as preservatives and antioxidants. Making burgers yourself enables you to use lean mince (or buy lean meat and mince it yourself at home) and mix it with finely diced fresh vegetables such as onion, carrot, celery and tomatoes, which not only make the meat further but add flavour and fibre.

Some butchers do provide burgers free from additives (see MEAT), but if you want a change from meat burgers there are a growing number of vegetarian products that offer protein without the saturated fats of meat. Vegetarian burgers are available as dry mixes or made up into burgers and sold frozen. They can be made

	Suggested serving	Dietary fibre	Fat	Sodium	Total sugar	Energy
	g	g	g	mg	g	Kcal
Bran cereal	40					
Bran flakes	30					
Cornflakes	30					
Toasted rice cereal	30					
Sugar-coated cornflakes	30					
High-protein cereal	30					
Puffed wheat	16					
Sugar-coated puffed wheat	30					
Wheat-flake biscuits	38					
Muesli	60					
Shredded Wheat	45					

Source: Produced for Nabisco's *Healthy Eating* booklet which features Shredded Wheat.

Typical Nutritional Analysis of Breakfast Cereals

Burgers

from a variety of ingredients such as soya proteins, or tofu (a soya-bean curd used in Chinese and Japanese cooking) or from beans and pulses. Alternatively they may be based on grains like wheat, millet, rye, etc., and include nuts (like a traditional nut cutlet). You can, of course, also make these at home in the same way as meat burgers, but if you want a quick meal straight from the freezer, chill cabinet or store-cupboard shelf, these non-meat mixes are every bit as convenient as their meat counterparts. (You can also use the mixes to stuff vegetables, add to pasta sauces, etc.)

What is Tofu?

Tofu is a soya-bean curd made by coagulating soya milk in a process similar to that of making cheese. The result is a soft white curd virtually fat free and very high in protein. It is very versatile, as Japanese cooking demonstrates, and it is also used in Chinese cooking under the name of beancurd.

Frozen vegetarian burgers

Vegeburger, from *Realeat*, is the market leader, and claims 2 per cent of the total burger market. It is the most widely available brand and is free from sugar and additives. The frozen Vegeburger contains only 5–6 per cent fat and has 4–5 per cent fibre. It is suitable for vegetarians and vegans. Available in one basic flavour.

Sunrise vegetarian quarter-pound burgers are made by *Soya Health Foods* and are made of soya proteins, rusks, palm oil, sea vegetables and tamari, and are flavoured with herbs and spices. They claim a 6 per cent fibre content and a total fat content of 4.7 per cent. Can be fried or grilled from frozen.

Nutriburger is made by *Care Foods* and is a soya-based burger in Plain, Onion or Herb flavours. Free from animal fat, but contains hydrogenated vegetable oil. The burger can be cooked straight from frozen. It is made from textured soya flour, hydrogenated vegetable oil, wholewheat rusk, soya flour, oats, modified starch, stabilizers (potato starch), hydrolysed vegetable protein, sea salt and mixed herbs.

Haddington's burgers are free from additives and animal products. They have 6 per cent total fats from vegetable sources and the fibre content is 4 per cent. They are based on soya protein. Their No Meat Grillburgers are available as quarterpounders or in 2 oz (55 g) size. (They also do savoury sausages and wholemeal sausage rolls.) All their products are kosher.

Fresh chilled vegetarian burgers

Tofu burgers are made with *Paul's Tofu*; the flavours include Curry, Herby and Nutty. They are packed in pairs and are free from additives and animal and dairy products, making them eminently suitable vegan fodder! Available in health-food shops in London and the south-east.

Tofu burgers from *Haldane Foods* are sold under the *Soyboy* brand name. They are free from additives and animal and dairy produce, and are available in Savoury Herb or Chilli flavours. Mainly sold fresh chilled but may be sold frozen. *Hera* (part of Haldane) also offer *Tofeata* tofu burgers. The flavours include Okara Patties, Spicy Burgers and Savoury Burgers. They come in packs of two quarterpounders and are made with tofu or okara, herbs and spices.

Cauldron Foods have Vegetable Chilli and Nut burgers which are free from additives and animal products. They contain about 16 per cent protein, 11–12 per cent fat and 1 per cent fibre.

What is Okara?

Okara is the pulp left after pressing the soya milk from the beans. It is high in fibre, unlike soya milk, and is often roasted to make a crunchy high-protein food. Not widely available as a raw ingredient, but can be found in health-food shops with fridge and freezer counters.

Burgers

Packet vegetarian burger mixes

Vegeburger claims to have more protein and less than half the fat of the equivalent burger made from meat. It is availabe in Herb and Vegetable, Chilli and a No Salt varieties. The burgers are mixed by adding egg and water. The mix is based on sesame seeds, oats, soya flour, wholemeal rusk, dried vegetables and yeast, and herbs for flavour in the no-salt version. Vegeburgers are free from additives and sugar, contain 4–5 per cent fibre and are low in fat (around 5 per cent). Suitable for vegetarians and – if mixed with water only – vegans.

Boots Vegetable Burger Mix is based on soya protein, rusk and dried vegetables. It is high in fibre, containing 23 per cent fibre, which works out at around 5.7 g a burger. It is also low in fat at 4.2 per cent and free from added sugar. The stabilizer used is naturally derived cellulose. Generous-size packs, too, with each pack making about eight burgers (most brands make only four). Needs only water to mix.

Hera burgers are made by health-food experts, *Haldane Foods*. Their range of high-fibre burgers are all free from sugar and additives and low in fat (3–5 per cent). The oil in the products is cold-pressed sunflower oil and all except the Shawburgers (which contain dehydrated Cheddar cheese) are suitable for vegans. The fibre basis of burgers is cereal brans and grains, with textured soya protein, mixed dried vegetables, sesame seeds, wholegrain flours and whole grains. They have a much more 'natural' ingredients listing than many of the products on the market. Available in Spicey, Savoury, Barbecue, and Shawburger (Yes, after G.B.S.!) varieties. Needs only water to reconstitute.

Other vegetarian store-cupboard meals

There are several other dried packet mixes that make up into 'alternatives to meat' and can be used as healthy convenience foods. The ingredients are free from additives and they are usually high in fibre from their vegetable or grain content. (So long as they are not relied on to the exclusion of fresh foods they can make a convenient addition to a healthy diet which is made up from a wide range of foods.)

Here is a selection of vegetarian main meals from the store-cupboard.

Hera do a large range of soya-protein packet-mix foods, including Vegetable Supreme, a mix of dried vegetables that reconstitutes in a creamy sauce by adding water; Vegetable Stew and Dumpling and Couscous with Vegetable kofte – two sachets that make up into the kofte and one that contains the couscous. Other products include a Vegetable Cottage Pie and a vegetable Bourguignonne Mix. A couple of Pizza Mixes and Meatball and Meatloaf mixes are also available. Fibre content is from 2 to 8 per cent, fat from 2 to 13 per cent (but all from vegetable sources).

Boots have a wide range of convenience vegetarian foods, including Country Cereal Mix, based on oats, sesame seeds and soya that can be used to make burgers or stuff vegetables, etc. A Textured Vegetable Protein Mince is equally versatile and is also based on soya. Vegetable Sausage Mix is another soya-based product for use in recipes that usually use sausage meat and Harvest Nut Mix and Farmhouse Lentil Mix offer other sources of natural vegetable protein.

Prewett's Main Course is a range of dried packet mixes available in Bacon, Beef, Chicken, Sausage, and Brazilian flavours. The mixes can be made up into a wide variety of dishes; they are based on soya, wheat bran, sesame seed and dried mixed vegetables and are free from additives and animal and dairy product. The fibre content is around 10 per cent and fat around 12 per cent (from vegetable sources).

Footnote

Various ranges of textured vegetable-protein products available in health-food shops provide a substitute for meat, but the products above are a little more imaginative and effective than the

Burgers

chunks and 'minced meat mimics'. After all, most vegetarians have given up meat and don't necessarily want to find other foods to mimic it, but some of these savoury mixes might be used in a regular diet to make meat go further, or as an alternative to meat for a change, or as a way of cutting down on meat for those who do like it.

BUTTER

Butter is also dealt with under MARGARINE, where the main points of the butter *v.* margarine debate are discussed. But if you want to know more about butter itself, then read on here.

Butter producers are keen to point out how natural butter is. It has no additives, and apart from salt in salted and slightly salted versions it is made simply by churning cream, the fat globules of which stick together to form grains, which are then drained of the buttermilk and worked to a solid mass. At that stage salt is added. It takes the cream of 18 pints of milk to make 1 lb of butter.

There are two types of butter – sweet butter and lactic butter. Sweet butter is made from milk that is 'aged' at a low temperature. Salt is used as a preservative in this type of butter. Lactic butter is made from milk cultured with lactic bacteria which ripen the cream at about 20°C. The lactic acid produced by the fermentation acts as a preservative, so these butters need not be salted. Sweet and salted butters contain about 2 per cent salt and slightly salted butters, 1.5 per cent.

Examples of sweet butters are *St Ivel*, *Golden Meadow*, *Kerrygold* and *Anchor*, and of lactic butter, *Wheelbarrow*, *Lurpack* and *Longboat*.

Using unsalted butter will help you achieve the long-term goal of cutting down on salt in the diet.

By law, butter is at least 80 per cent fat, and current medical advice is that we should all cut down on the amount of fat we eat (see MARGARINE).

Cakes

> **My choice**
>
> Unsalted butter or margarines high in polyunsaturates for spreading on toast and bread – preferably margarines devoid of hydrogenated fats. For cooking I prefer cold-pressed vegetable oils or soft, high-in-polyunsaturates margarine.

CAKE MIXES
See also CAKES.

Good news for those addicted to packet cake mixes – there are now 'healthier' versions available, although some still contain animal fats and additives. Additive-free home baking is better still, but if this is not your scene, here are the best of the cake mixes. (Incidentally there is no additive-free cheesecake mix.)

Greens of Brighton have a Fruit and Nut Wholemeal Cake Mix which has no salt added and is free from preservatives, colour and flavourings. The flour is wholemeal and the sugar is raw cane. Currants, raisins, dates and hazelnuts supply the fruit and nuts.

Viota Fibremix has not gone as far as that of Greens. The flour is still white with added bran, but Bran Crumble Mix uses only vegetable fat and is free from additives. It needs water to mix. Wheat 'n' Bran Scone is mixed with milk and contains hydrogenated marine oils, plus sugar, syrup, stabilizer E466 and emulsifiers E471 and E481.

Country Basket, by *Newform Foods*, available in health-food shops and chemists, make a wholewheat cake mix for diabetics – you just add eggs and water.

CAKES
See also CAKE MIXES.

Cakes

This is an area where you will most likely have to make your own if you want low-fat, low-sugar and high-fibre cakes.

Generally speaking, the better choices are something like a wholemeal scone (so long as you do not overload it with cream and jam), or perhaps a wholemeal teacake or teabread. Banana cakes and date and walnut cakes, or a fruited malt loaf, all of which could be wholemeal, are other options.

Some own-label wholemeal cakes are appearing in supermarkets and there are often seasonal good buys such as *Waitrose* wholemeal hot cross buns and some wholemeal mince pies. *Marks & Spencer* have a range a wholemeal cakes which are made with Allinson's stoneground 100 per cent wholmeal flour and are free from additives (Allinson's own baked wholemeal goods are not always additive-free). The ingredients, for example, in the Date and Honey Cake are: 33 per cent dates, plus egg, 14 per cent flour, hydrogenated vegetable oil, 6 per cent honey, invert sugar, brown sugar, modified starch, almonds, dried skimmed milk and wheat gluten. You will see from this that it is high in sugar and some other refined ingredients, despite being wholemeal. *Lyons Bakery* have also introduced *Wholemeal Recipe Cakes*.

The health-food chain, *Holland & Barrett* has a range of 'home-made' cakes made without preservatives, or artificial colourings or flavourings. Carob Brownies and Carrot and Banana Cakes come in trays of six bars, and they are all iced with raw cane sugar and a vegetable margarine mixture. Typical ingredients are wholemeal flour, vegetable margarine, raw cane sugar, skimmed milk powder, low-fat soft cheese, natural vanilla essence and carob powder.

Soreen Wholemeal Fruit Malt Loaf is an additive-free loaf with raisins, a high-fibre alternative to tea-cakes and scones, etc. Unlike many 'wholemeal' products all the flour is wholemeal, not a mixture of white flour with some wholemeal added. The ingredients are wholemeal flour, water, vine fruit, malt extract, black treacle, whey protein, vegetable fat, dried fermented whey, salt, yeast. Suitable for vegetarians, but not for vegans.

Local health-food shops and bakeries are often a better bet for 'healthier' cakes.

CANNED FOOD

Buying cans

- When buying food in cans it is important to check that they are not rusty or damaged, distended or leaking. Check the sell-by date and read the ingredients panel.
- Store in a cool place and use them in the order you bought them, or in the order of the sell-by dates.
- Once opened, transfer the contents to a non-metallic container and store, covered, in the fridge. Use as soon as possible. (Cartons have an advantage here over cans because opened cartons can be used to store things in for up to ten days.)

A general guideline to the shelf-life of cans is:

Baby food	up to 2 years
Fish in oil	up to 5 years
Fish in sauce	up to 2 years
Fruit juice	up to 2 years
Fruit	up to 2 years
Vegetables	up to 2 years (new potatoes 18 months).

CANNED FRUIT AND VEGETABLES

See CANNED FOOD for general notes on buying food in cans; see also BAKED BEANS, FRESH FRUIT AND VEGETABLES and FROZEN FOODS.

Canned foods have suffered from a poor image in the shopper's mind for some time, possibly because they think some manufacturers may use less-than-top-quality ingredients and add colourings and flavourings or flavour enhancers to make them palatable. They have also been regarded as nutrionally inferior because the heat treatment which is used to sterilize the products in the can destroys some vitamins, and others leach out into the liquid in the can, which is not always used. Those which are especially vulnerable are vitamins C and B_6 through heat-sensitivity, and folic acid

Canned Fruit and Vegetables

(often low in our diet) through the altered alkalinity (folic acid is destroyed by a neutral or alkali environment). However, the fibre, fats, proteins and carbohydrates are virtually unchanged by the process and fruit and vegetables canned within a few hours of harvesting have been demonstrated to be as good a source of vitamins and minerals as fruit and vegetables from the greengrocer, which may have been sitting around on the shop shelves for some time. (Green Giant sweetcorn canners claim there may be as little as 45 minutes between harvesting and canning.) Fresh fruit and vegetables deteriorate during distribution, and some of their vitamins and minerals are lost during storage. Bruising and injury will also destroy vitamin C, and bacteria and fungi in the atmosphere start the process of putrifaction, especially if the product is damaged.

Canning makes seasonal fruit and vegetables available all year round and provides a more convenient form of beans which otherwise require long soaking and slow cooking — kidney, haricot, butter and borlotti beans and chick peas, etc. It also makes exotic Chinese vegetables like bamboo shoots and water chestnuts, or Caribbean fruits, more widely available.

Canning without additives

But, and here comes the rub, it is often difficult to find products that are simply cooked and canned without the addition of salt and sugar, and additives too. Yet there is a growing number of products canned without these additions, and these are listed below.

A survey by Mediterranean Growers (who can the Valfrutta brand) found that 'housewives' thought fruit canned in natural juice tasted better than fruit canned in syrup. Their survey of 1,400 women revealed that half those who bought canned fruit were buying less, but more of what they were buying was canned in natural juice. Forty-six per cent of those asked bought fruit canned in natural juice, which now accounts for nearly 20 per cent of the UK canned fruit sales.

Canned Fruit and Vegetables

The same general advice applies to buying canned fruit and vegetables as to other processed foods. Read the label and decide if the additives contained are ones you want to eat. Unfortunately, labelling laws still list the ingredients only in descending order by weight, which does not give any indication of how much salt or sugar has been added, so it is best to stick with the brands that can in water or natural juice. The natural juice brand are less likely to harm teeth and they are also lower in calories than the typical peaches in heavy syrup, for example, which contain about five teaspoonfuls of added sugar per 425 g can.

When shopping for brands without added salt and sugar don't pop the can in your basket without reading the ingredients panel. Even if the label does scream 'No Added Salt, No Added Sugar', if it does not also scream 'No Additives' the chances are it will contain other things. For example, some canners make 'No Added Salt' peas, which contain sugar. Some say 'No Preservatives' on the label, but contain colourings and flavourings. This device comes in many variations, so always read the small print as well as the advertising blurb on the label.

Now here is the pick of the bunch – can-openers at the ready!

Fruit canned in its own juice

These products are also free from added sugar and artificial additives.

John West	Pears Grapefruit segments Pineapple cubes Pineapple rings	Mandarins (in orange juice) Apple slices (no added juice)
Red Sail	Grapefruit segments Pineapple slices Crushed pineapple	
Del Monte	Pineapple Grapefruit segments	
Valfrutta	Mandarin orange segments	

Canned Fruit and Vegetables

Safeway   Grapefruit segments
              Canned pineapples

Sainsbury's Grapefruit segments
              Orange segments
              Pineapple pieces
              Satsuma segments

Waitrose   Apricots (plus apple juice)
              Peaches (plus apple juice)
              Pears
              Pineapple
              Grapefruit
              Mandarin orange segments

Fruit canned in natural juice

These products are also free from added sugar and artificial additives.

John West   Apricots in apricot and apple juice
              Peaches in peach and apple juice
              Blackberries in apple juice
              Black cherries in apple juice
              Guava halves in guava and apple juice
              Prunes in apple juice

Red Sail   Apricots in apricot and apple juice
              Peaches in apple juice and peach juice
              Pears in apple juice and pear juice

Pickerings Prunes in apple juice and pear juice

Chivers   Black cherries in apple juice
              Blackberries in apple juice
              Prunes in apple juice (with citric acid, vitamin C)

Del Monte   Peach slices in fruit juice
              Peach halves in fruit juice
              Pear halves in fruit juice
              Apricots in fruit juice

Canned Fruit and Vegetables

Valfrutta	Pear halves in grape juice and pear juice Peach slices in grape juice and peach juice Apricot halves in apple juice and apricot juice Prunes in prune juice and grape juice Black cherries in apple juice
Lockwoods	Blackcurrants in apple juice Blackberries in apple juice
Safeway	Peach slices in grape juice Peach halves in grape juice Pear halves in grape juice Pineapple rings in grape juice Pineapple pieces in grape juice Mandarin segments in grape juice
Sainsbury's	Apricot halves in fruit juice (may be apple or grape) Pear quarters in fruit juice Prunes in fruit juice Blackcurrants in fruit juice Raspberries in fruit juice Strawberries in fruit juice
Waitrose	Raspberries in apple juice

Fruit cocktails may also appear in the natural-juice ranges, but although most of the fruits are free from additives, as are the other contents, the canned cherries invariably contain the synthetic colouring E127.

Canned strawberries and raspberries may also be in natural juice, but they contain the synthetic colourings E127 and E124 respectively.

Canned blackcurrants in some ranges contain the colouring E132.

Fruits canned in water

Red Sail	Apple slices (with added vitamin C)
Dietade	Apricots Peaches Pears

Canned Fruit and Vegetables

        Pineapple
        Fruit salad (but this contains E127 in the cherries).

Vegetables canned without added sugar and salt

Green Giant   Sweet corn niblets
                4 corn on the cob

The rest of the Green Giant range of sweet corn and canned asparagus is canned in very little water and has very little added sugar and salt. The sugar content is 9 g per 100 g compared with 2 g for boiled fresh corn on the cob, and the salt content is increased by only 1 mg. Green Giant steam their corn for only 7 minutes and so no vitamins and minerals are leached into cooking water; the corn is then sealed in the can in a vacuum.

Del Monte   Cut green beans
              Whole carrots
              Sliced carrots
              Garden peas and golden sweetcorn (contains sugar).

Del Monte say that their no-added-salt canned vegetables contain 1–50 mg sodium per 100 g compared with 230–400 mg in drained vegetables canned in salted water.

John West   Tomatoes in tomato juice
Cirio   Chopped tomatoes in natural juice
              Tomato purée and paste
Lockwoods Garden peas (but these contain sugar and artificial additives).

Vegetables canned in water

Lotus Brand do a range of Chinese vegetables canned in water and free from artificial additives. These include bamboo shoots and water chestnuts.

Vegetables in cartons

Cirio   Passata – sieved tomatoes (with a trace of salt)
                 Pomi – strained, crushed tomatoes (0.6 per cent salt)
Napolina   Creamed tomatoes.

CAROB
See under SNACK FOODS.

CEREAL BARS
See also BISCUITS, FRUIT BARS and SNACK FOODS.

It all started with *Jordans* Original Crunchy Bars only a few years ago and now it is a £10m plus business. Before the 1980s cereal bars were unheard of in Britain, but by 1982 we were crunching our way through 55 million and in 1985 the estimate was 160 million.

They originated in the United States, where they are better known as Granola bars. President Reagan lunches on a 153 calorie crunchy snack bar called the President's Lunch. It is a high-fibre product and contains pollen and kelp (seaweed). Granola is a toasted form of muesli (see BREAKFAST CEREALS) and is a mixture of oats and other grains, nuts, sugar and honey or other sweeteners and dried fruit.

Since the launch of Jordans Original Crunchy Bar, there have been many others, some crunchy and some chewy and moist. *Quaker's* Harvest Crunch now claims to have 65 per cent of the market but their product is not listed here because it contains several additives including one of the most worrying, BHA.

Weight watching
When buying cereal bars look out for the sugar content because some versions contain no less than five sweeteners, or different forms of sugar. Harvest Crunch, for example, contains brown

Cereal Bars Compared

	Calories	Weight	Sucrose	Total sugars (g)	Dietary fibre (g)	Fat (g)
Jordans Original Crunchy Bar						
Honey and Almond	135	33	n.a.*	8.9	4.6	6.6
Apple and Bran	135	33	n.a.	9.6	4.6	6.6
Coconut and Honey	135	33	n.a.	7.5	4.6	6.6
Orange and Carob	140	33	n.a.	10.0	4.3	7.0
Fox's Natural Crunch						
Honey and Oats	91	21	n.a.	n.a.	1.8	4.3
Fruit and Nut	94	21	n.a.	n.a.	1	4.3
Chocolate Chip and Almond	96	21	n.a.	n.a.	0.8	4.5
Cluster						
Chewy						
Apricot and Chocolate Chip	115	30	3.5	13.2	4.5	4
Apple and Hazelnut	114	30	11.1	12.4	3.3	4.17
Crunchy						
Hazelnut and Raisin	125	30	5.9	10.1	4.1	5.13
Peanut and Almond	139	30	5.9	8.1	4.7	7.02

Boots

Crunch Bars				
Honey	139	25	1.3	6.1	1.2	5.5
Coconut	148	25	1.3	5.9	2.3	8.8
Seed Bars				
Poppy	139	30	5.4 + 0.6 g honey	1.4	5.6
Sesame	139	30	5.6 + 2.6 g honey	1.2	1
Sunflower	139	30	5.6 + 2.6 g honey	1.1	6.9
Grizzly Bars				
Apricot and Honey	108	25	0.4	2.5	3.5	6.4
Muesli and Honey	115	25	0.4	2.5	2	6.2
Fruit 7 and Honey	110	25	0.4	2.5	3.1	6.4
Barbara's Bakery Granola Bars				
Coconut and Almond	183	35	no added	3.4	4	14.1
Cinnamon and Oats	170	35	sugar	5.3	2.9	10.8
Lucy Foods Granola Bars				
Grain and Fruit	231	56	no	17.2	3.4	8.2
Grain and Nut	239	56	added	16.8	3.4	9.4
Granola Bar	176	40	sugar	10.1	3.3	5.8
Shaw's Biscuits Northumbrian Bars				
Bran Flake and Honey	130	30	17.25	n.a.	1.86	5.4
Carob Chip Crunch	131	30	17.2	n.a.	1.74	5.9
Coated Carob Crunch	155	33	21.52	n.a.	1.87	6.9

Cereal Bars Compared (continued)

Nutrients per Bar

	Calories	Weight	Sucrose	Total sugars (g)	Dietary fibre (g)	Fat (g)
Allinson's						
Fruit Crunch	119	28	5.6 + 1 g honey		4	17.4
Carob Crunch	150	32	6.5 + 1.2 g honey		3.3	20.8
Braycott Wholesnack Bars						
Fruit and Coconut	114	25	n.a.	5	1.25	4.8
Half-coated Muesli	158	33	n.a.	6.6	1.5	7
Honey and Hazelnut	114	25	n.a.	5	1.1	5.5
Castaway Carob Topped Bars (with organic oats)						
Original	197	40	n.a.	7.7*	2	10.8
Banana	212	40	n.a.	7.4†	2.2	11.2
Apple/Hazelnut	200	40	n.a.	7.7†	2.1	10.8

* n.a. = not available.
† Includes carob coating.

sugar, sugar, glucose syrup, honey and malt, which adds up to a total of 25–27 per cent sugars. In fact, most cereal bars are high in sugar, but they do offer a more nutritious 'confectionery' than a bar of chocolate or other types of confectionery and they are lower in sugar than a Mars bar, for example, which is around 65 per cent sugar. *General Mills*, the American food giants, have launched their cereal bar Jump on the UK market. This product contains 100 per cent 'natural' ingredients, but it also contains five types of sugar: glucose syrup, dextrose, sugar syrup, raw sugar and honey (cheaper and more refined ingredients than those in some of the wholefood bars).

When buying, check for the number of sugars on the label, and for the additives. Often the sugar is not listed on the nutritional information given on these products; it is hidden away under the heading of carbohydrates so that you cannot really see how much there is in the bars. Always check the weight too. There is a big difference between Jordans Original Crunchy Bar at 33 g and Quaker's Harvest Crunch at only 18 g. What appears to be cheap by comparison is, perhaps, not so cheap.

The bars listed in the table are included because they are free from additives and the fat in them is of vegetable origin, so they are suitable for vegetarians, if not always for vegans.

> **My choice**
>
> Jordans Original Crunchy Bars for flavour, high-quality ingredients and value for money. Lucy Granola Bars and Boots Seed Bars are also good.

CHEESE

In the infancy of the science of nutrition, cheese was categorized as a high-protein food for building and repairing muscles in the body and for protection against ill health – it contains vitamin A and D. During the Second World War the Ministry of Food endorsed this, praising cheese as a concentrated form of energy. Unfortunately, these ideas have stuck. Today, nutritionists are trying to

Cheese

re-educate us, to see cheese mainly as a high-fat food rather than a high-protein food.

It was the fat content that led the Ministry of Food to call cheese a concentrated form of energy, which it is because fat is very high in calories. Today, however, we are eating too much fat, so we should cut down on fatty foods and use high-fibre carbohydrate foods instead for our energy. We also know now that the best sources of protein are low-fat sources.

Cut down on cheese

So where does that leave cheese? Far from being the essential food for energy or protein (or even vitamins A and D, which are present in many other foods in our Western diet), cheese should be regarded as a treat. (We would do better to get our vitamins from fresh green leafy vegetables than to eat cheese daily.) In fact, we could do without cheese altogether. In the East, in China and Japan, people have lived very healthy lives for thousands of years without dairy produce; Western influence has recently made dairy products more popular and the Japanese government is trying to encourage people not to desert their healthy traditional diets for Western diets high in dairy produce (and hence fat).

If we want to continue to enjoy cheese it would be healthier to change the way we regard it – not to nibble on cheese or eat large chunks of it or use it as an extra course to a meal, but to regard it as a main ingredient, and make a little go a long way in conjunction with other ingredients. This may sound rather killjoy to cheese lovers, but it is not saying 'never again' – just use it like butter or margarine, sparingly.

Cutting down on cheese will also help with weight control. You would be amazed at the weight you could lose in the long term if you thought twice every time before nibbling cheese. When shopping look out for the lower-fat versions of hard cheese, or buy mature cheeses, with lots of flavour, such as Farmhouse Cheddar. They may be more expensive, but they save money in the long run, because a little goes a long way. With the stronger-flavoured cheeses you can cut down the amount you use in

Cheese

cooking too – Gruyère and Parmesan are good for cooking because they have a lot of flavour.

Vegetarian cheese

The usual way to make cheese is to curdle milk with rennet, which is a form of rennin, an enzyme taken from the stomach of slaughtered calves. (It helps them digest milk.) The rennin clots the milk, which is then drained of its whey, cut, pressed and salted, and left to mature in a cool place. Vegetarian agents for clotting milk are plant enzymes such as extracts from figs, or fungi. Lactic acid and bacteria can also be used. Health-food shops with chill counters often sell vegetarian cheese made from non-animal rennet and an increasing number of supermarkets do too (see list below and the table on p. 397).

Additives in cheese

Most hard cheese is made without additives using 'natural' processes, because it is strictly controlled by law. Traditional Cheddar, Cheshire, Leicester, etc., do not contain additives. Sorbic acid (E200) is allowed in hard cheeses, but it is not normally used. However, Edam and Gouda usually contain two additives some people might prefer to avoid, sodium nitrate (E250) and sodium nitrate (E251). The rinds of these cheeses (and others) also contain colourings but the rinds are not edible. Other cheeses that contain colouring are Double Gloucester, Red Leicester and other coloured hard cheeses, but the colours are naturally derived vegetable dyes like annatto (E160b) or carotene, or their synthetic equivalents, which may be also used to give cheese a marbled effect.

Proposals for revising the Cheese Regulations issued in 1986 will mean, if they are accepted, that more additives will be allowed in hard cheese. Other sorbates – E201 sodium sorbate, E202 potassium sorbate and E203 calcium sorbate – and 234 nisin, would be allowed in hard cheese (and all other cheese). More preservatives will also be allowed in cheeses, except Cheddar,

Cheese

Cheshire and soft cheese, and these include the nitrites and nitrates used in Dutch cheese, plus E252 potassium nitrate, and E249 potassium nitrite. A lot of other additives will be allowed, but these are mainly for use in processed cheese and cheese spreads.

Processed cheeses, cheese spreads and 'flavoured' cheese spreads are made by heating the cheeses and then blending them, sometimes with the addition of flavourings. Emulsifying agents, lactic and acetic acids and salt are also added to these cheeses. The cheese is 'fixed' by heating, so it cannot mature or change, ensuring a consistent product. The ingredients labels of these cheeses are worth reading before you buy.

Low-fat cheeses

These are made from skimmed milk and do not contain rennet; the milk is curdled by using natural souring agents like bacteria or lactic acid, so they are suitable for vegetarians. The curds are cut, drained and sometimes washed in single cream. These naturally low-fat cheeses are:

	Fat content (%)
Cottage cheese* – made from skimmed pasteurized milk	2–4
Ricotta – made from a mix of whole milk and skimmed	5–10
Curd cheeses – made from a mix of whole milk and skimmed	5–10
Quark – made from skimmed milk	5–10
Fromage blanc – as above	5–10
Skimmed milk soft cheese	5–10

* Cottage cheese usually contains preservatives and other additives but additive-free versions are available in health-food shops, specialist cheese shops and some delicatessens. Eden Vale's natural cottage cheese is free from additives, and so is Marks & Spencer natural. Lebne (Lebna/Lebnie) is similar but is more of a strained yoghurt than a cheese.

Cheese

Reduced-fat cheeses

These are low-fat versions of traditional hard cheeses.

Plain varieties

	Fat content (%)	Type
Sainsbury's 14% fat cheese	14	Cheddar
Tendale Cheshire type	14	Cheshire
Marks & Spencer Lite	15	Cheddar
Slimcea 15% fat cheese	15	Leicester
Prewett's Reduced Fat Vegetarian Cheese	15	Cheddar
Tendale Cheddar type	15	Cheddar
Light, by Kerrygold	15	Cheddar
Anchor Freeway	15	Cheddar
Shape	16	Cheddar
Scottish Pride	17	Cheddar
Co-op's Good Life	17	Cheddar
Blue Tendale	17.5	Blue Stilton

Flavoured varieties

The *Ilchester Cheese Company* have produced four Cheddar-style cheeses with half the fat of ordinary Cheddar and only a two thirds of the salt content.

	Fat content (%)	
Ilchester Abbeydale	15	(with onions and chives)
Ilchester Penmill	16	(with peppercorns)
Ilchester Grosvenor	16.5	(with mixed herbs)
Ilchester Albany	17	(with celery seeds)

Vegetarian cheeses

These are the most widely available vegetarian cheeses, and can be obtained from health-food shops and supermarkets. There are

Cheese

also small regional dairies producing vegetarian cheese so ask at your local health-food shop.

	Type
Marigold Vegetarian	Cheddar, Cheshire, Gouda
Prewett's	Cheddar, Cheshire, Bleasdale, Wensleydale, Double Gloucester, Lancashire
Farm Maid	Cheddar, Cheshire, Double Gloucester, Red Leicester, Wensleydale
St Ivel	Cheddar
Safeway	Cheddar
Sainsbury's	Cheddar

Other cheeses

Raines Dairy Food make a natural cottage cheese using only natural gums. They also make flavoured varieties; the additives used are E412, E415, E410.

Soderasens Vegetarian Vegetable Oil Cheese. This cheese is made in the same way as conventional cheese but using pasteurized skimmed milk and sunflower and soya oils. It is therefore unusual in being high in polyunsaturated fats. There are vegetarian and animal rennet versions, available in supermarkets.

Dutch cheese

Edam and Gouda are naturally lower in fat than many hard cheeses. They are 25–30 per cent fat respectively – Cheddar is about 34 per cent fat – but they contain the preservatives sodium nitrate and sodium nitrite. This will be declared on the outer rind of whole cheeses or on the pack of prepacked cheeses.

Blue cheese

In recent years there has been an increasing concern about mycotoxins in foods. These are moulds and other similar substances; research is continuing into their effect on health, but it has been strongly suggested that any mould on food could be harmful and mouldy food should be discarded. The spores in the food penetrate much deeper than the surface, so it is not enough simply to cut away the mould. Moulds produce the blue veining on cheese and the white crust on Brie and Camembert, but cheese experts say that these moulds are harmless, unlike moulds such as the aflatoxins found on peanuts. See PEANUT BUTTER.

Vegetarian rennet

If you want to make your own cheese, vegetarian rennet is sold in health-food shops or from specialist cheese-equipment suppliers such as: R. J. Fullwood and Bland Ltd, Rennet Works, Ellesmere, Shropshire (069-171 2391).

Organic cheese

There is very little organic cheese available and most of it is made on a small scale from goat's and sheep's milk. It is usually only available in the area of production or from specialist suppliers. See ORGANIC FOOD.

Cheese spreads

There are an increasing number of 'low-fat' cheese spreads around, some of which make 'health' claims; read the ingredients panels closely – they usually contain emulsifying salts, preservatives and flavourings.

Cheese desserts

Buttermilk and low-fat soft cheese desserts flavoured with fruit and fruit purées, imported from France and Germany, are similar to yoghurt, but with less tang. Some, such as *Petit Chambourcy Dessert*, contain only low-fat soft cheese, natural flavour and sugar. Others contain artificial additives. Read the label to check.

Cheese

> **Bread and Cheese**
>
> If you have a cheese course during a meal, or a Ploughman's Lunch, don't bother with the butter or margarine. Britain is probably alone in Europe in eating butter with cheese and biscuits or bread. This adds another source of fat to an already fatty food, and it also detracts from the flavour of the cheese. If you like butter eat bread and butter. If you like cheese eat bread and cheese.

Fat Content of Popular Cheeses (see also 'Low-fat Cheeses', p. 207)

	Fat content (%)
Mozzarella (pizza cheese)	25
Edam	25
Brie	26
Camembert	27
Gouda	30
Parmesan	30
Danish Blue	30
Wensleydale	31
Caerphilly	31
Double Gloucester	32
Leicester	32
Cheshire	32
Sage Derby	33
Cheddar	34
Stilton	40
Lymeswold	40

> **My choice**
>
> I buy a mature cheese with lots of flavour and make a little go a long way – that cuts costs and cuts down the amount of fat you are eating too. Farmhouse or mature Cheddars are useful, or, for cooking, Gruyère and real Parmesan. Generally I buy only a small amount – the amount the recipe calls for; then I am not tempted to nibble at the cheese.

CHUTNEY

The original Indian chutneys were often fresh relishes, but in Britain chutney is a preserve using sugar and vinegar. Some varieties are made without added sugar. Many of the standard chutneys contain additives, but some of the Indian ones and *Sharwood* relishes are free from additives. *Rayner & Co.* is another company specializing in relishes and sauces, and they also have a couple of additive-free chutneys in their range, *Mango Chutney* and *Goodfare Chutney*.

Down to Earth make a range of four no-added-sugar chutneys which are also salt-free and made with organic cider vinegar, apple juice and spices. They include Mango and Orange, Apricot and Date, Lemon and Apple and Pineapple and Ginger, and are available from health-food shops.

Organic Beetroot Chutney is sugar-free and is available at selected health-food shops. It is made by *Branton Kenton-Smith*, son of beauty writer Leslie Kenton. He makes it from vegetables grown on his organic market-garden in Wales.

Wendy Brandon's chutneys are also available through health-food shops and they are free from added sugar. They are made with fresh and dried fruit and vegetables, apple juice and organic cider vinegar. The varieties are: Apricot, Aubergine and Sweet Pepper, Mango, Date, Banana, Spicy Apple, Gingered Fig, Kashmiri Apple and Hot Fig. Also from Wendy Brandon are Apple Butter and Plum Butter, made with organic cider vinegar and apple juice. (These don't contain butter – they are reductions of fruit.)

Eden organic chutneys are imported from Holland. *Thursday Cottage* chutneys, like all their preserves, are made with raw cane sugar and contain no additives. *Culpeper* the herbalists make additive-free mango chutney and lime pickles.

Chutney

> **My choice**
> Down to Earth – paradoxically, they are heavenly, and so are Wendy Brandon's.

CLINGFILM

Although not a food, this is relevant to shopping for health. Clingfilm has been the subject of much-publicized scares after reports that a plasticizer called DEHA in the film was found to be causing cancer in mice. The use of films containing DEHA has been banned in Italy on fatty foods like cheese, where the molecules are more likely to 'migrate' into the food, and an EEC Working Party is looking at the evidence.

There are government plans to tighten regulations about use of chemicals which might migrate, and manufacturers have stated that they are not using these substances any longer. Although there is 'no concern' over the use of clingfilm, the government has warned against using it in microwave or conventional ovens. While the experts deliberate, your food is going dry in the fridge. There are some products which claim to be free from the problematic plasticizer, but they are not so clingy, because it is the clingy one that is giving the problems. One such product is *Glad Wrap*, which is made from polyethelene and is available from grocers; another, called *Purecling*, is sold by Woolworth's, Cullens and other grocers.

If in doubt about clingfilm why not wrap food in greaseproof paper or use sealed containers in the fridge. Limit the use of clingfilm to the tops of basins, etc., where it does not come into contact with the food, but can still prevent some moisture loss, keep the food sealed and stop it absorbing foreign odours in the fridge.

COFFEE

Only twenty years ago the British were drinking six cups of tea to one cup of coffee; today we are drinking two cups of tea to each cup of coffee, and 90 per cent of the coffee drunk is instant.

The only other country drinking such a high percentage of instant coffee is Japan – traditionally another tea-drinking country. Although we don't link tea with caffeine, it contains almost as much as coffee, but it seems to act differently. The caffeine in tea has its effect about fifteen minutes after being drunk, whereas that in coffee is effective almost immediately.

Instant Coffee

To make instant coffee the beans are first selected, then blended, washed and percolated to a strong liquid concentrate which is either spray-dried or freeze-dried to powder or granules. Freeze-drying makes a better flavoured instant coffee.

Decaffeinated coffee

Whether or not coffee is good for us depends on whether we are sensitive to its many effects, whether we are hooked on it and how much we drink. The main effects are a direct result of the caffeine. It seems that the nations who drink the most coffee must be aware of the bad points because they also drink the largest percentage of decaffeinated coffee. In America 30 per cent of the coffee drunk is decaffeinated, and in West Germany 10 per cent. In Britain it is estimated that only 3 per cent is decaffeinated, but this is the fastest-growing sector of the coffee market – there has been a 70 per cent increase in volume since 1983.

Decaffeinated coffee can be bought as instant coffee, either in powder or granule form, or it can be bought ready ground; it can also be bought as beans. The brand leader in decaffeinated coffee is *Café Hag* which is imported by *General Foods* from the manufacturers in West Germany. Other names in the game

Coffee

include Rombouts, Jacqmotte, Melitta, Gold Blend (from *Nestlé*), and *Champneys* from *Calypsa Foods*.

Several methods can be used to remove the caffeine, but they can be divided into three main categories: chemical solvents, the water process and the carbon-dioxide method. The last two are sometimes lumped together as one process.

By law not more than 0.3 per cent of caffeine residue is allowed in decaffeinated coffee and in fact typical analyses reveal that about 0.02 per cent is left. There is, incidentally, no law about how much caffeine should be in regular coffee – it depends on the bean used to make it.

Chemical solvent

Three chemical solvents are commonly used: methylene chloride, ethylene acetate and dichloromethane. First the beans are washed and steamed and then the solvent flushed through to carry out the caffeine. The beans are then washed several times to remove the solvent before being dried and roasted.

Carbon dioxide (CO_2)

This involves placing green beans in an extraction vessel to which pressurized carbon dioxide and water are added. The contents are kept under pressure for several hours and then the decaffeinated beans are separated from the carbon dioxide and water.

Water processing

The 'Swiss water process' is used by Nestlé, who say no chemical solvent is used – the beans are steamed and then have warm water flushed through them a number of times. This removes the caffeine and some of the coffee components which give flavour and aroma. The mixture containing the caffeine and coffee components is then passed through filters of charcoal penetrated with sucrose and formic acid which take out the caffeine and leave the coffee components, which are then returned to the partially dried beans.

Another water process, used by other companies, involves soaking the beans in a mixture of water and coffee components

Coffee

Who Does What

Instant coffee	Process	Type
Café Hag	CO_2	granules and freeze-dried
High Blend Maxwell House	CO_2	granules
Sainsbury's Gold Choice	CO_2	freeze-dried
Nescafé Decaffeinated	water	freeze-dried
Nescafé Gold Blend	water process	freeze-dried
Boots	methylene chloride	granules and freeze-dried
Twinings	methylene chloride	freeze-dried
Presto Gold Roast	methylene chloride	freeze-dried
Tesco Gold	methylene chloride	freeze-dried
Waitrose	methylene chloride	freeze-dried
Prewett's	methylene chloride	granules
Douwe Egbert's Moccona	Dichlorine methylene	granules

Ground coffee	Process
Café Hag	CO_2
Champneys	chemical solvent
Nescafé Gold Blend	water process
Jacqmotte	dichloromethane
Kenco	methylene chloride
Langford Brothers	chemical solvent/switching to water process
Melitta	chemical solvent
Nairobi Pure	methylene chloride
Nairobi Pure Kenya	Secoffex water process
Rombouts	water process
Waitrose	methylene chloride
Twinings	methylene chloride

Coffee

for several hours until 97 per cent of the caffeine is removed. The coffee components help prevent substances other than caffeine being leached from the beans, which therefore retain their flavour and aroma. The caffeine-rich mixture is combined with methylene chloride which draws off the caffeine. The mixture is then steamed to remove the methylene chloride and is afterwards collected and used to decaffeinate more beans.

Which method is best?

Some years ago chemical-solvent and cancer scares in the US put a lot of people off decaffeinated coffee because of the fear of chemical residues, but the offending chemicals are no longer used and residues of the present ones are minute.

The chemical solvent method is said to remove more caffeine, but has some residues. The water/CO_2 processes have no residues but they do not remove the caffeine as effectively as chemicals.

Buying decaffeinated ground coffee

As with all coffee, the quality of the beans and the skill of the blender and roaster determines the flavour. Some brands declare on their packaging what type of bean is used. Usually manufacturers are keen to boast about Arabica beans because they are considered the finest; they are also relatively low in caffeine. Arabica is grown mainly in Kenya and other parts of East Africa.

> **My choice**
>
> Café Hag and Nescafé Gold Blend decaffeinated instant coffees; Café Hag, Nairobi Pure Kenya and Kenco decaffeinated ground coffee.

Organic coffee

As far as I know there is only one supplier of organically grown coffee beans; *Wholefood* of Paddington Street, London. Their organic roast coffee beans are 100 per cent Costa Rican Arabica beans in 250 g vacuum packs; they are supplied by the French organic specialists Le Maire.

Coffee

Why decaffeinated?

If you are wondering why there is so much fuss about caffeine and think that it is only troublesome because late-night coffees keep you awake, you might be interested in the other reasons for finding an alternative to replace at least some of the caffeine-rich drinks taken during the day.

1. Caffeine is a stimulant that works directly on the brain, prompting enhanced perception, inspiration and alertness. It is used in anti-soporific medicines and drugs, and in pick-you-ups. If it's that powerful, it should not be used all the time as a drink, because it can cause anxiety, nervousness, tension and sometimes nausea and palpitations if it is used too much.

2. One of the most popular reasons for drinking coffee is because it stimulates the gastric juices after dinner, but caffeine taken throughout the day in coffee, tea, cola and other drinks (and chocolate and sweets) is not such a good thing.

3. Caffeine is a diuretic, and quite a strong one, so it stimulates the kidneys and causes the body to excrete more fluid than might be necessary, thus depleting the body of water-soluble vitamins such as vitamin C and the B complex vitamins.

4. Some trials have shown that caffeine can raise blood fat levels, especially cholesterol. One Norwegian study suggests that giving up coffee can lower cholesterol more effectively than a low-fat diet. American research has also shown that five-cup-a-day coffee drinkers are more likely to have heart disease.

5. Expectant mums should cut caffeine intake to two cups of coffee a day at most, says the Health Education Council.

6. Coffee can stimulate the adrenal glands to release substances that in turn release stored energy from the liver into the blood. This demands insulin from the pancreas and can result in the ups and downs of blood sugar levels experienced in hypoglycaemia (low blood sugar); the effect is similar to that of sugary sweets and snacks. It's a vicious circle of lifts and slumps that the coffee addict knows well!

Coffee

7. Caffeine can also be a cause of cystic breast disease (lumpy and painful breasts, especially prior to menstruation); by avoiding caffeine, mainly in coffee, but also in tea and cocoa, the symptoms can be alleviated in some cases. The methyxanthines (stimulants) in the caffeine encourage binding of the hormone prolactin to the breast, causing the lumps.

And those are just seven of the reasons why you might be interested in decaffeinated coffee!

Alternatives to coffee

If decaffeinated coffee is not to your taste there are several other drinks that either mimic or replace coffee. Many are based on chicory, dandelion or roasted cereals. Some of the most popular (and acceptable!) are listed below. You will find them in health-foods shops and chemists.

Barleycup is a caffeine-free cereal drink without any artificial additives. It is made from roasted barley, rye and chicory ground to a powder. Make it with hot water or cold, and take it with or without milk.

Bambu is a Swiss coffee substitute made with chicory, figs, wheat, malted barley and acorns. It is made to a recipe by the famous Swiss naturopath Dr A. Vogel (of Vogel bread fame). It is processed using only pure mountain water and is (of course) free from additives.

Caro is a caffeine- and additive-free substitute for coffee made from roasted malted barley, chicory, rye and sugar beet. The instant version is dissolved in water; Caro Extra can be used with hot or cold water or milk.

Dandelion coffee is available in several brands, for example Symingtons Instant Dandelion Coffee, which is made from lactose and soluble solids of dandelion root. The specially cultivated root is dried, roasted and made into granules.

Carob drink can replace drinking chocolate and cocoa, which both contain added sugar, salt and some additives. Carob is a stimulant-free alternative to chocolate; it is available as an instant powdered drink for use with milk or water – for example, Carob Cup from *Survival Foods*, Carob Drink (with raw sugar, milk and skimmed milk) from *Healtheries* and Carob Night Time Drink (with dried skimmed milk powder, carob powder, raw cane sugar, guargum and vanilla) from Prewett's. (See SNACK FOODS, 'Carob', for more information about carob.)

> **My choice**
>
> Don't compare them with coffee and you might develop a taste for Bambu or Symington's Dandelion Coffee.

COOKING FAT
See under MARGARINE.

COOKING OIL
See OILS.

CREAM

In a book about healthy eating you might think it rather absurd to be including cream. Well, this book is not intended to tell you what to eat, but to give you the information that will enable you to make the best choices for health; that includes knowing the comparable fat and calorie contents of cream, so that when you are not buying it you will know why! If you can't resist it altogether, buy it in smaller amounts and buy it less frequently.

Obviously you don't have to remember exact calories and fat content of the various types of cream; it is enough to know which is highest in fat. The table overleaf gives a visual reminder of the degrees of 'naughtiness'.

Cream

	Minimum fat content (%)	Maximum fat content (%)	Calories per 100 ml
Half cream	12	18	
Whey cream*	18		
Single cream	18	35	212
Soured cream†	35		270
Whipping cream	35	48	332
Double cream	48		447
Clotted cream	55		577
Devonshire cream	55		577

* Whey cream is a newly created cream under the regulations. It is part of the cheese whey that is rich in fat and has been separated by skimming or other cheese-making process.

† Not specified in the Revised Cream Regulations, part of the Fat Content Labelling Regulations, 1986; figures given by dairies.

Apart from calories and cholesterol cream has little to offer in the way of nutrients. Even the dairy industry takes the 'naughty, but nice' approach, and they are now looking for new ways to rid themselves of the cream lakes which result from over-production and the boom in skimmed milk – adding it, for example, to ice-cream (see ICE-CREAM).

> **Strained Yoghurt**
>
> Originally imported from Greece, strained yogurt is now also imported from Cyprus and made in Britain too. It has a thick texture like cream and makes an excellent substitute for spooning cream, toppings to desserts and baked potatoes. It can also be made into a delicious piping cream to replace whipped double cream (see YOGHURT – where I have given a recipe for home-made yoghurt cream).

UHT and sterilized cream

They may contain many food additives and they are, of course, heat-treated, which changes their flavour and probably their protein structure. Read the labels if you buy them.

Cream

Soured cream
This will contain natural bacterial agents or rennet to sour it, or acids such as E260, E270, E330, E338, 507 or 575.

Whipped cream
This may contain E400 alginic acid or a mix of 500 sodium hydrogen carbonate, E450(a) and alginic acid (another version of E400), E466 carboxymethylcellulose, E471, E472(b) (see 'Aerosol Cream' below) and nitrogen.

Whipping cream
This is free from additives and a little lower in fat than double cream. Whipping cream (and whipped cream) sold for use to caterers and food manufacturers may contain many additives.

Aerosol cream
Cream in aerosols is UHT (heat treated). It contains a propellant such as nitrous oxide to allow it to be squirted from the aerosol, and it may also contain other additives such as E401 sodium alginate, E402 potassium alginate, E404 calcium alginate, E407 carrageenan, E410 locust bean gum, E412 guar gum, E415 xanthan gum, all natural gelling agents. It may also contain 500 sodium bicarbonate, E450(a) tetraSodium diphosphate, E400 alginic acid, sodium, and E471 and E472(c), fatty substances of animal or vegetable origin used as stabilizers.

Loseley Extra Thick Jersey Single Cream
This is made from homogenized single Jersey cream which gives it the 'spoonability' of whipped double cream with only the calories of single.

My choice

Loseley's Extra Thick Jersey Single Cream, soured cream for treats or strained natural yoghurt.

Cream

Cream substitutes

These have recently appeared on supermarket shelves and in dairy chillers. They often claim to be lower in calories and lower in fat than standard cream. They look similar to cream and are packed in the same sort of cartons, often with the same colour coding, i.e. red for the equivalent of single cream and blue for the equivalent of double cream. Most are also cheaper than regular cream, giving the shopper an incentive to buy. But they may not be quite what you think they are.

Incidentally, packing which might lead shoppers to mistake a cream substitute for cream is not allowed by law, and some of these products could easily mislead. Real cream is controlled by law (how much fat it must contain, etc.) These substitutes have not been included in the Revised Cream Regulations, but they are covered by general food controls. They can be called cream so long as it is clear on the label that they are made with non-dairy cream; their fat content will have to be declared under the new fat-content labelling regulations.

Elmlea

Described on the carton as 'the real alternative to cream' this is available as *Elmlea* Single and Elmlea Whipping. The ingredients are: vegetable oils (palm kernel, coconut – but these are subject to variation), butter, buttermilk powder, stabilizers E410, E412 (from vegetable sources), colour E160(a).

	Single	*Whipping*	
Calories	195/100 ml	330/100 ml	Sizes: 142 ml (5 fl oz)
Fat	19 g/100 ml	34 g/100 ml	and 284 ml (10 fl oz)

Comment: The oils used are high in saturated fats and the product is also high in cholesterol, so what's the benefit over real cream?

Equal

Equal is made by *Brooke Bond* and need not be kept refrigerated before opening. It is free from milk fat and the ingredients are: water, hydrogenated vegetable oil, sugar, sodium caseinate,

Cream

emulsifiers E471, E322, stabilizers E401, E466, E407, acidity regulators E340, E339, salt, colour E160(a).

Calories   283/100 ml (566 per carton)   Size: 200 ml
Fat   29 g/100 ml

Comment: Although the fats are all vegetable in origin, they are hydrogenated and will have the same effect in the body as saturated fat. So again there is no real benefit over cream in the type of fat. There are also lots of additives to consider.

Marks & Spencer Lite

This is described as a 'dairy topping' for use as a substitute for cream. It has a much lower fat content and far fewer additives than many of the comparable products. The ingredients are: skimmed milk, cream, modified starch, skimmed milk powder, gelatine.

Calories   135/100 ml   Size: 284 ml (10 fl oz)
Fat   9 g/100 ml

Comments: It is one of the varieties with less 'objectionable' additives; it is high in animal produce, however.

Sainsbury's Non Dairy Cream

This cream may be whipped and it can also be frozen. It is recommended for whipping and pouring, but not for cooking or for coffee. The ingredients are: water, sugar, salt, flavouring, colourings E102, E110, E160 (a), emulsifier polyoxyethlene, sorbitan monosteareate, stabilizers E401, E465, hydrogenated palm kernel oil.

Calories   280/100 g   Size: 284 ml (10 fl oz)
Fat   26 g/100 ml

Comments: This product is made with hydrogenated palm oil, so the fat will have the same effect on the body as saturated fats even though it is vegetable in origin. The product is also high in sugar and salt and contains quite a few additives.

Cream

St Ivel Shape

Shape single and double 'creams' have half the fat content of their regular counterparts. The ingredients are: skimmed milk, butter oil, and vegetable fat, plus emulsifier. The double cream also contains skimmed milk powder and colour.

	Single	*Double*	
Calories	104/100 g	250/100 g	Size: 142 ml (5 fl oz)
Fat	8 g/100 ml	24 g/100 ml	and 284 ml (10 fl oz)

Comment: This one has a lower fat content than some of the others and it is thickened by the addition of skimmed milk (which is how most yoghurts are thickened), so it does not use so many additives and is a more 'natural' product.

> **My choice**
>
> Natural strained yoghurt; see also cream choice above.

CRISPBREAD AND CRACKERS

See also BISCUITS.

Crispbread originated in Scandinavia where it was baked from a fermented dough, generally made from rye flour. Today that process is not always used. Ryvita, for example, have a different process which gives a lighter product: the 100 per cent wholemeal rye flour is mixed with water and salt or malt or bran (depending on the recipe) and chilled to a thick paste which is beaten well and aerated with compressed air to make a foam. This is spread on a cotton conveyor belt dusted with flour and a pattern is dockered on to it; the crispbread is then baked in an oven twice as hot as a domestic oven.

Crispbread is good value for money compared with other 'processed' foods and many brands are free from artificial additives (choose from the brands and products outlined below). They are also high in fibre, low in calories and fat and sugar and they have a long shelf-life.

Crispbread and Crackers

Ryvita was probably the first to introduce crispbreads to Britain back in the 1920s. The range is free from additives and added sugar and fat. All, except Crackerbread, which has 1 per cent skimmed milk power, are suitable for vegans.

Ryvita Original contains only wholemeal flour and 0.5 per cent salt;

Ryvita Swedish-style Brown contains a wholemeal rye, 1 per cent salt and 0.5 per cent malt;

Ryvita High Fibre contains wholemeal rye, 30 per cent wheat bran, 0.5 per cent salt;

Allinson's Wholemeal Crispbread (made by Ryvita) contains wholemeal wheat flour and 1 per cent salt;

Salt-Free Allinson's Wholemeal Crispbread contains only wholemeal wheat flour;

Crackerbread is the only one not made with wholemeal flour – it also contains 1.25 per cent vegetable oil, 1 per cent skimmed milk powder, 1 per cent salt.

Scanda Crisp is a slim, dark rye crispbread from Finland. It is double baked to make it extra crisp and is free from additives; it contains wholemeal rye, flour, salt and yeast.

Kalvi do the *Primula* range of additive-free crispbreads including Primula Rye Crispbread made from whole rye flour, wheat and salt;

Primula Extra Thin Crispbread made from whole rye flour, salt;

Primula Rye Bran, thick and extra thin, made from whole rye flour, bran wheat and salt.

Kalvi have also put their own name to three new products:

Muesli Crispbread, made from whole rye flour, wheat bran, oats, wheat, barley, rye, millet and salt;

Crispbread Fingers, which contain whole rye flour, wheat bran and salt;

Crispbread Wafers which contain whole rye flour and salt.

Each pack contains twelve individual wrapped packs of four crispbreads to keep them fresher longer, making them useful for packed lunches, etc.

Crispbread and Crackers

The *Ryking* range of crispbread is from Crawfords, part of United Biscuits; it is also free from artificial additives. The range is based on wholemeal wheat and rye flour (except *Ryking Goldenwheat*, which is not all wholemeal).

Ryking Fibre Plus contains 55 per cent wholemeal, 40 per cent wheat bran, vegetable fat, yeast, salt and the emulsifier E322 (lecithin);

Ryking Brown Rye contains 70 per cent rye wholemeal, sifted rye flour, yeast, salt;

Ryking Light contains 98 per cent rye wholemeal, salt;

Ryking Crispbread Snack contains rye wholemeal, cheese powder, vegetable fat, sifted rye flour, yeast, skimmed milk powder, salt and E160(c), a natural plant colouring;

Ryking Golden Wheat: 90 per cent wheat wholemeal, sifted wheat flour, raising agent ammonia bicarbonate, skimmed milk powder, whey powder, hydrogenated vegetable fat, dextrose, soya protein, emulsifier E322 and salt.

Energen Crispbread has changed from a starch-reduced crispbread to a high-fibre, low-calorie product range which is free from additives except for caramel, used as colouring in the Brancrisp. The range includes:

Wheatcrisp made from wholemeal flour, bran, salt, skimmed milk powder, sugar, hydrogenated vegetable oil;

Brancrisp is similar, but made from brown flour and free from added sugar;

Cheesecrisp is made from wholemeal flour and bran, plus refined vegetable fibre, cheese, salt and autolysed yeast;

Ryecrisp is made from rye flour, wheat bran, vegetable fibre, salt, hydrogenated vegetable oil, wheat flour, dried whey powder.

Ideal is a range of Norwegian wholegrain crispbreads, all 'thin' and free from artificial additives. Ideal Bran is made from wholewheat flour, rye flour, barley flour, wheat bran, salt and yeast and has added sesame seeds; there is also a wholegrain salt-free version.

Crispbread and Crackers

GG Scandinavian bran crispbread is made in Norway from unprocessed wheat bran, rye flour and salt and is imported by Scandinavian Suppliers (London) who also import the *Ideal* range and *Siljan*. GG is 85 per cent bran and is free from additives. Siljan is a large traditional wheel crispbread with a hole through the middle, wrapped in colourful paper.

Other brands worth trying – found in health-food shops and free from additives – are *Slymbred* and *Country Basket*.

Rice crispbread is especially useful for those on a gluten-free diet or those avoiding wheat. It contains rice flour (87 per cent), rice bran (10 per cent), skimmed milk powder (2 per cent), and peanut oil (1 per cent). Each slice has twenty calories and the product is free from additives, added sugar and salt. Made by *Healtheries* and available in health and wholefood shops.

> **My choice**
>
> Ryvita Original or Swedish Style, or the 'real thing', Siljans from Scandinavian Suppliers.

Organic crispbread

Two sorts of organic rye crispbread are imported from Holland. They are available from Infinity Food (for address see ORGANIC FOOD).

Other products
Crisprolls

Crisprolls are toasted, halved, wholegrain bread rolls imported from Scandinavia. They are like rusks for grown-ups and are becoming increasingly popular! The bread rolls are halved and dried out to make them crispy and golden. The two available brands, *Pogens* Krisprolls and *Scanda Crisp*, are made from wholegrain breads and are free from additives. *Marks & Spencer* also do crisprolls which are wholegrain and free from additives.

Crispbread and Crackers

Matzos

Rakusens, who produce kosher foods, make Rye Matzo Crackers using wholemeal flour, Tea Matzo and Matzo Crackers, plus a Superfine Matzo without added salt. All are free from artificial ingredients and dairy or animal ingredients. They also make, from brown flour and water, Hi Lo Crackers. All the flour used is unbleached.

Oatcakes

These are a natural food which has been a staple for centuries in Scotland. They are as useful as crispbreads and have the added advantage of containing soluble oat fibre (see BREAKFAST CEREALS, p. 180, for an explanation). Many brands of oatcakes are free from artificial additives and added sugar; a widely available brand is made by Paterson-bronte and sold under the *Paterson's* brand name. This range includes: Oatcakes (with added bran), Rough Oatcakes, Oatcake Farls and Farmhouse Oatcakes.

CRISPS

See SNACK FOODS.

CUSTARD POWDER

Real custard is made with milk, sugar (or honey if you are making it at home) and eggs. The eggs give the colour and thicken the sauce.

Most custard powders are made from refined starches, sugar, skimmed milk powders, fat and colourings such as tartrazine – the 'demon yellow peril'.

Boots have replaced tartrazine with carotene, and artificial flavours with natural vanilla, to produce Boots Custard Powder, which contains only maize starch, vanilla and natural colour. It is used in exactly the same way as standard custard powders.

Canned custard is available, but also needs watching! One

additive-free canned custard made from soya milk is available from health-food shops under the *Golden Archer* brand name.

Mr Merry Instant Custard Mix, made by Modern Health Products, is available in sachets from health and wholefood shops. It contains raw cane sugar, guar gum, carageenan, lecithin, natural vanilla and annatto, and each sachet makes up with 1 pint (600 ml) milk to produce pouring custard which will set on cooling.

DRIED FRUITS

Dried fruits make a great substitute for sweets for both children and adults. Dried apricots, pears, peaches and figs, and prunes, sultanas and raisins are especially good. They are naturally sweet and also contain vitamins and minerals.

The best type to buy are sun dried, because these do not undergo any heat treatment to speed them on their way and they are not (usually) coated with mineral oils to give them a gloss and stop them sticking to the packaging. This cosmetic sheen does nothing for the nutritional value of the fruit and nothing for our health, being mainly liquid paraffins – too much of which is not a good thing! If you do like fruit to have a sheen then look out for fruit coated with vegetable oil rather than mineral oil.

The new no-need-to soak and ready-to-eat prunes and other fruits have had some of the water put back and may contain potassium sorbate or sulphur dioxide to stop them going mouldy or 'sugaring'. They are moist and less chewy.

Dried fruit is also often treated with sulphur dioxide to preserve its colour. The use of sulphites as preservatives on fresh fruits and salads has been curbed in America (see Table 1) and there is some concern about the effects it has, especially as it is in such widespread use. It has triggered asthmatic attacks and caused allergies and it destroys vitamin B_1 and vitamin C, although we probably do not eat it in large enough concentrations for it to destroy the body's own supplies. Dried fruit without sulphur dioxide on it may be found in health and wholefood shops.

Dried Fruits

Glacé cherries

Glacé cherries also contain artificial colourings, but natural glacé cherries are now available under the *Epicure* brand from Petty, Wood and Co. They are a burgundy shade which is nearer to the colour of fresh, ripe cherries than the traditional scarlet colour. They are imported from France; the colouring used is anthocyanin, made from crushed grape skins.

DRINKS

See COFFEE, FRUIT JUICE, MILK, SOYA MILK, TEA, WATER, WINE and YOGHURT ('Yoghurt Drinks').

EGGS

Almost all the eggs we eat today are produced by battery hens, but there are alternatives such as barn-laid eggs, nest-box eggs and free-range eggs. These are increasingly being found in supermarkets and other high-street chains. There are many humanitarian arguments against the battery system, rather beyond the scope of this book, but it is worth commenting that healthy food comes from healthy animals and hens confined in the battery system are more likely to need drug treatment and medication than those allowed to move around, behave naturally and exercise properly.

The feed for battery hens contains dyes to produce eggs with a consistently deep yellow yolk – this dye may be tartrazine, which is particularly problematic for hyperactive children and is known to cause adverse reactions. Antibiotics are also routinely used in hens' feed as a preventative against ill health, because the conditions in which battery hens live encourage disease and lower resistance. Free-range eggs contain more B vitamins than battery eggs.

Eggs

The colour of the shells has nothing to do with the nutritional value of the eggs, as far as we know; it depends on the breed of chicken. What follows is a brief description of each of the types of egg production.

Free range

Hardly any birds are kept under genuinely free-range conditions as epitomized in our romantic conceptions of the traditional farm yard. There have been court cases in Britain over the use of the term 'free range' and one crown court judge decided that the term should apply only to birds kept no more than 150 to the acre and deriving a significant amount of food from the natural herbiage.

In July 1985, however, the EEC introduced a new set of descriptions for the terms you will see printed on egg boxes (but not on eggs sold loose from trays, at market stalls, at the farm or door-to-door):

Free range: the hens have continuous access to open-air runs during the day with not more than one hen to each 10 sq m of available ground.

Semi-intensive: these hens must also have daytime access to open-air runs, but they are more intensively farmed, with not more than one hen per 2.5 sq m.

Deep litter: these hens live indoors with not more than 7 hens per sq m of available floor space.

Perchery and/or barn eggs: these hens live indoors with no more than 25 hens per sq m and at least 15 cm of perch space for each bird.

My choice

Free-range every time, but do make sure that the box states the words 'free range'. Often descriptions like 'country fresh' can imply eggs produced in the open air, but they are just blurb – they are not legal descriptions of free-range eggs.

Eggs

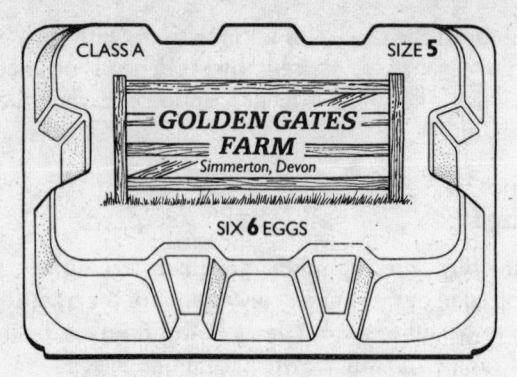

Explanation of the Labelling on an Egg-box

Class

This refers to the quality of the egg:

Class A. The egg must have a clean and normal shell. The airspace must not exceed 6 mm. The white must be of a gelatinous consistency and the yolk free of blood spots. The egg must not have been refrigerated below 8°C (46°F) or treated with preservative. It must not have been cleaned in any way.

Class B. Again, the egg must have a clean and normal shell. The airspace must not exceed 9 mm. There is no definition as to the consistency of the white. Grade B eggs may be washed or cleaned. They may also be refrigerated or undergo other preservative treatments such as being oiled, stored in gas or even in waterglass.

Class C. Includes all other eggs, but they must go to an egg processing plant for the manufacture of pasteurized egg products.

Size

This is given by a number from 1 to 7 and is a measure of weight.

Grade 1	70 g	Grade 5	50–55 g
Grade 2	65–70 g	Grade 6	45–50 g
Grade 3	60–65 g	Grade 7	40–45 g
Grade 4	55–60 g		

Eggs and health

The discovery that eggs contain cholesterol led to a panic move away from eggs, but they do also contain lecithin, the natural emulsifying agent (which helps control unwanted cholesterol deposits), B vitamins choline and inositol (which are 'fat fighters' and cholesterol controllers) and some minerals. However, eggs *are* quite fatty and should be kept to a minimum in the diet – probably no more than four a week. To make matters worse, one of the most popular ways of cooking them is frying, usually in animal fats or highly saturated oils – it is better to poach or boil them instead, or scramble them without fat.

Whether you buy free range or not is a matter of personal choice but they are now becoming more freely available in supermarkets (see SUPERMARKETS), as well as health-food shops.

FISH

Fish is an excellent food and we are not eating enough of it! Fresh fish consumption fell by 5.5 per cent in 1984; the number of fishmongers has declined from 8,000 to 3,000 between 1970 and 1984 and there are only 400 supermarkets selling fresh fish.

Market research indicates that young people do not know how to prepare fresh fish, having been brought up on canned and frozen fish products. In one survey, only 37 per cent of younger women, compared with 70 per cent of 55–64-year-olds, bought fresh fish.

Fresh fish is one of the best convenience foods we have (if we don't batter and fry it!) – it takes only 5–10 minutes to grill a piece of fish or 12–15 minutes to poach it, and it is extremely versatile. Briefly it is a good food because it is a low-fat form of easily digestible protein; oily fish in particular contain a high level of polyunsaturated fatty acids together with some special marine oils that have been shown to be useful in preventing heart disease. Recent research has also shown that the 'old wives' tale' that fish is

Fish

good for the brain is actually true, because another substance found in fish oils is taken up by the brain.

So come on – let's stop the decline of the fishmonger and make more use of fish – after all we are living on an island and surrounded by seafuls of the stuff!

How to buy fish

Here are a few pointers of things to look for when choosing fish:

- Make sure the flesh is firm.
- Look for clear, shiny eyes on whole fish.
- Ensure the fish has a 'clean smell' – any hint of ammonia indicates that it's off.
- Avoid gluey or watery fleshed fish.
- If there are any gills they should be red in colour.

When to buy fish

Most foods are now available year-round and some fish are on the fishmonger's slab at most times of the year. These include cod, coley, haddock, rockfish (huss), sole, plaice and whiting. These are all white fish; the first four are sold in fillets and steaks – sole, plaice and whiting may be sold whole or in fillets as they are smaller. If you haven't tried whiting do give it a go, because it is a very delicate fish.

Oily fish like mackerel, herring, and trout are also available most of the time. Fish farming has made trout a common fish and salmon farming is increasing the supplies of salmon.

The table on p. 237 lists some of the fish you might not have tried, together with some idea of when they are available and what to do with them! There are lots more exotic ones around too, especially in areas with high ethnic populations.

How much to buy

The quantity will depend on whether it is a main course or a starter; the average main course portion per person is:

whole white fish	10 oz (285 g)
whole oily fish	8 oz (225 g)
gutted fish (white or oily)	8 oz (225 g)
filleted fish	6 oz (170 g)

Fish farms and additives

Ten years ago most of the fish we ate was caught from the sea or rivers, but the last decade has seen an explosion of fish farms in the UK. There is as yet no official register, but there are thought to be around 450 commercial fish farms, mostly producing trout, with about eighty-five producing salmon and a couple producing carp for Chinese restaurants.

Fish farming has brought prices down, and the more fish eaten in place of higher-fat meats the better, but there could be some risks involved in this form of animal farming. In the wild, trout and salmon are carnivores eating plankton and fish-fly larvae. On fish farms they are given a manufactured diet of pellets made mainly from fishmeal and other animal protein like blood. This is enriched with fish oils to boost the vitamins and energy value. Trace elements and synthetic vitamins are also added. Fish meal is made from 'trash' fish, the small bony fish that fishermen cannot sell, plus the carcasses of waste fish gutted and filleted at sea which previously would have been made into fish 'flour' for export to Third World countries for use in human food. The additives used in fish feed are preservatives and colouring to make the flesh of the salmon and trout pink (in the same way that dye in hens' feed gives battery eggs a deep yellow yolk). Preservatives are used to prevent the pellets going rancid due to their fish-oil content.

Hormones and drugs

Hormones are used in a form of genetic engineering to produce either all female or sterile fish. This is done because the fish must reach a saleable weight before they reach sexual maturity, when they lose colour and plumpness. Sexless fish also grow better and are less aggressive.

When illness occurs, as it often does in overcrowded fish tanks,

When to Buy Fish

White fish	JAN	FEB	MAR	APR	MAY	JUN	JUL	AUG	SEP	OCT	NOV	DEC	
Brill	X	X	X	X									Usually grilled
Turbot	X	X	X	X	X	X	X	X	X	X	X	X	For a special occasion – steaks are very good with a sauce
Flounder	X	X	X	X					X	X	X	X	Roll the fillets and fill with fruit or veg, then poach
Whiting	X	X	X	X	X	X	X	X	X	X	X	X	Delicate flavour; grill with lemon juice or poach
Halibut	X	X	X	X				X	X	X	X	X	Stands up to casseroles or Mediterranean-style grilling with a robust sauce
Sea bream						X	X	X	X	X	X	X	Pretty pinkish flesh; poach or grill
Bass		X				X	X	X					Poach or grill
Skate	X		X						X	X	X	X	Only the wing is used; suitable for grilling

Oily fish

Red mullet	x x x x	Fill with fennel sprigs and grill or barbecue
Sardine	x x x x x	Another good fish for barbecues or grilling
Grey mullet	x x x x x x x	Delicious baked Caribbean-style with lots of freshly ground black pepper
Smelt	x x x	Simply grill
Carp	x x x x x x x x	*The* fish for Chinese food fans

Fish

antibiotics are used under the direction of a vet. Fish farmers say that indiscriminate use of antibiotics is unlikely because they are very expensive, but the presence of antibiotics in water effluent from fish farms is a cause of anxiety for the water authorities. To prevent fungal disease the trout are treated with a malachite green dye which has an antibacterial effect. The dye shows up in rivers and inland waterways, indicating that fish-farm effluent is present and possibly spreading disease among the natural fish population.

Feeding animal protein to fish to produce more animal protein is, of course, a wasteful exercise – it is estimated that up to 1½ tonnes of fishmeal results in one tonne of trout and research at BP has as yet failed to come up with an alternative feed.

Codes for the organic farming of fish have been drawn up by the Soil Association but as yet there are no guidelines about producing fish without chemicals, nor are there any specified conditions laid down for organic fish husbandry.

Shellfish

These are a good source of protein; they contain cholesterol, but we eat them in relatively small amounts and the type of cholesterol they contain is considered to be less harmful than that in some saturated fat products. Shellfish are also high in minerals, but are rejected by some people because they are scavengers and filter feeders eating a less than delectable diet.

Mussels

The best ones are heavy, with tightly closed shells. Reject any that are broken or open. Scrape the shells well in cold water, then scrub them and pull off the beards. They will open as they cook and need very little cooking. An excellent convenience dish.

Frozen and fresh chilled additive-free recipe dishes are available in *Marks & Spencer*'s and in other supermarkets under the *Starfish* brand name.

Fish

Scallops

These are expensive and they are fiddly to prepare, but they are often sold ready-prepared either in plastic see-through trays or on the shells in fishmongers'. Only a few are needed and there is no waste, so they are really good value for money. A little goes a long way. Delicious with wild and brown rice which adds fibre to the meal.

If you are preparing them yourself hold the shell with the flat side uppermost and slip a long-bladed knife into the saucer-shaped bottom shell, keeping the blade close to the line of the shell, which can now be opened. Remove the 'frilly' matter from the edges and cut away the black bag and the dull feathery gills beneath the orange part. Now wash well under cold running water to remove any grit. To remove the scallop from the shell slip the blade of the knife beneath the scallop.

Oysters

For the connoisseur a fresh oyster service offering delivery to the door is now available should the local fishmonger fail to come up with the goods, but you need to give twenty-four hours' notice and the minimum order is a hundred oysters. The 'shore to door' service is operated by *Starfish* of Ipswich, who rush Pacific oysters from Northern Ireland *Cuan Sea Fisheries*, via Securicor to your door. Starfish Oyster Service (SOS) (0473) 626527.

Frozen oyster recipe dishes from *Cuan Sea Fisheries* are available in supermarkets and food halls and some specialist food stores.

Crabs

Like mussels, crabs should be 'heavy' for their size; reject any light ones that seem small. The fishmonger will loosen the body from the main shell, remove the stomach sack and pull off most of the gills. Then all you have to do is scrape the flesh from the inside of the shell and, using a skewer or crab/lobster pick, remove the white meat from the cracked claws and body area – a hammer and board are needed for this job. A sharp knife will open the body to remove flesh there.

Fish

Prawns

These are most popularly sold frozen and ready peeled. They are glazed with ice-glaze – water – to speed the freezing process, and to prevent them drying out in the freezer or getting freezer burn. This ice-glaze can be an expensive way for the shopper to buy water, so when buying prepacked frozen peeled prawns chose a variety that states the weight as 'defrosted weight', otherwise you may end up with a thawed bowl of water, not prawns. *Starfish* and *Youngs* both state defrosted weight on their frozen peeled prawns.

Smoked fish

There is debate over the health value of smoked fish and some people prefer not to eat it because the hydrocarbons found in it have been linked to stomach cancer in Iceland. But it is worth noting that on further investigation this was found to be mainly because of home-smoking – commercially smoked foods have a lower concentration. Interestingly, in Japan, where little smoked food is eaten, the incidence of stomach cancer is very high and has been blamed on salt.

In Britain we eat little smoked food so it is probably a harmless addition to the variety of our diet. If you do like smoked fish here are a few pointers.

Avoid additives

Choose varieties free from additives. Smoked fish can be produced with synthetic colours and by adding synthetic flavourings rather than smoking the fish. The colours and flavours used to do this are among the most noxious of additives. So read the labels and avoid those with added colour and flavour.

Choose traditional products

Finnan haddock is a good choice because this is usually free from added colouring and flavouring. The fish has a pale colour and delicate smoked flavour which comes from the real process.

Arbroath smokies are also traditionally smoked. They are small whole haddock (as opposed to the large opened Finnan haddock);

Fish

they are hot-smoked to a brown colour without the use of additives. Hot-smoked fish are ready to eat.

Smoked trout are usually produced without the addition of colour and flavour, but again check the packet label or ask the fishmonger.

Manx Kippers from the Isle of Man are free from colouring because Manx Kipper Rules 1983 disallow any additives.

Some colours are OK!

More supermarkets are now offering some smoked fish which is free from artificial colours tartarzine, Yellow 2G (107), Sunset Yellow and Brown FK (154). They include *Safeway*, *Waitrose*, *Asda*, *Fine Fare* and *Tesco*.

Natural colours are often used instead by supermarkets, so read the label before disregarding all brightly coloured fish. Annatto and crocin, natural colours, can produce bright yellow fish, and *Marks & Spencer* and *Sainsbury's* use these colours – the labels state if this is the case.

Among the fish processors *Youngs* also use natural colours on their kippers, kippered mackerel and smoked fresh cod, and *Bluecrest*'s smoked haddock fillets do too.

Smoked cod's roe

This is a useful product if you like taramasalata – the Greek dip sold in delicatessens as a pink soapy substance. The real thing can be made at home from smoked cod's roe liquidized or blended with lemon juice, a little butter, margarine or olive oil (or make it fat free), plus some wholemeal breadcrumbs. It is (thankfully) nothing like the shop stuff. Smoked roe is available all the year round and freezes well.

Frozen fish

Although fresh-fish consumption is in decline, the amount of frozen fish we eat has increased by 57 per cent in the last few years. If you buy frozen fish steaks and other products remember to check the packet for additives.

Fish

The majority of frozen recipe dishes contain some additives, especially preservatives, e.g. most *Birds Eye* products; *Marks & Spencer* frozen fish dishes are free from additives, as are some of *Waitrose*'s, *Safeway*'s and *Sainsbury*'s.

Also check the labels for polyphosphates because these chemicals allow water to be added to the product to increase its weight and who wants to buy frozen water when they intend to buy fish? (For a fuller explanation see 'Prawns', p. 240.)

> **My choice**
>
> Fresh fish once or twice a week – or maybe fresh once and shellfish once. If you can only get frozen, avoid the battered and breadcrumbed varieties.

Canned fish

See CANNED FOOD for general information on buying food in cans.

Canned fish has enjoyed increased popularity in recent years at the expense of fresh fish. Consumption has risen by 90 per cent since 1978, with salmon increasing its market share to 52 per cent of the canned fish market and tuna 25 per cent.

Most fish are canned either in oil or in tomato sauce; both contain salt. A recent innovation is fish canned in brine. While this is lower in calories, because no oil is added, it is higher in salt because of the brine, so it becomes a question of your particular health priority as to which you choose – if any.

The oil used will not be fish oil; it is usually described on the can either as edible oil or vegetable oil if there is a choice, vegetable oil sounds the best as it is more likely to contain at least some polyunsaturated fats, unless it is 'hydrogenated' vegetable oil. The oil can of course be drained off before the fish is eaten.

This table from John West illustrates the difference in calories between fish canned in oil and fish canned in brine (The table does not take into account sodium content.)

Fish

	Average per 100 g			
	Calories	Fat	Protein	Carbo-hydrate
Sardines in brine (drained)	150	8	20	–
Sardines in oil (drained)	197	11.8	22.9	–
Sardines in tomato sauce	196	11.6	17.0	–

One nutritional advantage of canned fish is that the heat process involved softens the bones and makes them edible (e.g. sardines) and this will boost calcium intake as well as that of other minerals. In Japan where dairy produce was not used until recently, calcium deficiency was a problem and much was obtained from sea vegetables and from small smoked fish eaten with the bones.

Which canned fish?

John West produce a wide range of canned fish in all mediums which are free from any artificial additives (apart from their skippers – brisling – which contain 'liquid smoke' for flavour). Now available in brine are tuna chunks, tuna steaks, mackerel steaks, mackerel fillets, pilchards and sardines.

Plumrose have a smaller range but all are either in edible oil or are free from additives.

Berisford's Pink Rainbow Trout is canned in its own natural juices and free from additives. The trout comes from freshwater farms in Scotland.

When buying

- Check the type of oil used.
- See whether the fish is in oil or brine.
- Look for the ingredients of the sauce if the fish is in tomato sauce, etc.; it may contain starches and sugars.
- Check for additives. Skippers have been mentioned already; canned prawns and shrimps seem to attract a liberal use of flavour enhancers like monosodium glutamate.
- Tuna is a popular canned fish and Skipjack is the most common

brand of tuna. *Sainsbury*'s have a range of tuna from Fiji called Yellow Fin. This is a less sociable fish; and is fished with a pole. (Other types of tuna are trawled in nets which also catch dolphin; these are then needlessly slaughtered.)

> **My choice**
>
> Tuna canned in brine; Yellow Fin if you can get it. Canned trout makes a nice change.

FISH PASTES AND SPREADS

By law, fish pastes have to contain a certain percentage of fish: 10 per cent for crab and lobster and smoked salmon, 20 per cent for bloater, kipper and smoked herring, 25 per cent for salmon, buckling and sardine, 40 per cent for smoked roe, pilchard, herring and brisling. Preservatives, antioxidants, colours, emulsifiers, stabilizers, flavourings, sweeteners and miscellaneous additives are permitted in these products.

Shippam's fish pastes and spread have introduced nutritional labelling to point out that their products do not contain artificial additives such as preservatives and colouring and that they are free from lactose (milk sugar). The ingredients for Shippam's Sardine and Tomato Spread, for example, are sardines, tomato purée, other fish, water, rusks, olive oil, salt, sugar, soya-protein products, malt vinegar, natural flavour, yeast extract powder; the minimum fish content is 70 per cent.

FISH-FINGERS

Around £100m worth are sold each year and although the market is growing in value for the food manufacturers, it is declining in nutritional value for the shopper. When fish-fingers first appeared they were around 80 per cent fish – now the average is about 56 per cent, but the government is considering new regulations which will ensure that all fish-fingers contain a standard amount of fish.

The regulations would also, hopefully, result in less use of polyphosphates; these are allowed in fish (and meat) products to retain water and so increase the weight of meat and fish without increasing its nutritional value, thus making shoppers pay for water when they thought they were buying fish.

In the meantime there are also changes going on in some products to remove the synthetic yellow colouring – tartrazine – from the bright yellow breadcrumb coating of fish-fingers. This is one of the additives most troublesome to hyperactive children and in response to consumer pressure, some manufacturers have already removed it.

Findus have introduced a range of cod fish-fingers in wholemeal breadcrumbs using 100 per cent stoneground wholemeal flour; this product is free from colourings.

Safeway, Sainsbury's, Tesco and *Waitrose* have also introduced colouring-free fish-fingers.

Of the frozen food centres, *Lakeland* and *Iceland* have followed suit with additive-free fish-fingers. *McCain Foods* have also introduce an 'all-natural' fish-finger without additives.

> **My choice**
>
> Fresh fish – or home-made fish-fingers using fresh fish. They can be made in batches and frozen. If you do need to buy ready-frozen fingers, choose the ones without additives and with wholemeal crumbs.

FLANS AND QUICHES

If you buy frozen flans and quiches there are two brands that use vegetable margarines and shortenings and wholemeal flour in the pastry.

Dorset Foods have three varieties of unbaked savoury wholemeal flan made with White Flora (a blend of sunflower oil and veg-

Flans and Quiches

etable fat). There are four 5½ oz flans in each box. The flavours available are: Cottage Cheese and Smoked Salmon, Broccoli Cheese and Smoked Bacon, and Farmhouse (with corn, apple, ham and chicken). The range is free from additives, although modified starch is used,

St Nicholas Wholefoods make a range of frozen pastry-based wholefoods, including samosas and Vegetable Pie and Courgette and Soufflé Flan. They are all unbaked and made with St Nicholas 100 per cent wholemeal English flour. The fat used is vegetable shortening and margarine; the flan contains an emulsifier E471 from the margarine and E450(a) in the baking powder. Suitable for vegetarians, but not vegans.

Prewett's make both unsweetened and sweetened wholemeal pastry cases – available from health-food shops.

> **My choice**
>
> Quite frankly, I don't think these frozen flans are ever a hundred per cent successful, but the two mentioned above are better than most and have the advantage of being made from wholemeal pastry.

FLOUR

If we are aiming to increase the amount of fibre in our diet then switching to wholemeal flour is a good move. Not only does it contain more fibre than white flour but it also contains other nutrients too. If we look at the way flour is milled we will see why.

When white flour is milled the outer layers of the grain are removed – this means the bran, including the aleurone layer, which contains a high proportion of the grain's protein and vitamin B_3. The wheatgerm, which contains vitamin E and wheatgerm oil, is also removed, along with the other major B vitamin of grains, B_1. The centre of the grain is then crushed, and trace minerals are lost here too. Wholemeal flour, on the other hand, is made from the whole grain, all of which goes into the flour.

Traditionally, wholemeal flour was made by crushing the grain between two millstones. This gave equal distribution of all the grain contents, so that the wheatgerm oil was spread evenly throughout the flour even when the bran was sieved out. Also, millstones ground the flour slowly and stayed cool, whereas modern roller mills are made of metal and they turn very fast, creating heat, which destroys some of the vitamins. Roller mills shear off the outer layers and crush the endosperm, leaving most of the oil in the flour, rather than spreading it throughout.

Because it is naturally a grey/yellow colour due to the wheatgerm and oils in it, white flour is bleached. After bleaching some of the nutrients will have to be put back by the miller. This has been required by law since 1963 and, despite recent moves, vitamin B_1 and B_3, iron and calcium are put into white flour to bring it up to the nutritional level of 80 per cent extraction flour. These do not have to be declared as listed additives on the label.

> **Extraction Rate**
>
> 100 per cent wholemeal flour contains the whole grain; 81 per cent, contains 81 per cent of the grain, most of the bran having been sieved out; the extraction rate of white flour is around 72 to 74 per cent.

It is still possible to buy wholemeal flour that has been ground by millstones. It will state 'stoneground wholemeal flour' on the bag. The bag will also state whether the flour is plain or self-raising. There will be no additives in wholemeal flour because they are not allowed by law. The nutrients which have to be added to white flour by law do not have to be declared on the label, but any other additives do.

Usually additives are put only in the flours that go to bakers for special jobs such as making biscuits or pastry. Below is a list of the additives allowed in flour. If they are added to the bags of flour you buy in the shops, they will be listed on an ingredients panel.

Flour

Additives permitted in flour – except wholemeal

E170	Calcium carbonate
E300	L-ascorbic acid
E341	triCalcium diorthophosphate
516	Calcium sulphate
920	L-cysteine hydrochloride
924	Potassium bromate
926	Chlorine dioxide
927	Azodicarbonamide
	Alpha-amylases
	Proteinases
	Benzoyl peroxide

Permitted only in white and brown

E150   Caramel

Permitted in flour for the manufacture of biscuits or pastry

E220   Sulphur dioxide
E223   Sodium metabisulphite

Permitted in flour for the manufacture of cake

925   Chlorine

Permitted in flour for the manufacture of biscuits

920   L-cysteine hydrochloride

Permitted in self-raising flour, and in flour for buns and scones

E336	monoPotassium L-(+)-tartrate
E341	Calcium tetrahydrogen diorthophosphate
E450(a)	diSodium dihydrogen diphosphate
500	sodium hydrogen carbonate
541	sodium aluminium phosphate, acidic
575	D-Glucono-1,5-lactone

Wholemeal and brown flour

Whether it is wholemeal, brown or white, most of the flour used in Britain is wheat flour, but there are others as well that can add fibre and variety to your diet and cooking. A rundown on some of the types of flour available and their uses follows:

Wholemeal

Wholemeal flour (100 per cent extraction) contains all the grain – it has the highest fibre content of all the flours. It can be milled by modern roller mills; if it is milled by old-fashioned millstones, it will be labelled 'Stoneground Flour'. Most 100 per cent wholemeal flour is plain flour. Organic wholemeal stoneground flour is sold in health-food shops.

Brown

Brown flours, can be 85–90 per cent extraction rate. Most are labelled 85 per cent flour, although some are called 'brown flour'. The term 'brown flour' legally covers all flours which have a minimum of 0.6 per cent fibre but are not wholemeal flours; 85 per cent extraction flour is usually the product of modern roller mills. It will be lighter in colour than 100 per cent wholemeal because it will have had 15 per cent of the wheat extracted – most of the bran in fact. However there are some stoneground varieties, such as *Allinson's* 85 per cent available (plain and self-raising). Eighty-one per cent extraction flour is again mostly roller milled, but *Allinson's* produce an 81 per cent Farmhouse Flour which is stone ground. This odd percentage was chosen because, by law, as we have seen, vitamins, calcium and iron have to be added to any flour of below 80 per cent extraction rate. To provide a 'white' flour that was unbleached and had nothing added to it, but did not have all the bran of 100 per cent wholemeal flour, 81 per cent extraction flour was developed.

Granary flour

Granary flour is the brand name of a brown flour produced by *Rank Hovis McDougall*; it is based on brown flour to which malted wheat grains have been added. Malted grains are grains which have been moistened, germinated and then roasted. Similar flours containing malted wheat, rye or other grains are available, and are described on their labels as 'malted flours'.

Flour

Hovis

Hovis flour has less fibre than Granary flour, although there is now a Hovis wholemeal flour too.

White flour

White flour has an extraction rate of around 72–74 per cent and has been fortified with vitamins, iron and calcium. 'Strong' flour is flour which is high in gluten, the protein in wheat that gives the flour elastic strength. Strong flour is used for bread-making because it allows the dough to stretch without breaking; pasta and yeasted pastry (e.g. pizza, puff pastry, croissants, etc.) also need a strong flour. Ordinary household flour, plain or self-raising, is more suitable for cakes and biscuits, where you don't want elasticity, but you do want softness. Soft flours may also be described as 'sponge flour' or 'cake flour', etc.

Which to choose?

The most versatile of all the flours is 100 per cent wholemeal flour. It has the highest fibre and the natural nutrient content; it tastes a lot better and performs well. Which brand you choose is a matter of personal preference – whether you like a finely ground wholemeal flour or a coarser one, whether you want a strong flour or a softer flour depending on the jobs you want the flour to perform. You may want an organically produced flour, or you may be happy with the ordinary 'run of the mill . . .'

You can add baking powder (either regular or salt free) to turn it into self-raising flour, adding the exact amount you want – not taking what comes from the miller. You can also sieve out the bran if you don't want so much in a particular recipe and you can double-sieve it if you want it nearer white.

Special-purpose flours

Semolina

Semolina is available in wholemeal forms, which give a richer flavour and colour to dishes. It can be made into milk puddings or added to cakes and biscuits, etc., to produce a short, crisp texture; it cannot be used on its own because it is not high in gluten – it is mainly the starchy endosperm of the flour.

Fine oatmeal

Oat flour, or fine oatmeal, is mostly used for making porridge and for oatcakes and pastry. Up to one third oatmeal can replace ordinary wheat flour in pastry, and it is traditionally the only flour used in oatcakes. (You can make your own by putting porridge oats in the liquidizer or blender to produce a flour.)

Buckwheat

This is made from the small dark grain widely used in eastern Europe. The flour is wholemeal and grey/brown in colour. It makes delicious pancakes and is traditionally used in Brittany where *crêperies* serve Breton *crêpes* made from locally milled *farine de blé noir*. From health-food shops.

Rye

Another east European grain. The flour is not usually wholemeal and is of quite a light extraction. Can be used in breads and crispbreads with wheat flour.

Best buys

There are many brands of flour, and many supermarkets and other stores have own-label wholemeal flours; some of the more interesting and individual flours are given below. They are available in health-food shops or in the area of their production where this is given.

Allinson's produce a range of wholemeal flours and 85 and 81 per cent extraction flours, all stoneground; also self-raising.

Prewett's produce a range of wholemeal and other extraction-rate flours; organic stoneground wholemeal is also available, and self-raising.

Flour

Jordans are family millers; their flours are ground by slow-moving rollers, which minimizes the loss of vitamins. They produce 100 per cent wholemeal and other extraction rates, and self-raising.

Loseley produce 100 per cent and 85 per cent wholemeal flours produced from organically grown grain.

St Nicholas are family millers; stoneground flour (Thanet, Kent).

Doves Farm are family millers; all stoneground and some organically grown flour (Marlborough, Wilts.).

Marriages are family millers; stoneground flours (Chelmsford, Essex).

Pimhill are family millers; organic flours sold loose and prepacked (Shrewsbury).

Rushall Farms produce organic and stoneground flours (Pewsey, Wilts.).

Millers Damsel produce stoneground flours (Isle of Wight).

Fibre in Flour

Flour	Fibre content (g per 100 g)
Wholemeal	9.6
Brown	7.5
Granary	8*
White	3.5
Barley	1
Buckwheat	1.6
Rye	0.5–2.5
Maize/corn	1
Semolina	9.6
Soya	2.5
Oat flour/fine oatmeal	7

*Rank Hovis have no specific figure for Granary flour, but Granary bread contains 6.4 g/100 g and it is estimated that Granary flour would contain about 8 g/100 g.

Nutrients in Flour: Wholemeal and White (per 100 g)

	Wholemeal	White
Fibre (g)	9.6	3.4
Calories	318	350
Potassium (mg)	360	130
Calcium	36	150*
Iron (mg)	4.0	2.2
Zinc (mg)	3.0	0.9
Vitamin B_1 (mg)	0.46	0.31*
Vitamin B_2 (mg)	0.08	0.03
Nicotinic acid	5.6	2.0
Vitamin E (mg)	1.6	trace
Vitamin B_6 (mg)	0.5	0.15
Folic acid (mcg)	57	22
Pantothenic acid (mg)	0.8	0.3
Biotin (mcg)	7	1

*Fortified by law.
Source: McCance and Widdowson, *Composition of Foods*, HMSO.

FRESH FRUIT AND VEGETABLES

See also CANNED FRUIT AND VEGETABLES, DRIED FRUITS, ORGANIC FOOD and FROZEN FOODS.

It's all very well knowing that we should be increasing our intake of fresh fruit and vegetables to up fibre in our diet, but many people complain that fruit and vegetables do not taste like they used to, which is hardly surprising considering that the majority of growers do not have taste high on their list of priorities.

They are more concerned with meeting cosmetic marketing requirements that mean the produce has to be free from blemishes and that it will fit the packaging designed for it and fall within the weight bands laid down for each grade of produce. Its length, breadth, weight and shape are more important than the nutritional or culinary requirements.

By now most people are aware of the campaigns of groups such as Friends of the Earth to alert us to the dangerously high levels of

Fresh Fruit and Vegetables

pesticide residues in our food. The use of pesticides, herbicides, chemical fertilizers and other sprays is necessary to meet the packers and marketing requirements, and produce large crops cheaply.

Shoppers have no real way of knowing what sprays have been used on the produce they are buying or whether they have been – in the case of citrus fruit and others – coated with fungicides or waxes to improve their shelf-life. When I once asked a top executive of a national supermarket chain whether he was happy with the use of these his reply was that he and his family never used the zest of lemons or oranges in cooking or drinks because he knew what went on to them. He used only the green-skinned lemons because at least they would not have been sprayed to encourage them to go bright yellow.

If you buy from a greengrocer you can try to look at the boxes in which the produce is packed, because this often declares what fungicides have been used on the citrus fruits, and some are considered safer than others. For example E233 and 234 (thiabendazole and nisin respectively) are considered safer than E230, E231 and E232 (biphenyl and diphenyl; 2-hydroxybiphenol and orthophenylphenol; sodium biphenyl and sodium orthophenylphenate respectively) which are synthetic benzoates.

With most fruit and vegetables, there is no way of telling what has been used in its production. Rather than dwell on the alarming finds of public-health analyses of produce, which have shown pesticide levels to be way over the top, let's concentrate on what we *can* do as shoppers. It is sometimes possible to find a local supplier of organically grown produce – produce grown without the use of chemical fertilizers or chemical sprays to control pests. Instead, organic fertilizers are used and standards are regulated by an independent body called the Soil Association, which awards its symbol of quality to growers who reach the required standards (shown below). The Farm Verified Organic symbol also indicates organic produce. See ORGANIC FOOD.

An increasing amount of organic produce is now available both from British growers and from the Continent. A complete list is beyond the scope of this book, but Alan Gear, Director of the

Henry Doubleday Research Association, an organic research establishment, has produced a book called *The New Organic Food Guide* published by J. M. Dent. It lists producers or retailers throughout the UK and outlines the basis of organic production and its standards.

There is an organic warehouse in Feltham, Middlesex, called *Organic Farm Foods* which has cash and carry facilities for organic produce. (See ORGANIC FOOD for other addresses.)

I have often been asked whether washing fruit and vegetables will remove the pesticide residues, and as far as I know this is not possible. However, some analyses of cabbage leaves did find that a certain amount of lead was removed from the outer leaves by scrubbing them. There is no procedure that will remove all residues of lead or of the chemicals used in modern farming, but washing and scrubbing, where appropriate, should nevertheless be carried out because it will help to remove some things sprayed directly on to the fruit or vegetables. Boiling may remove some too.

Health hazards and sensitivity to these residues will vary from individual to individual, but there have been no really scientific trials to examine the effect these substances are having. Some are thought to be carcinogenic, and these have been found on a wide variety of fruits and vegetables. Friends of the Earth's Campaign for Pesticide-free Food is based at 377 City Road, London EC1V 1NA, (01-837 0731).

Exotic fruits

What one person calls exotic may of course be everyday to someone else. Exotics are seen as a growth area in the fruit and vegetable market and the trade press has estimated sales will double over the next five years.

At one time avocados were thought of as exotic, but since 1978 they have shown a 152 per cent increase in sales; and mangoes are tipped for the next boom in the £3,000m UK fruit and veg market (1984).

Although aubergines, peppers and courgettes are also now

common or garden vegetables, we still stick to our firm favourites in the fruit line with apples being the most popular followed by oranges and bananas.

FROZEN FOODS

All methods of food preserving will incur some loss, but frozen foods stand up well in the nutrition stakes. Frozen-food manufacturers like to point out that frozen peas are likely to have more vitamins than tired peas on the greengrocer's shelf because they are picked and frozen within hours. They do not undergo long journeys, wilt in the sun and heat, etc.

Contrary to popular belief they are not dyed, either. The fresh green colour comes from the blanching process they undergo before freezing – those who freeze their own will be familiar with this change in colour. The same applies to other frozen fruits and vegetables; unless the ingredients panel states that additives have been used, they will be free from additives. The blanching process inactivates enzymes which would cause a further breakdown in nutrients.

If you buy frozen fruit and vegetables, do read the labels. You will find that most are free from added salt, sugar, etc., unlike most canned products. It is usually only products in sauces and/or fruits in syrups that contain added ingredients and chemical additives.

Frozen foods can bring variety to the diet, especially in winter when frozen raspberries, blackcurrants and other summer fruits are especially welcome for a treat. Vegetables tend to be more everyday foods, and peas and spinach are probably the most useful to have in the freezer.

Organic vegetables

A 10 oz pack of mixed frozen organic vegetables produced by *Sunrise* is sold in health-food shops with freezer sections. The mix varies according to what is seasonal at the time of freezing.

FRUIT
See DRIED FRUITS, CANNED FRUIT AND VEGETABLES, FRESH FRUIT AND VEGETABLES and FROZEN FOODS.

FRUIT BARS
See also CEREAL BARS and SNACK FOODS.

These are often a good bet for a snack because they can be free from added sugar and come in a wide range of flavours. They are based on dried fruit and nuts, and they are soft-textured, weighing around 25–40 g. Honey is a common sweetener and malt is also used. There is a high-fibre content from the fruit and nuts; some also have added bran. The fat content is low.

Shop around for your favourite, but beware of the 'high-energy' bar which may look like a fruit or cereal bar but is a vehicle for 'instant' energy in the form of glucose and other sugars.

There are too many bars to list here, but some of the brand names and companies making fruit bars are mentioned below so you can look out for them. These are made from 'wholefood' ingredients, generally without additives.

Bellis Fruit Bars
Patent Bran Bars
Dekama Foods Fruit Bars
Granose Fruit Bars
Holly Mill Fruit Bars
Neilsons Fruit Bars
Plamil Carob Fruit and Nuts
Prewett's range of eight fruit bars
Real Foods range of bars
Shepherdboy range of fruit bars.

Another snack similar to a fruit bar is the traditional Spanish fig cake now sold in health-food shops. This is just compressed dried figs, sometimes with added almonds or ginger, sold wrapped in 'slices'.

Fruit Bars

Carob

A variety of carob-coated fruit and nut bars and carob-coated nuts, raisins and confectionery is sold in health-food shops. Carob is the natural alternative to chocolate. It is free from caffeine, theobromine and phenylethylamine stimulants and migraine triggers found in chocolate. Carob is naturally sweeter than cocoa and so usually has less sugar in the things made from it. It contains vegetable fats rather than saturated dairy fats. It is also free of oxalic acid which is found in chocolate and can bind with minerals like zinc and calcium, making them unavailable for the body. A deficiency of these minerals is associated with acne-type problems such as the spots often associated with eating too much chocolate, especially in young people, who have extra requirements for these minerals. However, that does not give *carte blanche* for eating as many carob snacks as you like!

FRUIT DRINKS

See under FRUIT JUICE.

FRUIT JUICE

Orange juice is Britain's favourite fruit juice, and although all the cartons lined up on the shelves and in the chill cabinets look the same there can be quite a big difference between what is actually inside them.

Juice is often labelled 'Pure Juice' or 'Fruit Juice' and is the nearest you will get to fresh juice squeezed from the fruit. There are several categories of fruit juice stipulated by law:

juice squeezed from the fruit, only flesh allowed, no pith or peel
concentrated fruit juice made by evaporating off the water so the juice is reduced by at least 50 per cent
reconstituted juice made from concentrated fruit juice
dried fruit juice, again concentrated, but this time to a powder or granule.

Because all of these different types of product can call themselves 'Pure Fruit Juice' or 'Fruit Juice', you will have to read the label

Fruit Juice

carefully to find out just which of the above you are getting.

There is a big difference between the freshly squeezed juice of oranges and the orange juice made up from concentrates, although some of the more expensive concentrates now contain orange 'cells' to make them more like fresh orange juice. (The cells are the little bits of orange that you find in freshly squeezed juice.) Look out for the words 'Made with Concentrated Orange Juice' on the pack – this indicates that the juice has been reconstituted. The fresh juice products are rare, although *Sainsbury's*, *Tesco* and *Marks & Spencer* do them; the higher price will usually prevent any confusion.

St Ivel has launched a blend of juice made from 51 per cent freshly squeezed juice and 49 per cent concentrates called *St Ivel Real Premium*; available in orange and apple.

Liquid Gold is a juice made from Jaffa oranges and imported from Israel where it is freshly pressed and packed.

The other two types of juice – concentrated fruit juices and dried fruit juices – are easy to distinguish between.

Additives

Up to 15 g (½ oz) of sugar per litre is allowed without it having to be declared on the label. For greater amounts than that the juice must say 'Sweetened' on the label and state the maximum amount of added sugar in grams per litre – up to 40 g per litre may be added as glucose, syrups or fructose.

Orange juice may also contain up to 10 mg per litre of the preservative sulphur dioxide (E220) without it being listed on the ingredients panel.

Natural preservatives are allowed in fruit juice. For example, citric acid (vitamin C) is permitted in orange juice and it may also be used in grape juice, peach nectar, apple juice and pineapple juice. Lactic acid is allowed in apple juice, pear juice and pear nectar, and malic acid is allowed in peach nectar, pear nectar and pineapple juice.

Other additives allowed are sulphur dioxide in grapefruit,

Fruit Juice

apple, pineapple, lemon, lime and grape juices and in juice concentrates. Pineapple juice and juice concentrates may also contain dimethylpolysiloxane at the rate of 10 mg per litre. Benzoic acid and its derivatives are allowed in fruit juices and nectars as a preservative. Watch out for them on the labels. (Sulphur dioxide used in preserving fruit or fruit concentrate need not be listed on the label.)

What the packs can tell you

Most of the fruit juice we buy is either in long-life cartons such as Tetra Pak or Combiblocs or in the shorter shelf-life tall gable packs. I mention the packaging first because it is connected with the way the juice is processed and hence might influence your choice of product.

Tetra Pak contains long-life juice which is packed under aseptic conditions with juice being pumped into a machine that forms the carton blocks as they are filled and sealed. The juice is flash pasteurized and immediately cooled before it is put in the cartons.

Combibloc cartons are pre-formed and flushed with hydrogen peroxide mist. Sterile air blows the mist out (0.1 part per million is the residue of the peroxide). The pasteurized juice is put into the cartons and steam is injected into the area between the juice and the seal to create a partial vacuum.

Gable packs are the type used by local dairies, supermarkets and food stores for their two-week shelf-life juice. The juice is pasteurized after the concentrate has been diluted and it is then put into the containers and stored in chill cabinets.

You will now see why we are talking about packs rather than brands. There are too many brands to mention individually, but looking at the type of packing they all use gives an idea of the content of the juice in each.

All of the juices mentioned above will most likely have been made from concentrates which are diluted with tap water.

Fruit Juice

Fluoride and your fruit juice

Virtually all of the juice we drink is made from imported frozen concentrates which are thawed, diluted and packed here. The juice is diluted with tap water and in fluoridated water areas that means you are getting extra fluoride in your juice. This may sound a good thing to you but there are very serious unanswered health-risk questions about fluoride and not everybody is happy to drink fluoridated water. If you know your local tap water does not contain it then the chances are your fruit juice from the milkman or local dairy will not either, but the juice you buy may have been packed in an area where the water is fluoridated. The other chemicals added to tap water in the area of packing will also end up in your fruit juice.

Juice without fluoride

However, there are some fruit juice concentrates that are diluted using demineralized water or natural spring water. These are imported from the Continent where people are a lot more fussy about the content of fruit juices – in Britain they are a relatively new drink and we do not have the legislation to control them as strictly as on the Continent, where they have been drunk for many years.

Stute fruit juices, for example, are reconstituted with water from 1,000 ft deep artesian wells on the site of the German factory.

Volonté fruit juices, imported from Belgium, are made up with demineralized water.

Vitamin C

Few brands make any claims about vitamin C, although this is particularly relevant to orange juice. The only brands to mention it are those where it is added. It is difficult to make claims about a natural substance like vitamin C because it differs from orange to orange let alone from batch to batch of juice. Pasteurization will

Fruit Juice

destroy some of the vitamin C in most of the orange juices made from concentrates, and once they are opened and oxygen enters more will be lost.

The table below gives the results found when several different types of orange juice were taken to a London analyst to determine vitamin C levels. These results are interesting, as one of the most common reasons for drinking orange juice (apart from liking it) is that it provides vitamin C. (It is a good source of vitamin C, especially when compared with orange squashes and orange drinks.)

	mg per 100 ml
Bottled	37.3
Canned	44.3
Combibloc	30
Frozen concentrates	40.3
Gable pack	30.4
Hypa pack	30.7
Tetra Pak	39.1
Fresh orange	44.1

Canned and frozen concentrates retain most vitamin C but it is lost when the pack is opened. Bottled juices lose more because of exposure to light, and fewer manufacturers are using bottles for juices. Cartons cut out loss from light. The loss is least in the shorter-life gable packs of juice because they have only a two-week shelf-life, and cannot continue to lose vitamin C over many months as long-life products do.

Fruit drinks – don't be confused!

Because fruit drinks are often packed in the same way as fruit juices, either in long-life cartons or in gable packs in chilled cabinets, it is easy to be fooled into buying what looks like a fruit juice but turns out to be a highly sweetened mixture of juice and sugar with, possibly, some additives thrown in as well. If you want to avoid these products, avoid fruit drinks. The key is the word

Fruit Juice

'drink' because it is a sure sign that it will have sugar added. It may still be made with concentrated fruit juice but it could also contain colourings, emulsifiers, flavourings and miscellaneous additives.

Fruit nectars

Again, nectars have added sugar – up to 20 per cent, so they have more than most fruit drinks. They also contain added water and although they may be made from fruit juice (or fruit juice concentrates and fruit purées, etc.) they will have only 25–50 per cent fruit juice in them. The rest is sugar and water. They may also contain the additives allowed in fruit drinks (see above). Citric, malic or lactic acids may be added to nectars.

Fruit syrups

These are relatively new to Britain but will have been known to Continental holiday makers for several years. Fruit syrups are being marketed in Britain on a 'natural' ticket because they are free from colourings and preservatives and so on (which is good news), but they are very high in sugar; although they may be preferable to some fruit squashes, fruit concentrates are even better – these are purely concentrated fruit juices without added sugar and are available in health-food shops. As yet there are no regulations covering these new syrup imports. They are around 60 per cent sugar, although this is, of course diluted when you add water. *Anchor* and *Dauphin* are two brands.

Fruit squash

This is attractive to mums because it is cheap and manufacturers keep the price down because the ingredients are pretty cheap and nutritionally not particularly brilliant. Squash is a concentrate and has to contain in its concentrated form 25 per cent citrus concentrates, but non-citric fruit squash need contain only 10 per cent fruit juice. When the water is added to the squash the fruit

Fruit Juice

content is down to about 2 per cent. Sugar or saccharin is used to sweeten squash drinks and a minimum of 22 lb of sugar to 10 gallons of concentrate is required by law.

There has been a lot of activity in the area of squash drinks recently as manufacturers have tried to meet criticism from hyperactivity groups concerned about links between behaviour problems in children and colouring in their food and drink.

Some squashes now contain more juice. These include *Robinson's Original High Juice* in orange and lemon which contains 40 per cent fruit juice and no artificial colours, flavours or sweeteners, but it still contains sugar and preservatives. The ingredients are: orange juice, sugar, water, oranges, citric acid, preservatives E211, E223, natural flavouring. *Robinson's Special R* is a range of low-sugar drinks in orange and orange and pineapple flavour with 'No tartrazine or similar artificial colour'. The ingredients list reads: water, oranges, glucose syrup (5.9 per cent), pineapple juice, citric acid, acidity regulator (E331), preservatives E202, E223, artificial sweeteners (aspartame, sacharin), stabilizer E466, flavourings, vitamin C, beta carotene.

St Clement's has a similar range of drinks. *Schweppes* have introduced *Rose's High Juice* range which is being reformulated without azo dyes, and a *Low Sugar Orange Kia-Ora*, partially sweetened by aspartame.

Safeway have removed tartrazine E102 and Sunset Yellow E110 from their squash drinks. *Sainsbury's* is also removing them and has a High Juice squash free from artificial colours; *Waitrose* removed tartrazine in 1985.

However, squashes are not a good idea if we want to bring up youngsters without a taste for sweet drinks. Far better to give them diluted orange juice, or buy fruit concentrates which do not have added sweeteners.

Fruit crush

This is a ready-to-drink product containing 5 per cent fruit-juice concentrate. It is sweetened with sugar or saccharin; if sugar is used it contains 4½ lb/10 gallons at a minimum.

Barley water

In its ready-to-drink version it has a minimum of 3 per cent citrus-fruit concentrate so it is not much better than squash and, like squash, it is sweetened with sugar or saccharin to the same degree as crush (above). Barley water before it is diluted has to have a minimum of 15 per cent concentrated fruit juice in it.

'Health drinks'

Many squash or crush drinks are now labelled 'health drink'. The cynical shopper will realize that this is probably not quite what it means! While they may have added vitamin C and possibly some other vitamins, virtually all of them contain additives and sugar. For example, one 'Orange Squash Health Drink' has an ingredients panel that reads: '(after dilution) [notice that they do that so water comes before sugar]: water, sugar, orange juice, citric acid, ascorbic acid, flavouring, preservative E223, E211, natural colour E160(a)'. Perhaps they are promoting the additives as the health-giving factor? Who knows? Whatever is intended you would be better off with straight orange juice.

What to buy

If you want to go one step further (and better) than the fruit juices that are standard to all shops you might be interested in the juices made from organically grown fruit.

Organic juices
Aspall Apple Juice is made from fresh English apples (not imported concentrates or chill-stored apples). The apples are crushed and the juice is pasteurized. The juice is produced at

Fruit Juice

Aspall Cyder House, in Suffolk, where the Chevallier Guild family have been established since 1728. The regular juice is packaged in cartons and blends include apple/blackcurrant and apple/pear. Aspalls also produce a bottled juice made from organically grown apples. Available from health-food shops and selected stores.

Copella Fruit Juices are also made from freshly pressed English fruit, not from concentrates. No sweeteners are added and no artificial additives are used, so the juice is flash pasteurized before being bottled or put in cartons. Vitamin C is added to preserve the juice at the rate of 19 mg/100 ml for apple, 29 mg/100 ml for pear with apple, 49 mg/100 ml for blackcurrant/apple, 9 mg/100 ml for morello cherry/apple. Also available are apple and carrot, apple and strawberry and apple and guava, in 690 ml bottles.

The apples used are mainly Cox's Orange Pippin, blended with other varieties. There is also a Discovery blend. Copella is run by the Peake family, who also bottle *Peake's* Organic Apple Juice made from their own organically grown apples. Available in health-food stores, some restaurants, motorway service stops, etc.

Infinity Foods, the Brighton cooperative health-food shop and wholesaler plus cash and carry, also import Dutch organic juices and sell them under their own label. Varieties include: grape (red and white), pear, apple/pear, apple/blackberry, pear/plum, pear/strawberry, apple/elderberry, apple/red currant.

Sparkling fruit juices

If carbon dioxide has been added to make the fruit juice fizzy, this will be described as 'carbonated' on the label.

Martlet, the health division of Merrydown Wine Company, produce a Pure Sparkling Apple Juice made from English Coxes and Bramleys. It is free from added sugar and artificial additives, and is sold in one-litre bottles.

Kiri is a sparkling apple juice made by Bulmers. It is 100 per cent apple juice with a touch of carbon dioxide and is free from additives. It is available in pubs, hotels, off-licences and high-street shops.

Fruit Juice

Orangina is well known to those who holiday in France, and it is now imported to Britain. It is made from orange concentrates diluted with demineralized water and it contains real orange pulp and juice. It is free from additives, too.

Francère is a range of French sparkling juices in several varieties: red and white grape and apple. They are free from additives and are available in supermarkets.

Appletise is another additive-free sparkling apple juice made with concentrated apple juice and carbon dioxide. It is free from added sugar and preservatives, etc., and is widely available in shops and pubs.

Stassen Sparkling Juices are imported by Leisure Drinks from Belgium; they include unusual blends of apple juice with either strawberry or apricot juice and an apple juice with low-alcohol cider (under 0.3 per cent alcohol).

Other products

Drink 10, despite its name, is free from added sugar. It is a blend of ten fruit juices with added vitamins; it is made by Eckes of West Germany and is sold in brown bottles. Available from health-food shops.

Stute Daily Dozen is a similar mixed-fruit drink with twelve fruit juices and a range of added vitamins and minerals; it is free from artificial additives.

Waitrose have an own-label 10 Fruit Juice Cocktail in a long-life carton and a Fruit Juice Cocktail of apple, orange, grapefruit, pineapple and lemon.

Juice concentrates

These are made by evaporating off the water from the fruit juice and then capturing and returning the aromas and volatile oils. Nothing is added to them and they keep longer than fruit juice because they are a concentrate and need to be diluted to drink. They make a better alternative to squashes and crushes because

Fruit Juice

they are not too sweet and are free from colourings, etc. Some of the brands available are: *Martlet* Concentrated Apple Juice, *Western Isles* Concentrates and *Harmony* Fruit Concentrates. Available from health-food stores in many different varieties, mostly mixtures of apple and other juices.

Culpeper Lime Juice. Culpeper the herbalists produce a natural lime juice free from additives and containing freshly pressed limes. It can be diluted to make a drink or used in cooking, etc.

Vegetable juice

Vegetable juices can be as refreshing as fruit juices and are often useful for convalescents, but you don't have to be ill to have them. They offer a savoury drink to those who do not like sweeter fruit drinks and they can also be useful for slimmers and those who like to undertake naturopathic fasts. They have the advantage of being made from freshly pressed juices and not from concentrates.

Organic vegetable juices

Biotta. These juices are made from organically grown vegetables including beetroot, celery, carrot and potato, and a Vegetable Cocktail and Breakfast Drink. They are imported from Germany by Vessen and are available in health-food shops. They are sold in brown bottles.

Eden is another imported German range of organic vegetable juices. Bottled; available from health-food shops.

Rabenhorst Tomato Juice is a biologically grown bottled juice made from tomatoes (of course!). Biologically grown is a Continental category very similar to organically grown.

Campbells V8 Tomato and Vegetable Juice may be less esoteric than the others, but it is more widely available and is free from additives, though it does contain salt. It is sold in cans and is a blend of tomato, carrot, celery, beetroot, parsley juices, plus salt, lettuce, watercress, spinach and spices. Also sold in handy individual serving Tetra Paks with a straw.

Prewett's Country Blend is a combination of six vegetable juices: tomato, carrot, celery, onion, celeriac, mushroom and spices. It is free from additives and has no added salt, which is a bonus. Available from health-food shops.

Stute Tomato Juice and Vegetable Juice are not made from concentrates, but from fresh juices, and they are free from additives. Available in health-food shops and supermarkets.

Sungold Pure Vegetable Juice is free from additives. It is packed in a long-life carton and contains tomato juice, celery, carrot, beetroot, kale, cucumber, onion, basil, parsley, paprika, lemon, salt, pepper and vitamin C.

> **My choice**
>
> All the above are good buys. If I am feeling extravagant I buy freshly squeezed juice such as Marks & Spencer clementine or Sainsbury's orange. Otherwise Aspall and Copella apple juices and M & S jaffa orange juice, grapefruit juice or mango and apple. Of the others Stute and Volonté are good on taste, and for sparkling juice I prefer Orangina and Appletise or Kiri.

ICE-CREAM
See also SORBETS.

Despite our British weather we love ice-cream and we spend a cool £460 million a year on it. According to Wall's, each of us manages to eat an average of 5.3 l a year. If you think that's a lot of ice-cream the Americans eat 24 l a head, the Australians 19.4 and the Swedes and Danes 10.2 and 8.3 respectively.

With such fiery passions for the cold stuff it seems rather hopeless to point out that it is one of those high-fat, high-sugar foods that we should eat only in moderation and should certainly be cutting down on. But perhaps we should at least look at some of the 'healthier' alternatives.

Because sugar and fat are needed to make ice-cream 'work'

Ice-cream

there can be no fat-free and sugar-free ice-cream, and indeed they must, by law, be present in ice-cream in specified amounts. It contains at least 5 per cent fat and 7½ per cent non-fat milk solids, which means skimmed milk (the non-fatty part of milk), plus sugar and artificial flavours and colours. One of the major ingredients is air – at least half of what you buy is air which is whipped in during the freezing process.

Supermarkets are now producing own-label ice-creams that are free from artificial colours because of the hyperactivity associations of artificial colouring. They have made much noise about reducing the additives in ice-cream, fish-fingers and squash drinks.

The 'healthy' alternatives to ice-cream have had to dream up other names for themselves because they do not contain the dairy products and fat required by law if they are to be called ice-cream. They are shown below.

Nevertheless, ice-cream is lower in calories, etc., than some other favourite puddings, so it is not such a bad choice if you are eating out or are 'obliged' to have a pud, and there is no fresh fruit salad or low-calorie pud available.

		Calories
Ice-cream	Non-dairy	165
(two scoops)	Dairy (5 per cent milk fat)	167
	Ice-cream made with dairy cream (Campaign for Real Ice Cream)	200
Favourite puds	Coffee/brandy soufflé	297
(average	Pineapple/hazelnut pavlova	387
portion)	Chestnut meringue nests	436
	Black Forest gâteau	516

Dairy ice-cream

Only 'dairy ice-cream' has to contain milk fat, although this need not be cream – its can be cheaper butter or butter oil (butter from which the water has been removed). Even if the ice-cream pack says 'contains cream' or 'made with cream' this can be a very small amount – some estimates put it at three teaspoonfuls in a litre block.

Cornish ice-cream

This is a generic name for a more 'buttery' ice-cream than normal – though the buttery taste can come from synthetic flavouring. It doesn't mean that the ice-cream comes from Cornwall or is made with West Country cream.

Non-dairy ice-cream

If the fat is not milk fat, butter or butter oil then the ice-cream becomes 'non-dairy ice-cream' and on the label it will say 'Contains vegetable fat' or 'Contains non-milk fat'. These are usually cheaper fats such as coconut oil and palm or palm-kernel oils, or hydrogenated groundnut, soya or rape-seed oils, which are all high in saturated fats, so vegetable fat does not mean that the ice-cream is made from healthier fats.

Camric ice-cream

This ice-cream carries the Campaign for Real Ice Cream's logo of two cows and an Ice-cream sundae between them, above the motto 'Ice-cream made with dairy cream'. The Milk Marketing Board is behind the campaign. Eight manufacturers use the quality mark, indicating that they add double dairy cream to their ice-cream. At least 10 per cent butter fat, half of which must be English or Welsh double cream, has to be used to qualify. The ice-creams in the scheme are made by *Dayvilles*, *Thayer's*, *Mor-Isis*, *Thorntons*, *Ashfords*, *De Marco*, *Pollards* and *Classic Ices*.

There are several ways of looking at the CAMRIC ice-cream. First, as a move back to the traditional taste of ice-cream – and the flavour is certainly better. Second, it could be seen as a jolly clever ploy by the MMB to get more cream used – our new health consciousness has meant a move to skimmed milk, and expanding butter mountains and cream lakes are a problem to the MMB.

Ice-cream

Third, it reminds us of the presence of cholesterol and saturated fats – though this does not mean that CAMRIC ice-cream has a greater saturated-fat content than other ice-creams. Fourth, it is useful to vegans who will want to choose ices that are free from animal fats.

Alternative ice-creams

There are several ice-creams available that use additive-free recipes and traditional dairy ingredients, and there are also others that are based on soya milk and so free from dairy products and low in fat.

'Healthier' ice-creams

Loseley Ice-no-Cream
The main ingredient is skimmed Jersey milk, plus fruit and raw brown sugar. It has the consistency of dairy ice-cream but less than 0.3 per cent milk fat and is free from artificial flavours and colours, etc.
Flavour: passion fruit.

Milk Ice
Made by *Blackburne & Haynes*, is a skimmed-milk alternative to ice-cream; it is free from artificial flavourings and colourings in all eight flavours except blackcurrant, which contains colouring.
Flavours: blackcurrant, kiwi, mango, grapefruit, papaya, raspberry, toffee and vanilla.

Scrummi Iced Confections
These are made from tofu (soya-bean curd), honey and fruit whipped together to make an 'ice-cream' consistency. They are made by *Vegetarian Feasts*, producers of frozen foods (see READY MEALS).
Flavours: banana and honey, apricot.

Sojal Frozen Desserts
These cannot be called ice-cream because they do not contain cow's milk products. They are made from soya milk sweetened

Ice-cream

with honey, polyunsaturated vegetable oils, natural flavours, soya lecithin and guar gum. They are free from cholesterol and higher in polyunsaturates than ice-cream, with only 100 calories per 100 ml.
Flavours: Light Carob, Light Hazelnut, Light Strawberry, Light Vanilla. Suitable for vegetarians.

Sunrise Soya Milk Ice Dream
Again, free from cow's milk, hence the 'Ice Dream' name. Vanilla flavour Ice Dream is made from soya milk, corn-syrup solids, soya-bean oil, fructose, vanilla, vegetable gums, natural colours; hazelnut is the same except that it uses nuts instead of vanilla. Suitable for vegetarians and vegans.
Flavours: hazelnut, vanilla.

Vive Frozen Desserts
Free from all dairy produce and with an excellent texture and good flavour this is more like 'real ice-cream' than many alternatives. It is made by Allied Food's Ice Cream Company and contains sugar, coconut oil, modified starch, glucose syrup, soya protein isolate, and strawberry purée or cocoa and carob where appropriate for the flavour. Being free from dairy produce, it is also low in cholesterol and saturated fat, only 2.2 g per 100 g (total fat 6–8 g/100 g). The stabilizers used are 'natural' gums (carageenan is one) and the emulsifier is of vegetable origin. Suitable for vegetarians and vegans.
Flavours: chocolate, strawberry, vanilla.

Dayvilles N'Ice Day
Dayvilles, who brought American razzamatazz to high street ice-cream, now have a soya-based ice-cream available through supermarkets and other shops. The following ingredients are common to the range (which comprises strawberry, vanilla, hazelnut and pistachio–almond), but of course the main flavour changes: soya milk, raw cane sugar, corn syrup, vegetable oil (palm), soya protein, natural flavour, natural stabilizers (guar gum and carob gum), lecithin and natural colouring.

Luxury dairy ice-creams

These ice-creams are made with more real cream than most. They are generally additive-free and are made from high-quality ingredients, and although they are higher in cholesterol, they are more satisfying for an occasional treat than many of the cheaper ice-creams.

Loseley Dairy Ice-Cream
This contains 21 per cent Jersey double cream and is sweetened with raw cane sugar. It relies on the natural flavours and colours of the ingredients and is additive-free. The enterprising list of flavours includes: Acacia and Honey, Brazilian Mocha, Country Strawberry, Montezuma Chocolate, Old Fashioned Vanilla, Stem Ginger, and Woodland Hazel.

Wall's
An 'all-natural' range of dairy ice-cream called *Alpine* have been introduced by Wall's; the flavours are vanilla, strawberry and chocolate. The ice-creams contain skimmed milk, double cream, butter, egg yolks and gelatine (making them unsuitable for vegetarians and vegans). They also contain natural flavours in the vanilla and strawberry varieties.

Cricketer St Thomas
This is made on the Cricket St Thomas estate in Somerset, known to viewers of the *To The Manor Born* TV series. There are thirteen flavours in the range, made with double cream, raw cane sugar and natural flavours; some do contain artificial colours.

Blackburne & Haynes
Another range of dairy ice-cream made with full fat Jersey milk and double cream and sweetened with raw cane sugar.

Ice lollies

Although the majority of these are cocktails of colourings and flavourings, there are now some companies producing iced lollies that are based on fruit juices and free from additives.

Lyons Maid Juice Bars
These are made from fruit juice and glucose syrup and are available in grapefruit, orange and pineapple flavours.

Co-op
Co-op Natural Ice Lollies use only natural colours and are free from preservatives. The stabilizers are natural gums and 'safe' additives, and the emulsifiers are too. However, they are still high in sugar and saccharin is used in Strawberry Surprise, Laser Blazer and Little Menace (orange). There is animal fat in Sensation, Strawberry Surprise and Little Menace (milk). All except Little Menace (orange) contain dairy produce which makes that the only one vegans might consider (but it does contain saccharin).

Iceland Frozen Food Centres
Additive-free orange lollies made from fruit juice are available in packs of twelve.

> **My choice**
>
> Of the 'real' ice-creams I think Loseley is the best and their Ice-no-Cream is an excellent alternative. Of the soya varieties, I prefer the Sojal brand. Vive Frozen Desserts are also very good.

IRRADIATION

Irradiation of food has been heralded by the food scientists as the non-chemical answer to food preservatives that we have all been waiting for. This space-age technology may rid us of our worries about the use of preservatives in food, but whether this is a matter for celebration or concern is another matter.

At present irradiation is still illegal in Britain, although practised in several other countries, but it is expected that the government will soon make it legal, especially since the publication in April 1986 of the *Report on the Safety and Wholesomeness of Irradiated Foods* by the Advisory Committee on Irradiated and Novel Foods, set up by the government in 1982, which concluded

Irradiation

that irradiation is safe. Many companies are ready to start irradiating food – they already have the specialist equipment in operation for the few areas where it is legal, sterilizing food for laboratory animals and astronauts, and sterilizing medical equipment.

So what exactly is irradiated food? Food irradiation is carried out by placing the food on a conveyor belt which passes through a special chamber containing highly radioactive cobalt 60. The gamma rays given off by the cobalt 60 irradiate the food, rendering it sterile. The food is usually pre-packed before it enters the chamber. Gamma rays do not make food radioactive because they are a different form of energy from alpha or beta rays – they are not like the radioactive rays of uranium.

Although irradiation does not make the food radioactive, the problem is that it changes the chemical components of the food to make radiolytic products. These are substances that were not present in the food before it was treated. Scientists say that these compounds are also produced during other processes, such as pasteurization, and that the changes are so subtle that it is not possible to detect them.

However minor changes in the chemical composition of food are, they still give rise to concern about the effects on our health, especially about the long-term effects that eating these new chemicals might have. And as well as creating new compounds in the food, some of which we know nothing about, irradiation also destroys some of the vitamins. It is true that pasteurization and sterilization also do this, but because irradiation is proposed for foods we think of as fresh – fruit, vegetables, meat and fish – we are in danger of losing more vitamins from our diet in the very foods that we think of as highest in these things.

The vitamins most likely to be affected are the heat-sensitive B vitamins (thiamin and pyridoxine, riboflavin, niacin and folic acid in particular) and vitamins A, C and E. These are also hit by other forms of food processing, but it is especially worrying if our staple foods such as flour, rice, oats and orange juice – as well as the fresh fruit and veg – are going to be treated, because this will leave the diet even more depleted.

Irradiation

Although food which has been irradiated will appear fresh, it may in fact be several months old, and will have lost the vitamins and enzymes we associate with freshness – the irradiation halts deterioration caused by bacteria and other micro-organisms, but it does not prevent nutritional deterioration.

Food manufacturers are keen to see irradiation introduced – it not only lengthens the shelf-life by making food appear fresh long after it would normally have gone off, it also relieves them of the need to maintain strict hygiene. Public-health inspectors see it as a good way of cutting down on outbreaks of salmonella food poisoning, because irradiation destroys all the spoilage bacteria. This approach also makes it less likely that salmonella infections caused by bad farming practices – potentially the most dangerous – will be tackled or corrected. So if people are not as hygienic as they might be in preparing and handling food, it can be irradiated and the bacteria removed. However, other researchers suggest that food is *more* susceptible to invasion after irradiation, because there are no natural enzymes left in the food to fight off the spoilage bacteria.

We also lack evidence about the long-term effects on our health of eating large amounts of effectively sterilized food. Once the enzymes and 'living' qualities of the food have been destroyed there will certainly be something lacking in our food. This difficult-to-define 'energy' or 'aura' may be regarded as unnecessary by scientists, but the long-term effects are unknown.

The advisory committee's findings

The government's Advisory Committee on Irradiated and Novel Foods has given irradiation the go-ahead on safety grounds. Its main findings were as follows.

Nutrition
The suggested average dose of irradiation 'will not have any special adverse effects' on food's nutritional content, even though the subcommittee admitted that 'much of the literature is incomplete and some reports appear to conflict', and that 'nutritionally

Irradiation

significant losses of polyunsaturated fatty acids can occur in irradiated foods'.

The subcommittee also pointed to losses in vitamin C, and the B vitamins thiamin and folic acid. Vitamin K and vitamin E are also easily destroyed. As potatoes are our main source of vitamin C, and they are a prime target of irradiation (to prevent sprouting), serious losses could occur.

Labelling

Although the panel saw no need to label for 'public-health reasons', because it is convinced of the 'positive benefits for the consumer' of irradiation, it recommended labelling foods as 'irradiated' to emphasize its beneficial effect, and because failure to label would imply 'positive concealment'.

Radioactivity

The National Radiological Protection Board told the panel that there would be some induction of radioactivity in irradiated food, but that 'the amount is extremely low and it is doubtful whether the incidence of radiation could be detected in the majority of irradiated foods'.

Bacteria, etc.

Even though irradiation is designed to kill all microbiological contaminants, because the ionizing radiation leads to chemical changes which kill or inhibit their growth, some organisms will survive and radiation mutation might produce even more dangerous strains.

These comments put in doubt the Advisory Committee's view of the main benefit – a large decrease in food-poisoning, especially from outbreaks of susceptible foods like chicken, meat and shellfish.

Toxicology

Irradiation produces chemical substances not naturally present in the food. These are called radiolytic products (food additives can also do this).

However, the Advisory Committee concluded that 'there are no significant differences between radiolytic products in irradiated food and the products of conventionally processed foods'.

What we should do

As shoppers we must demand that irradiated food be properly labelled if it is introduced. Experts argue that there is no need to label it because

(a) shoppers would not buy it if they saw it had been irradiated;
(b) food that has been sprayed with fungicides or pesticides is not labelled, nor are other methods of 'processing' explained. The answer is, of course, that they are in error for not giving us this information and that it is everyone's right to know what has happened to the food they have to eat. The very least we can expect is freedom of choice.

Irradiation

Irradiation 'works' because it kills all the bacteria and other microorganisms and pathogens that make food go off. In effect it sterilizes food.

Set dosages are proposed for it. They have to be big enough to be effective, but not too much because that would make food taste awful and cause natural fats and oils to go rancid. The bigger the dose of irradiation the more radiolytic products are produced (see text).

JAM, MARMALADE AND SPREADS

Jam is a preserve. It is a way of preserving a glut of fruit by boiling it with sugar. The concentration of sugar makes it impossible for spoilage organisms to live and so the fruit is preserved. When jam was first introduced, the amount of highly concentrated sugary food in the diet was lower than it is today. Although we are

Jam, Marmalade and Spreads

beginning to cut down on our jam again, it is still popular – we eat much more than is good for us.

The laws covering what is allowed in jam have now made provision for jams to contain less sugar and more fruit. So if you want to cut down on the sugar in your food one of these varieties of jam might suit you.

Jams may contain additives and many of the lower-sugar products do so, partly to overcome the problems of setting. Most jams can be made from sulphured fruit (sulphur dioxide is the most commonly used fruit preservative, particularly for retaining colour), and labels will not always tell you this because the sulphur is already in the fruit that the jam-maker buys. Because he does not add it to the fruit during his manufacturing process he does not have to state its presence on the label.

Just what you are getting in the different types of jam is listed below, so you can see which to buy for extra fruit and less sugar.

By law jam must contain 60 per cent added sugar and at least 35 per cent fruit (with some exceptions, listed below), but the total sugars will be higher because of the naturally occurring sugars in the fruit. Most jams are made with white sugar, but any of the following may be used: honey, cane sugar, molasses or brown sugar, fruit sugar, sugar solution, glucose syrup, extra white sugar, dried glucose syrup, dextrose monohydrate or dextrose anhydrous. Some health-food-shop jams use only raw cane sugar. This is still sugar but the products are usually free from additives and taste good!

What's allowed in each type

Jam

Basic ingredients
sweetening agents, fruit pulp, fruit juice, fruit purée
Composition
35 per cent fruit except raspberry and gooseberry – 30 per cent, black-currant, rosehip and quince – 25 per cent, ginger – 15 per cent, cashew apple – 16 per cent, and passion fruit – 6 per cent

Jam, Marmalade and Spreads

60 per cent sugars
Also allowed
sulphur dioxide
preservatives
permitted colouring
apple, rosehip or quince – vanilla, vanilla extract, vanillin, ethyl vanillin
quince jam – citrus peel and pelargonium leaves (as flavour enhancers)
raspberry, strawberry, gooseberry, redcurrant and plum jam – red beetroot juice, citrus fruit juice.

Reduced-sugar jam

If you want less sugar, then a reduced-sugar jam is a possibility but most brands contain artificial additives, sweeteners and preservatives because there is less sugar in the product to preserve it. Gelling agents are also allowed, but are mostly natural.

Basic ingredients
sweetening agents, fruit pulp, fruit juice, fruit purée
Composition
as jam, but 30–55 per cent sugars
Also allowed
sulphur dioxide
preservatives
permitted colouring
artificial sweetening agents
strawberry, raspberry, gooseberry, redcurrant and – plum jam – red beetroot juice.

No-added-sugar 'jam'

This is the 'jam' to choose if you really want to avoid sugar and have the taste of the fruit instead. It is sweetened with concentrated grape (or other) juices and has, in some cases, 100 per cent fruit content with only fruit juice and pectins added. The best varieties are free from additives, and manufacturers usually use grape juice, free from sulphur dioxide, with which to boil the fruit. The first variety made in Britain was *Whole Earth* 'jam', but because there is no category in law for such a product (the definition of jam being that it has to contain 60 per cent sugars) the manufacturer was taken to court and told not to call it jam.

Jam, Marmalade and Spreads

Despite changes in the regulations covering jams since then, there is still no provision for the growing number of products in this area, so there is still no legal definition of the product and some manufacturers who have since brought out similar products have called them no-added-sugar fruit spreads or a similar name.

These products are more expensive than standard jams because fruit is their main ingredient and this is more expensive than sugar, the main ingredient of jam. They also have a shorter shelf-life and must be kept in the fridge after opening. Some of these 'jams' may state that they contain no added sugar but they do contain honey – sugar under another name – so read the ingredients panels, as usual, before buying.

Fruit spread

Basic ingredients
carbohydrate sweetening matter, fruit, fruit pulp or purée
Composition
fruit percentage not specified
sugar content not specified
Also allowed
fruit may be treated with sulphur dioxide (up to 100 mg/kg)
preservatives.

There are not many fruit spreads around. They are made in a similar way to jam by heating together fruit, fruit purée or pulp and sweetener to produce a gelled product. They may be with or without additives and the fruit used can contain sulphur dioxide; other preservatives may also be used.

Preserves or conserves
These words may be used only to describe jam or extra jam.

Extra jam
If you are looking for a standard-type jam, but without additives, then extra jam is suitable. You get more fruit than standard jam but the same amount of sugar. The advantage of extra jam is that fruit treated with sulphur dioxide is not allowed, neither are the

Jam, Marmalade and Spreads

other additives such as preservatives, flavourings, colours, etc., found in many standard jams.

Basic ingredients
sweetening agents, fruit pulp
Composition
45 per cent fruit (except blackcurrants, rosehips and quinces – 35 per cent, ginger – 25 per cent, cashew apples – 23 per cent, passion fruit – 8 per cent, and 60 per cent sugars. (Strictly speaking, sugars in jams are measured by the amount of 'soluble solids' present. This explains the apparent discrepancy in the percentages, since some of the naturally occurring sugars in the fruit will add to the total.)
Also allowed
fruit treated with sulphur dioxide is not allowed, but the regulations allow for up to 10 mk/kg residual sulphur dioxide
apple, rosehip and quince jam – vanilla, vanilla extract, vanillin, ethyl vanillin
quince extra jam – citrus peel and pelargonium leaves
raspberry, strawberry, gooseberry, redcurrant and plum jam – red fruit juice
citrus peel.

Marmalade
Like jam this has to contain 60 per cent sugars, but its citrus fruit content can be lower at only 20 per cent. It must also contain 7.5 per cent citrus peel. The label has to say what type of cut the peel is, e.g. thick or thin.

Basic ingredients
sweetening agents, citrus fruit, pulp, purée, juice, peel, aqueous extract
Composition
20 per cent citrus fruit, 7.5 per cent citrus peel, 60 per cent sugars
Also allowed
fruit treated with sulphur dioxide
permitted colouring
essential oils of citrus fruit

Reduced-sugar marmalade
This contains 30–35 per cent sugars, like reduced sugar jams, and it may also contain other additives.

Jam, Marmalade and Spreads

Basic ingredients
sweetening agents, citrus fruit, pulp, purée, juice, peel, aqueous extract
Also allowed
fruit may be treated with sulphur dioxide
preservatives
permitted colouring
artificial sweetening agents
strawberry, raspberry, gooseberry, redcurrant and plum – red fruit juice and/or beetroot juice.

Jelly

The same basic standards of sugar and fruit content apply to jellies as to jams. They may also contain the same sort of artificial additives.

Basic ingredients
sweetening agents, fruit juice, aqueous extract of fruit
Composition
35 per cent fruit (except blackcurrants, rosehips and quince – 25 per cent, ginger – 15 per cent, cashew apples 16 per cent, passion fruit – 6 per cent) and 60 per cent sugars
Also allowed
fruit extracts may contain sulphur dioxide
permitted colouring
apple, rosehip and quince – vanilla, vanilla extract, vanillin, ethyl vanillin
quince jelly, citrus peel and pelargonium leaves
strawberry, raspberry, gooseberry, redcurrant and plum – red beetroot juice.

UK standard jelly

Basic ingredients
sweetening agents, fruit juice, aqueous extract of fruit derived from fruit, fruit pulp or purée not less than 35 per cent of finished product (except blackcurrants, rosehips and quince – 25 per cent, ginger – 15 per cent, cashew apples – 16 per cent, passion fruit – 6 per cent) and 60 per cent sugars
Also allowed
fruit treated with sulphur dioxide
permitted colourings.

Jam, Marmalade and Spreads

Extra jelly
Basic ingredients
sweetening agents, fruit juice, aqueous extract of fruit
Composition
45 per cent fruit (except blackcurrant, rosehip and quince – 35 per cent, ginger – 25 per cent, cashew apples – 23 per cent, passion fruit – 8 per cent) and 60 per cent sugars
Also allowed
fruit treated with sulphur dioxide is not allowed but regulations allow for sulphur dioxide residue of 10 mg/kg
artificial sweetening agents
apple, rosehip and quince – vanilla, vanilla extract, vanillin, ethyl vanillin
quince extra jelly – citrus peel and pelargonium leaves.

Reduced-sugar jelly
Basic ingredients
sweetening agents, fruit juice, aqueous extract of fruit derived from fruit pulp or purée not less than 35 per cent of finished product (except blackcurrant, rosehip and quince – 25 per cent, ginger – 15 per cent, cashew apples – 16 per cent, passion fruit – 6 per cent)
30–35 per cent sugars
Also allowed
fruit products treated with sulphur dioxide
preservatives
permitted colouring
artificial sweetening agents
strawberry, raspberry, gooseberry, redcurrant, plum – red fruit juice and/or beetroot juice.

Diabetic preserves

The usual requirements for added sugar do not apply with diabetic products and the bulk sweetening agent sorbitol may be used. Fructose or artificial sweeteners are also allowed, but the jam must contain 50 per cent less 'rapidly absorbable carbohydrates' than standard jams. Many of the no-added-sugar jams and reduced sugar jams are suitable for diabetics and they state this on their labels if it is the case.

Jam, Marmalade and Spreads

What to buy

No-added-sugar jams and marmalades

These should be refrigerated after opening and should keep in the fridge for three to four weeks.

Whole Earth (12 oz jar)
The original range of no-added-sugar jams is now available in several varieties: apple, blackcurrant, blueberry, black cherry, Hedgerow, Mixed Berry, raspberry, strawberry. Also orange marmalade. Made from fruit, grape juice and pectin.

Safeway (8 oz jar)
Safeway is the first supermarket to introduce its own range of no-added-sugar jams. The range is sweetened with grape and apple juice and set with pectin. Lemon juice is also added. The range includes: apple, blackcurrant, raspberry, strawberry and orange marmalade.

Country Basket (10 oz jar)
This range is made from grape juice, fruit and pectin and is available in: apple, blackcurrant, blackberry, raspberry, strawberry and orange marmalade.

Nature's Store (10 oz jar)
This range has honey added and it is made from fruit, fruit juices (grape or apple) and pectin. Range of four jams and three marmalades.

Ethos (10 oz jar)
The brand name of Health Stores Wholesalers who supply health-food stores; their no-added-sugar jams are sweetened with concentrated fruit juices and free from additives. Varieties include: apple, blackberry, blackcurrant, raspberry and strawberry, plus orange marmalade.

Meridian (10 oz jar)
Actually called 'all-fruit spreads', these are made with the relevant fruit juice, apple juice concentrate and fruit pectin. Varieties are:

Jam, Marmalade and Spreads

apricot, strawberry, raspberry, blackcurrant, morello cherry, blueberry, black cherry, mixed berry and Seville orange.

Life Cycle (10 oz jar)
This is the own-brand range of the chain of health-food shops; it includes blackberry, strawberry, raspberry, blackcurrant, apricot and marmalade made with oranges. The ingredients are just fruit and fruit pectin.

Saffron Whole Food Company (9 oz jar)
The range is made from fruit, apple juice and pectin, and contains 100 per cent fruit, with more than 3 lb fruit to each 1 lb jam. The range includes strawberry, raspberry, blackcurrant, black cherry, apricot and fine- and course-cut orange marmalade.

> **My choice**
>
> Whole Earth is the original and, I think, still the best, but Country Basket and Saffron have good flavour. Batches vary, so shop around to find the colour, texture and flavour you prefer.

Spreads

Whole Earth (10.5 oz jar)
The range is called *Sweet 'n' Fruity Spreads*, and like Whole Earth jams they have no added sugar, but are twice as sweet, as the jams are sweetened with concentrated apple juice and set with pectin.

The plums used are organic and more of the spreads will be switching to organic fruits in the future. Varieties are: apple, blueberry, strawberry, raspberry, blackcurrant, black cherry, peach, plum, blackberry and Arctic Fruits, plus orange marmalade.

Sunwheel (8 oz jar)
This is a range of pear spreads with no added sugar. Flavours include pear/apple, pear/apricot, pear/strawberry, pear/black cherry.

Robertson's (10 oz jar)
Robertson's Pure Fruit Spreads contain no added sugar. The

Jam, Marmalade and Spreads

ingredients are fruit, concentrated fruit juices and pectin. There are four flavours: apricot, blackcurrant, raspberry and strawberry, plus fine-cut orange marmalade.

Reduced-sugar jams and marmalades
De L'Ora (11.5 oz jar)
This is a range of exotic jams with 40 per cent sugar content, including varieties such as Fruits of the Islands (pineapple, banana and coconut), Fruits of the Forest (raspberry, strawberry and blackberry, elderberry and bilberry) and Kiwi and Peach. The range is certainly fruity, but the products do contain additives, although the colours are natural. There are also two marmalades, Grapefruit with Pineapple and Mediterranean Marmalade, which contain potassium sorbate as preservative, but no added colourings.

Streamline (2 lb tub)
Probably the highest proportion of sugar in any reduced-sugar jam. These have 53 g per 100 g, most others have 40–44 g. Streamline is sold in 2 lb resealable tubs and is imported from Denmark. There are no artificial colourings or flavourings, but there are preservatives E202 (potassium sorbate) and E211 (sodium benzoate), plus citric acid. The jam is set with pectin and is available in apricot, blackcurrant, black cherry, raspberry, strawberry and mixed fruit, plus orange marmalade.

Today's Recipe (12 oz/340 g)
From *Robertson's*, this range contains 40 per cent less sugar than standard jam and includes: apricot, blackcurrant, raspberry, strawberry and orange marmalade. The ingredients are: raspberries (for example), sugar, water, fructose, gelling agent E440(b), E341, DL-malic acid, natural flavouring, preservative E202, colours E122, E124, E110.

Energen (12 oz/340 g)
The *Energen* range uses pectin as a setting agent as well as tartaric acid; the preservative used is E211 (sodium benzoate). The range includes: apricot, blackcurrant, raspberry, strawberry. There is

also an orange marmalade and a lemon marmalade – these are set with pectin and contain E211, plus E220 (sulphur dioxide – another preservative) and orange and lemon oil respectively.

Raw-sugar jams and marmalades

These have been sold in health-food shops for many years and offer jams and marmalades made with raw cane sugars instead of white sugar. They do still, therefore, contain sugar and are the same in that respect as standard shop preserves. However, they are free from additives and have a slightly lower sugar content than standard jams. They also have more of the flavour of home-made, traditional products.

Thursday Cottage is one range of jams and marmalades made with raw cane sugar – they have also introduced reduced-sugar versions. Another is *Delicia*, which uses raw cane and Barbados sugar in its conserves. As these have more fruit than standard jams, they fall into the extra-jam category.

Saffron Whole Food Company is also introducing a range of raw sugar jams made with sugar from Mauritius.

> **My choice**
>
> Where the no-added-sugar varieties are unavailable or not liked, I would opt for Thursday Cottage.

MARGARINE
(and butter)
But see also the separate section on BUTTER.

The first thing to be said about margarine is that it is a fat. By law it must contain at least 80 per cent fat. Exactly the same can be said of butter – it also has at least 80 per cent fat in it. And whether we choose to eat butter or margarine we should use them sparingly. As we have seen, our diet is too high in fat and we would do well to

Margarine

cut our intake to about 2½–3½ oz (70–100 g) a day, which includes the visible fats, like butter and margarine, as well as the invisible fats in meat, milk, cheese, pastry, cakes and biscuits, crisps, etc.

Another thing to be said about butter and margarine is that they both contain virtually the same number of calories – butter is *not* more fattening than margarine. It is only the low-fat spreads which are less fattening, because they contain a lot of water, so if you spread the same amount you are getting fewer calories than you would with butter or margarine.

Some fats are necessary to our health; some are detrimental. Here is an outline of the fats found in margarine and butter:

Saturated fats
These have been linked with heart disease. In the past cholesterol has been singled out and incriminated, but it now seems probable that the total amount of saturated fats has a greater influence on heart disease than cholesterol alone. As far as we know, there is nothing in saturated fats that we need for our health which the body cannot manufacture for itself or get elsewhere in the diet.

Polyunsaturated fats
These are thought to give an element of protection against heart disease and they are essential for health because they contain substances we need from our food and which the body cannot make – the essential fatty acids.

Monounsaturated fats
These can also be described as 'neutral' fats. This is because they seem not to have any particularly beneficial or harmful effect on heart disease. Nevertheless they are still fats and as such are high in calories, contributing to the total fats in the diet.

Trans fatty acids
Also called trans fats, these are substances that result from hydrogenating or hardening vegetable fats. They occur in minute amounts in nature, but in large amounts in processed fats and

foods and are thought to have the same detrimental effects in the body as saturated fats.

Cis linoleic acid
This is one of the essential polyunsaturated fatty acids; it is needed in the body to make prostaglandins. These do many jobs in the body, one of the most important being to stop our blood getting too sticky and help prevent arteriosclerosis. It is the cis, or cis cis, linoleic acids, that are turned into trans fats during the hydrogenation of vegetable fats.

The fats in butter and margarine

Butter is made from cream; as animal fats are saturated, butter is virtually all saturated fat.

Margarine can be high in polyunsaturates, but it can also be high in saturates and trans fats, depending on what it is made from and how it is made. So, to make sure you get the one low in saturates and 'high in polyunsaturates' – look for those words on the packaging.

Hard margarine, such as block margarine, may be made from vegetable oils, but it will have been hydrogenated. The saturated fat content will be very similar to that of butter. If it is not an all-vegetable product it will also contain quite a lot of cholesterol.

Additives

Butter is a 'natural' product without additives, although all, except unsalted butter, contain some salt. Very few contain colouring and if they do the wrapper will say so.

Margarine is a highly refined product; even if it contains all vegetable oils, some will be hardened, or some naturally hard ones will have been used – otherwise the margarine would be liquid in the tub (i.e. oil). Margarine may contain vegetable oils, salts, hydrogenated oils, milk fat (up to one tenth), emulsifiers, stabilizers, antioxidants, colourings and added vitamins. Many of these additives may be 'natural' or naturally derived, but this depends

Margarine

on the brand. Margarines are also fortified with vitamins A and D by law to bring them up to the vitamin value of butter.

Which is best for our health?

Whether you choose to use butter or margarine, the opinion of medical science at the moment is that you should

- Cut down on total fats.
- Make a greater percentage of the fats polyunsaturated. Although official reports such as the COMA report on Diet and Cardiovascular Disease have recommended aiming for a ratio of .45:1 polyunsaturates to saturates, some health experts believe we should go further and recommend 1:1. Other advice, outside of mainstream medicine, has suggested a ratio of 2:1 (making two thirds of the fat we eat polyunsaturated) but this would be very difficult to achieve on a typical British diet. As far as we know only polyunsaturated fats are essential for health – we could get by without saturated fats. (See also pp. 10–12.)

In practical terms, if we are aiming to reduce saturated fats to one half or one third of our fat intake, we can prefer soft margarines which are high in polyunsaturates for general use and possibly save butter for spreading or in the occasional baked treats where it is essential for flavour and cooking characteristics.

Which margarines to buy

Confronted with the rows of margarine tubs in the supermarket it might seem that there is nothing to choose between them except the price and the pattern on the tub. But not all soft margarines are the same (and I am assuming you are going to choose soft margarine because it is more likely to be high in polyunsaturates).

However, the manufacturers don't always tell us the exact level of polyunsaturates in their brands, which would help us make our choice. The listings below will assist you here, and new labelling laws on fats may tighten up the situation and make a

Margarine

manufacturer declare the amount and type of fats in a product (see Chapter 2).

As shoppers we are up against the sophisticated processing that can make soft margarine which looks like the high-in-polyunsaturate margarines but is in fact made from saturated animal fats or from cheaper saturated vegetable fats. We have to look for the products which state that they are 'high in poly-unsaturates', because these will, by law, contain at least 35 per cent fat by weight, with at least 45 per cent of that being polyunsaturated and not more than 25 per cent saturated.

Below are some of the main brands to look out for. Many supermarkets have their own too.

Fatty Acids in Butter

Fatty acids in butter can vary widely from sample to sample, and different sources quote:

Polyunsaturates	2–3%
Saturates	55–63%
Other unsaturates	14–23%.

NOTE: The percentages given are percentages of the total product. The amount of fat in margarine is not less than 80 per cent – the rest is water, etc.

Vitaquell Extra
Polyunsaturates   40–44%
Saturates   20% (maximum)
Monounsaturates   16–20% (varies)

Ingredients: 15–20 per cent cold-pressed sunflower, maize-germ and wheat-germ oils, safflower, palm, palm-kernel oils, water, vegetable lecithin, lemon juice, vitamins A, D and E.

Comments: this is the only range that does not used hydrogenated vegetable oils and it is therefore free from trans fatty acids. Instead of chemically hardening the oils to obtain the right texture they are blended with naturally firm vegetable oils. No salt is added. The range uses the same oils consistently; other brands switch to whatever is cheapest at the time. The emulsifier used is lecithin,

Margarine

which is natural, and the acidity regulator is lemon juice. This margarine is free from animal and dairy products.

Vitasieg
Polyunsaturates   20–30%
Saturates   30–40%
Monounsaturates   30–40%
Ingredients: soya oil, palm oil, coconut oil, water, vegetable lecithin, lemon juice, vitamins A, D and E (natural).
Comments: see Vitaquell Extra. This margarine is specially formulated for cooking.

Vitazell
Polyunsaturates   50% (at least)
Saturates   19% (plus/minus 2%)
Monounsaturates   13% (plus/minus 4%)
Ingredients: safflower oil, sunflower oil, palm oil, palm-kernel oil, coconut oil, plus 15–20% cold-pressed sunflower, wheat-germ and maize-germ oils, water, vegetable lecithin, lemon juice, vitamins A, D and E (natural).
Comments: this is a dietary margarine using a higher proportion of vegetable oils (safflower and sunflower) to achieve an even higher polyunsaturated content. It is also suitable for vegans. For other comments see Vitaquell Extra.

Vitaquell Cuisine
Polyunsaturates   22% (plus/minus 2%)
Saturates   30% (plus/minus 4%)
Monounsaturates   31% (plus/minus 2%)
Ingredients: soya oil, palm oil, rapeseed oil, mustard oil, water, vegetable lecithin, lemon juice, salt, vitamins A, D and E (natural).
Comments: this is specifically for baking. It is cheaper than the spreading Vitaquells and is also firmer – not through hydrogenation, but because of blending techniques.

Vitaquell give the following analyses to illustrate the absence of trans fatty acids in their margarines:

Margarine

Vegetable Margarines – Trans Fatty Acids and Salt Content

	Trans fatty acids (%)	Sodium (mg/100g)
Golden Rose Vegetarian, unsalted	14.1	17.4
Granose Vegetable	14.2	435.9
Prewett's Safflower	12.1	873.8
Prewett's Sunflower	16.2	700.3
Rakusen's New Improved Vegetable	30.6	765.4
Rakusen's Pure Vegetable	17.8	713.1
Tomor Kosher	13.9	648.1
Vitaquell Extra	under 1	2.4
Vitasieg	under 1	1.8
Vitazell	under 1	2.4

Tests carried out by independent laboratories, October/November 1984.

Prewett's Sunflower Margarine
Polyunsaturates 40% (minimum)
Saturates 17% (maximum)
Monounsaturates 21%
Cholesterol no more than 10 mg/100 g
Ingredients: natural sunflower oil, natural vegetable oil, hydrogenated vegetable oil, water, salt, emulsifier (monoglyceride), natural colour (beta carotene), antioxidant, alpha tocopherol (vitamin E), natural flavour, vitamins A and D.
Comments: Prewett's use natural vitamin E as an antioxidant and monoglyceride as a natural emulsifier. The product is free from animal products.

Prewett's Safflower Margarine
Polyunsaturates 44% (minimum)
Saturates 14% (maximum)
Monounsaturates 20%
Cholesterol not more than 10 mg/100 g
Ingredients: natural safflower oil, natural vegetable oil, hydrogenated vegetable oil, water, salt, emulsifier (monoglyceride),

Margarine

natural colour (beta carotene), antioxidant, alpha tocopherol (vitamin E), natural flavour, vitamins A and D.
Comments: see Prewett's Sunflower Margarine.

Flora
Polyunsaturates   42%
Saturates   13%
Monounsaturates   25%
Ingredients: sunflower oil, other partially hydrogenated vegetable oils (i.e. soya, rapeseed), whey, salt, emulsifiers E471, E322, colour E160(a), E100, flavouring, vitamins A and D.
Comments: Flora is high in polyunsaturates and the oils used are subject to variation. Salt is added and hydrogenated vegetable oils are used. Whey solids are also used so the product is not suitable for strict vegetarians or for those on a milk-free diet.

Gold Cup Sunflower Margarine
Polyunsaturates   40.3%
Saturates   20%
Monounsaturates   20%
Ingredients: sunflower oil, hydrogenated vegetable oil, vegetable oil, whey, salt, whey solids, emulsifiers E471, E322, flavouring, vitamin A, colour E160(a), vitamin D.
Comments: this margarine is from Merseyside Foods, the makers of many own-brand labels of margarine. It uses 'natural' additives as colours, emulsifier and flavouring.

Kraft Vitalite
Polyunsaturates   43%
Saturates   13%
Monounsaturates   24%
Ingredients: sunflower oil, hydrogenated vegetable oil, whey, salt, whey solids, emulsifiers E471, E322, flavouring, colour E160(a), vitamins A and D.
Comments: the additives in this margarine are 'natural'. Salt is added, and it also contains milk products, so while it is suitable for vegetarians it is not suitable for vegans. Hydrogenated oils are used, too.

Margarine

Granose Vegetable Margarine (green pack)
Polyunsaturates   45%
Saturates   20%
Monounsaturates   not available
Ingredients: soya-bean oil (minimum 65 per cent), partly hydrogenated vegetable oils, water, salt, emulsifier, soya lecithin (E322), E471, citric acid, vitamins A and D.
Comments: a vegetable margarine high in polyunsaturates that is free from animal products, making it suitable for vegans. Uses 'natural' additives. Granose also do another vegetable margarine, in a red pack; this is based on soya and rapeseed oils, also with vegetable contents, but it contains a sweetener and is lower in polyunsaturates, at 23.4 per cent.

Suma Sunflower Margarine
Polyunsaturates   40%
Saturates   12%
Monounsaturates   30%
Ingredients: sunflower-seed oil, hydrogenated sunflower-seed oil, water, salt, emulsifiers (soya-bean lecithin, mono and di glycerides of vegetable fatty acids), vitamin A (beta carotene), vitamin E, vitamin B_{12}, vitamin D.
Comments: this is a totally non-animal margarine. The makers, a wholefood cooperative, give information on the vegetable origin of the monoglycerides used (see panel, p. 300). It is unusual in containing vitamin B_{12}, which is useful for vegetarians, who run the risk of shortage of this vitamin as it is found mainly in animal foods.

Marks & Spencer Sunflower
Polyunsaturates   40%
Saturates   15%
Monounsaturates   24% (plus/minus 1%)
Trans fatty acids 4.4%
Ingredients: sunflower oil, hydrogenated sunflower oil, reconstituted dried whey, salt, dried whey, emulsifiers E471, 492, colours E100, E160(b), flavouring, vitamins A and D.
Comments: this margarine is high in dairy content, which means

Margarine

it is unsuitable for vegans and those on a milk-free diet. However, the additives are all 'natural' ones.

Safeway Soft Margarine
Polyunsaturates   41–44%
Saturates   16–20%
Monounsaturates   19–23%
Trans fatty acids 3–7%
Ingredients: sunflower oil, vegetable oil, hydrogenated vegetable oil, water, salt, whey, sugar, emulsifier E471, lecithin E322, colour E160(a), flavouring, citric acid E330, vitamins A and D.
Comments: another margarine containing whey; the additives are 'natural'.

Sainsbury's Sunflower Margarine
Polyunsaturates   41%
Saturates   14%
Monounsaturates   25%
Ingredients: sunflower oil, hydrogenated vegetable oils, vegetable oil, reconstituted whey powder, salt, emulsifiers E322, E471, citric acid, lactic acid, flavouring, colour E160(a), vitamins A and D.
Comments: natural additives; contains milk products. Sainsbury's do a similar soya margarine, but the polyunsaturates content is only 30 per cent.

Waitrose Sunflower Soft
Polyunsaturates   44%
Saturates   18%
Monounsaturates   21%
Trans fatty acids 3–6%
Ingredients: sunflower oil, vegetable oil (sometimes soya), water, salt, whey, sugar, emulsifier E471, lecithin, colour (beta carotene), flavouring, citric acid, vitamins A and D.
Comments: this is the highest polyunsaturate in the Waitrose range of own-label margarines; it uses natural additives, but it does contain added sugar.

Where to buy

Of the above margarines some are available only in health-food shops: Granose, Prewett's, Suma and Vitaquell.

Blue Band is a margarine from Kraft; it has a guarantee that it is free from artificial additives, the only ones used being from naturally occurring materials. Consequently it is often recommended for the allergic or hyperactive. However, it is not high in polyunsaturates (containing 20 per cent) and the total unsaturated fat is 57 per cent. It is a vegetable-oil product. (Other margarines previously listed are also free from artificial additives.)

Salt-free margarine

Vitaquell and *Vitazell* are both free from added salt; they are listed in the main section.
Safeway's Sunflower Margarine is also available as a salt-free product; it has a 60 per cent level of polyunsaturates, but it does contain additives.
International/Gateway also does a salt-free sunflower margarine.

There are many other common brands of margarine but they have not been included because of their low polyunsaturate and/or high saturated fat content.

Kosher margarine

Tomor is a margarine from Van den Bergh which is free from all animal products. It is a kosher margarine and suitable for vegans. The vegetable oils used may be subject to variation, but they are usually palm, palm kernel, soya bean, rapeseed. The product is very low in polyunsaturates, only 6 per cent, with 31 per cent saturated fats – the rest will be monounsaturates.

Margarine

> **Additives in Margarines**
>
> Many margarines contain the following additives, which are derived from natural substances, or are nature-identical:
> E471 mono and di glycerides of fatty acids
> E322 lecithin.
> Both of these may be of animal or vegetable origin. Few manufacturers state which on the label, but most use vegetable products. Usually the label will simply state E471 or E322, but if, for example, it also says 'soya lecithin' then you will know it is of vegetable origin.
> Other additives often used are natural colourings E160(a), E100, E160(b).

Cooking fats

Soft margarines which are high in polyunsaturates may also be used for cooking, as may vegetable oils; most block margarines are designed specially for cooking, but they are high in saturated fats. One of the Vitaqell range is designed for cooking – see main listing. Generally stick to the polyunsaturates for baking and the vegetable oils for other cooking (and baking, if preferred). Remember that low-fat spreads like Outline and dairy spreads like Gold and Delight! should not be used for cooking because they contain a high percentage of water.

White Flora is intended specifically for cooking; it is 100 per cent vegetable fat and oil without additives. It is unusual among cooking fats in being high in polyunsaturates; it is made from sunflower, soya and rapeseed oils. Being free from animal products it is also useful for vegans and those who wish to avoid dairy products.

Polyunsaturates   46%
Saturates   18%
Monounsaturates   36%

Nut butters

Vegetable suet and nut butters are designed for vegetarian use, but they are hydrogenated and thus saturated. They are free from dairy produce, but they are *not* useful in achieving a change in the ratio of fats we eat.

Animal fats in cooking fat and margarine

Not all margarines are entirely made of vegetable products. There are some that contain fish oils and beef oils. Here is a list of some of the margarines and cooking fats that contain animal fats:

Krona
Krona Silver
Stork S B
Cookeen
White Cap
Spry Crisp 'n Dry Solid Cooking Oil
Summer County
Kraft Special Soft
Kraft Superfine

Low-fat spreads

Although butter and margarine contain the same number of calories and are equally 'fattening', low-fat spreads are lower in calories because the water-in-oil emulsion that makes up all margarines is 'stretched' to include more water and less fat. These spreads do not contain the statutory 80 per cent fat of butter or margarine. Like slimmers' products in general, they seem to attract more additives than standard products; hydrogenated fats are as common as they are in margarines. They contain milk solids, so they are unsuitable for vegans, and in the case of Outline, gelatine which vegetarians will want to avoid.

You might think that they are an expensive way of buying water and that it would be less costly to just spread half the butter or fat that you use at present on your bread or toast. Also, these

Margarine

products are less versatile because they are not suitable for cooking.

Slimmers' Gold

Fat content	39%, of which
saturates	25%
polyunsaturates	50%

Unlike most other low-fat spreads this spread from Merseyside Food Products qualifies as being high in polyunsaturates because 50% of the fat used is polyunsaturated. It is made from a blend of sunflower oils and other vegetable oils.

St Ivel's Gold

Fat content	39%, of which
saturates	27%
polyunsaturates	36%

This was the first low-fat spread, combining buttermilk with vegetable oils before the new generation of dairy spreads was launched (see p. 303). It contains 9 per cent milk protein from the buttermilk. It is not cholesterol-free and neither is it high in polyunsaturates. The ingredients are: skimmed milk, vegetable oil, hydrogenated vegetable oil, buttermilk, caseinates, salt, acidity regulators E325, E331, E339, emulsifier E471, preservative E202, flavouring, vitamins A and D, colour E160(a).

St Ivel's Unsalted Gold

Contains the same fat profile and ingredients as standard Gold, minus the salt and preservatives.

Outline

Fat content	40%, of which
saturates	33%
polyunsaturates	20%

Again this product is half the fat of butter. The ingredients are: water, vegetable oil, hydrogenated vegetable oil, buttermilk, gelatine, salt, E160(b), E471, E202, lactic acid E270, flavourings, vitamins A and D.

Margarine

Dairy spreads

These are products that look like margarine and are packed in the same sort of containers. They also spread straight from the fridge, but the difference is that they are made from cream and/or buttermilk and blended with vegetable oil to give the flavour of butter rather than margarine.

Their cholesterol levels are, on average, 15 per cent of that of butter and they have only half of butter's saturated fat, but they are not high in polyunsaturates.

The Butter Information Council has launched a poster campaign to try to iron out the confusion, with the slogan 'If it isn't called butter, it isn't.'

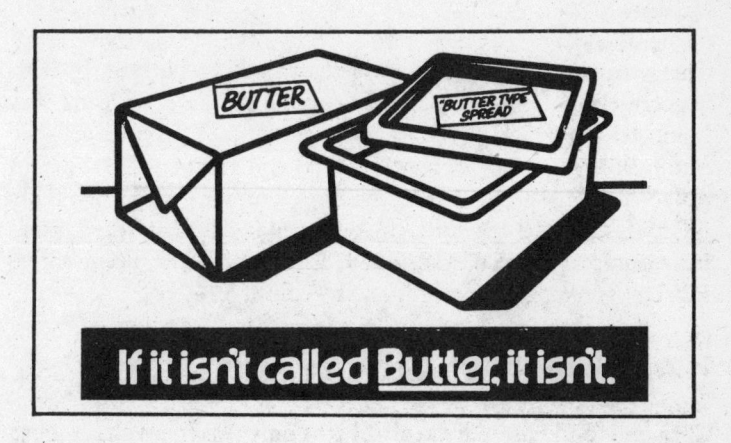

Clover
This is advertised as what butter lovers have been waiting for – butter that spreads from cold. It is made by mixing cream with vegetable oil and hydrogenated vegetable oil, plus salt, E471 and the natural colour E160(a). It will be high in saturated fats because of its cream content and it is high in fat – 75 per cent – with 682 calories per 100 g. It contains 1.7 per cent salt.

Margarine

Golden Churn

In a novelty pot shaped like a milk churn to imply butter, this is spreadable blend of vegetable oil with a minimum of 15 per cent butter. It contains vegetable oil, whey, butter, salt, emulsifier E471, E322, whey solids, flavouring, colour E160(a), (b), E100, and vitamins A and D.

Fats in Spreads (percentages)

	Saturated fat	Polyunsaturated fat	Other unsaturated fats	Water, etc.
Butter (80% total fat)	55	2	23	20
Block margarine (80% total fat)	50	10	20	20
Soft margarine (80% total fat)	25	20	35	20
Margarine high in polyunsaturates (80% total fat)	15	45	20	20
Low-fat spread (40% total fat)	10	10	20	60

Source: *Eating for a Healthy Heart*, JACNE.

MARZIPAN

Christmas and Easter are probably the only two times a year most people buy marzipan – which is a *highly* sugary product. Real marzipan is made with ground almonds and eggs from which it gets its colour. Most commercial marzipan is made from sugar syrups, almond flavouring and colourings. If the marzipan is yellow, be suspicious, because it will almost certainly contain colouring, which may be a synthetic azo-dye-based colouring.

If you do buy marzipan, look for white marzipan, which is made without colouring. *Whitworths* make one which is free from artificial additives and contains sugar, almonds and glucose syrup. *Sainsbury's* also do an own-label white marzipan.

Prewett's make a raw cane sugar marzipan, free from additives and available in health-food shops, as do *Ethos* health products.

> **My choice**
>
> I prefer the raw sugar varieties for their better colour and flavour.

MAYONNAISE, SALAD DRESSINGS

With the growing interest in healthier eating and the permanent interest some people have in losing weight, salads are on the menu more and more often – but are there any healthy salad dressings to go with them?

Salad dressings are easy enough to make at home with good-quality vegetable oil and good-quality vinegar for vinaigrette style dressings, and natural yoghurt also makes is also a good basis for replacing high-calorie mayonnaise. But what are the chances of buying a healthy salad dressing straight off the shelf?

By law, salad cream and mayonnaise have to contain vegetable oil and egg, so that makes life difficult for vegans, for a start. These two ingredients are also high in fats and most products don't say what type of oil they have used. Presumably, as no claims are being made about the high quality or the polyunsaturates they contain, they are poorer quality oils and probably high in saturated fats.

Many salad dressings also contain added sugar and salt and are made with cheap vinegar – to say nothing of the additives allowed in salad cream and mayonnaise, which are: antioxidants, colours, emulsifiers, stabilizers, flavourings, preservatives and miscellaneous additives.

Salad dressings for slimmers tend to contain a lot of additives and although the 'real' mayonnaises may be made from all natural ingredients, the emulsion of egg yolks and oil is very high in fat.

So, what do we look for when buying these products? As usual, the number one rule is to read the ingredients panel on the label,

Mayonnaise, Salad Dressings

but, to save you the trouble of ploughing through them all, here is a selection of products that might be of interest.

Real mayonnaise

Products sold under this category tend to be more expensive and the typical ingredients are: vegetable oil, egg yolk (or dried egg yolk), vinegar (spirit or lemon juice), sugar (and/or glucose syrup), salt, dehydrated lemon juice.

Very often they will be free from additives, but some contain antioxidants such as BHA and BHT. They will be high in fats and almost certainly high in saturated fats. Flavours tend to be much better than the cheaper products. Some real mayonnaises without additives are:

Ratcliffe's Real Mayonnaise
Safeway Real Mayonnaise
Cuisine Real Mayonnaise.

Proper Mayonnaise is made to a classic recipe: oils, fresh egg yolks, wine vinegar and salt and spices. The makers claim to use the best oils (28 per cent olive oil, plus vegetable oils) and make the product in the original chef's manner by whisking the oil into the egg yolk, not using mechanized processes. It is packed in an airtight container with a resealable lid. It is high in fat, but it is free from additives – if this is what you are looking for. Available from delicatessens and health-food shops.

Suma Mayonnaise is made by Suma Wholefoods, a cooperative in Leeds. The ingredients are: sunflower oil, free-range eggs, wine vinegar, real lemon juice, fresh mustard, sea salt and freshly ground black pepper. Available in health-food shops in the north.

Mayonnaise-style dressings

These are not called mayonnaise because they contain no eggs and animal products, making them the answer for the vegetarians or vegans. They are also useful for the rest of us because some of them are free from salt and sugar, and are high in polyunsaturates.

Crosse & Blackwell's Waistline range contains a reduced-oil mayonnaise based on sunflower oil. It does contain whey powder, sugar and modified starch, but the stabilizer is a natural gum and the colour is natural. Not suitable for vegans.

Life Low Sodium Mayonnaise Style Dressing; this is free from added sugar and salt and 'high in polyunsaturates' because half of the oil used is high in polyunsaturates. It is also lower in cholesterol because it is egg-free and has a 50 per cent oil content. The dressing is made by mixing tofu with vegetable oils, cider vinegar, skimmed milk, concentrated apple juice and natural gums, spices and flavourings, plus carotene for colouring (mayonnaise usually gets its colour from the egg yolks). Suitable for vegetarians, but not vegans. Available from health-food shops and chemists.

Prewett's Low Sodium Mayonnaise Style Dressing contains only about 5 per cent of the sodium content of standard brands of mayonnaise and is made entirely without additives and animal ingredients, making it suitable for vegans.

Salad cream

Life Salad Cream Style Dressing. Like the mayonnaise, this is free from additives, sugar and salt, and has the same type of oil content. In addition it is free from eggs, making it suitable for vegans. It contains only 25 per cent oil (50 per cent of which is high in polyunsaturates) which is much lower than regular products.

Prewett's Low Sodium Salad Cream Style Dressing, like the mayonnaise in the same range, has only 5 per cent of the sodium of standard products and is made entirely without animal products and additives, including eggs, making it suitable for vegans.

Both available from health-food shops and chemists.

Salad dressings

This includes the popular range of dressings like Thousand Island, French dressing, blue cheese and vinaigrette dressings. It is dif-

Mayonnaise, Salad Dressings

ficult to find a complete range of products free from additives – French dressings and vinaigrettes are most likely to be free from additives. Or they may contain 'safe' additives such as vegetable gum stabilizers, etc.

For example, *Ratcliffe's* French Dressing and Classic French Dressing fall into this category (although they do contain sugar). *Kraft's* Thousand Isle contains only E405, and their Classic French is free from additives, but both contain added sugar.

Specialist dressings

The *Duchesse* range includes Thousand Island, French dressing and Italian dressing, which are all free from additives and contain a minimum of 50 per cent polyunsaturated oils. They are low in added salt (0.7 per cent) and contain 2–3 per cent added sugar. The French and Italian dressings are suitable for vegetarians and vegans but the Thousand Island dressing is not suitable for vegans.

Martlet Salt Free French Dressing – 90 per cent of the oil is grape-seed oil and 10 per cent is olive oil, so it is high in polyunsaturates and has the flavour of olive-oil dressings. It also contains Martlet cider vinegar and natural herb extracts, plus guar gum as an emulsifier.

Duchesse also has a range that can be used as a dip or a salad dressing. It includes Tofu which is suitable for vegans, and an Avocado and Garlic one, which is suitable for vegetarians. Like other Duchesse products they are 50 per cent polyunsaturated oils and are free from additives. Each contains 0.9 per cent added sea salt and 3 per cent added sugar.

Tofu Soyannaise is a mayonnaise-style dressing made from tofu, cider vinegar, water, soya oil, honey, salt, yeast, guar gum thickener, soya lecithin emulsifier and yeast extract. It is available in health-food shops and has a slightly nutty flavour.

MEAT

More and more people are cutting down on the amount of meat they eat, according to surveys and polls conducted by independent companies and by magazines. The steadily growing number of vegetarians is also a witness to the trend.

There are several reasons: concern about health, concern about animal welfare, concern about our 'right' to eat meat, concern about modern methods of animal husbandry that result in residues of drugs and hormones in meat.

Antibiotics in meat

Although fresh meat may look natural and unadulterated, the animal is likely to have been given hormones and other drugs as a matter of routine. Since the Swann Report in 1969 the use of antibiotics should have come under much stricter control because it was realized then that not only were animal bacteria becoming resistant to antibiotics through over-use in farming, but resistance was also being transferred to bacteria in humans, who would then be at risk when antibiotics were needed in emergency medical situations.

Today the use of antibiotics still causes concern, especially in dairy herds where they are routinely used to combat mastitis, and so find their way into the milk we drink. Antibiotics are also added to the feeds of young animals to promote their growth – if livestock reach their market weight two weeks early then the farmer saves money on two weeks' animal feed. Many animal feedstuffs are labelled with warnings that they should be used only for young animals and not for breeding animals, which indicates that there are drugs and additives in the feed.

Drugs and additives

Antibiotics have a dual role. As well as promoting growth, they, and anti-fungal and anti-parasitic drugs, are used to control disease, which is rife in overcrowded modern farming conditions.

Meat

Additives are also used in animals' feedstuff because in these overcrowded conditions, where the animals do not get sufficient exercise, they lose their appetite and so flavourings and appetite stimulators are used – and appetite suppressants too sometimes. To keep the foods fresh, antioxidants are added, and the highly controversial BHA and BHT are among these. Binders and colourings are also used. Copper is added to pig feed to promote growth, but not for those that will be used as breed stock because it accumulates in the liver and would poison adult stock. Arsenic compounds are also used to promote growth because a short-term increase in weight is the aim; it is claimed that the long term does not matter as the animals will be slaughtered.

Hormones in meat

Hormones and anabolic steroids are used in animal feed to promote growth. They too give cause for concern: there are reports of Puerto Rican children developing secondary sexual characteristics and entering puberty before the age of five and younger, due to hormone residues in poultry. The public in France and Italy has also been vociferous against the use of hormones since baby deaths in Italy in 1980 were linked with hormone residues in veal-based baby foods.

After this tragedy the EEC rushed through legislation in the face of a veal boycott by French housewives. The hormones banned were stilbenes and stilbene derivatives; five others were permitted, three natural and two synthetic. In December 1985 the EEC decided to ban the use of hormones for fattening beef cattle and promoting growth; for a while Britain fought for an exemption for an extra year after the ban becomes law in the other eleven EEC countries, at the start of 1988.

The implant of slow-release hormone pellets, usually behind the animal's ear, is the commonest way of using hormones in controlling weight, size and leanness of the carcass (the ear is easily discarded after slaughter), but even butchers are now backing bans on hormone implants, not because they consider them dangerous but because they recognize shoppers' concern about them and think it is bad for meat sales.

Although nearly four million cattle are slaughtered for meat annually in the UK the Ministry of Agriculture tests only 300 for hormone residues, etc., so many think the ban will be unenforceable.

Organic meat

Winning back meat eaters who have rejected meat because of hormone and drug residues is going to be difficult. In other parts of the EEC there are strong moves to rid meat of hormones, but in Britain, according to bodies like the Consumers' Association, there is too much emphasis on defining the permitted levels of residues in meat and how to measure them, rather than on preventing them getting there in the first place.

Some farmers, however, have returned to more traditional methods to produce what is known as organically reared or organically produced meat, but distribution is uneven; the missing link is an organic meat wholesaler or national distributor. At the moment most farmers sell their livestock to abattoirs, which, by law, must slaughter the animals and then sell them to meat-market wholesalers, large butchers' chains, supermarkets, etc. Some chain stores and butchers' chains also have their own abattoirs and buy direct from the farmers. But until there is an abattoir specifically for organically produced meat, with a central or national distributor, availability will continue to be patchy throughout the country. The following is a basic guide to some suppliers:

Butchers

Wholefood Butchers, Paddington Street, London W1M 4DR (01-935 3924).

F. A. and J. Jones, Red House Farm, North Scarle, Lincolnshire (0522 277 224).

Hockeys Farm Shop, Newton Farm, Sough Gorley, Fordingbridge, Ringwood, Hampshire (0425 52542).

Richardsons, 42 Ashingdon Road, Rochford, Essex (0702 545712).

Meat

Soil Association meat producers
E. W. and J. C. Morrish, East Ackland Farm, Llandley, Barnstaple, Devon (0271 216).
H. Russell-Ross, Petlon Hall Farm, The Parsonage, Stone Street, Boxford, Colchester, Essex (020 636 210258).
A. C. Oakes, Howton House, Winsford, near Minehead, Somerset (064 385 245).

Soil Association butchers
F. A. and J. Jones, address above.
J. A. Hall, Church Farm, Northborough, Peterborough (0733 252224).

Books
The New Organic Food Guide (J. M. Dent) lists organic farmers and growers who produce organic and naturally reared meat.
David Mabey, *Jordan's Real Fool Guide* (Quiller Press), lists suppliers of traditionally cured ham (without nitrites and nitrates) and other 'real' foods.

See also ORGANIC FOODS.

Leaner meat

Apart from the concerns about drugs and farming methods, one of the other major health concerns is that meat is very high in fat. Even lean meat has a high proportion of 'invisible' fat in it (see also Chapter 1); when buying meat look for cuts of meat that are leaner.

Fine Fare, for example, has introduced a range of meat called *Extra Trim* with all visible fat trimmed off and lower-fat cuts of meat such as ground steak, diced beef, sirloin, frying steaks, kebab, etc.

Presto has introduced a similar service with *Supertrim* meat, indicated by the stickers on meat which has been trimmed of excess fat and gristle.

Although these may be more expensive per pound there is no waste from fat or bone, so they are good value. For healthier ways to prepare meat, see Chapter 4.

What Makes Organic Meat Different?

The Soil Association lays down strict rules that farmers must follow if they want to sell their meat as organic or naturally reared under the Soil Association symbol (see ORGANIC FOODS). Many non-symbol holders also follow their guidelines.

Foremost in their code is the rule that farming should be 'based on ethical considerations' that allow the animals to follow their natural behavioural patterns in a natural environment. This rules out cages, tethering and penning (except for a short time), and outlaws 'unsuitable' feeding, growth promoters, hormones and 'other interference with normal growth'.

Animal housing must allow free movement and provide as much natural light and fresh air as possible, and the animals must have access to the outside; permanent housing is against the rules.

Debeaking and fitting of spectacles to poultry, de-tailing and teeth cutting of pigs is outlawed, and castration for pork and bacon animals is not recommended.

Grazing has to be on organic land to Soil Association standards and feed must also be free from growth promoters (including copper for pigs), antibiotics and hormones. Some mineral additives such as rock salt, calcified seaweed, seaweed powder and steamed bone flour are allowed in the short-term as mineral supplements to make up for soil deficiencies. Vitamins should also be of natural origin, such as cod liver oil and yeast.

'Every effort should be made to avoid the use of synthetic amino acids, antioxidants, emulsifiers and chemical colourants that influence the colour of egg yolks.

'Feed containing animal manure is prohibited. Coccidistats and anti-blackhead drugs are allowed in the early stages of poultry rearing but the Soil Association recognizes that further research on this subject is necessary.'

The association recommends herbal and homoeopathic remedies for sick animals, but until research can come up with less harmful drugs it allows, 'for the time being', antibiotics and other drugs, anthelmintics for fluke, lung and gutwork infestation and vaccination with use being declared. Routine use of drugs is not allowed, neither are organo-phosphorus compounds for warble fly.

Meat

Poultry and game

Both poultry and game are recommended for healthier eating because they are lower in fat than other 'muscle' meats (as opposed to organ meats like liver and kidney). More of the fats in game and in free-range chickens are likely to be polyunsaturated, rather than the saturated fats found in confined animals that do not get exercise. Game is also less likely to contain hormone and drug residues.

The British Chicken Information Council says, 'To produce the 450 m chickens we eat every year on a free-range basis would require an area about the size of Wales, so it is not only impractical but would significantly increase the cost of chicken. The majority of free-range producers tend to be small and sell locally in fresh form, since they lack the technology for efficient and hygienic freezing.' However, more free-range poultry is becoming available in the high street (see SUPERMARKETS, table).

Marks & Spencer
M & S sell free-range French chicken. A special slow-growing breed is used and they have access to covered runs. Feed is free from growth promoters and fishmeal; anticoccidials are the one drug allowed.

Moy Park
This Irish-based poultry producer supplies stores in Britain with free-range Poulet Noir birds – a black-feathered strain of French stock with a gamy flavour. They also produce corn-fed chickens, reared on maize which is free from additives.

Frozen poultry

The addition of water to meat products has been criticized because it allows meat producers to sell us water rather than meat. Polyphosphates are used in some frozen poultry, in particular, because they hold water in meat. So when buying frozen poultry (and fish products and fish-fingers) watch out for polyphosphates on the label. There is, however, some control over the amount of water which is allowed to be added. The Poultry Meat (Water

Content) Regulation 1984 limits the amount of water contained in frozen chicken to 7.4 per cent.

Some water is bound to be contained in frozen poultry which is chilled with cold water to lower its temperature; the water is drained off before they are frozen, but some remains are inevitable. Newer methods of freezing mean that chicken do not have to be frozen this way. They can be air-chilled; the name to look out for on the labels is 'chill frozen' or 'dry chilled', which sometimes appears with the rider 'without addition of water either during or after chilling'. The process is apparently costlier than the water method so 'chill-frozen' birds are likely to be more expensive, but you will not be paying for water (unless it states polyphosphates on the label!).

Cooked flavoured chicken

These are often coated with artificially coloured breadcrumbs and the flavourings and colourings used to produce tandoori-style or Italian-flavoured products are often artificial. Pay particular attention to the labels of this type of chicken.

However, *Sun Valley* has introduced an additive-free fresh roast chicken; it is available from major multiples including Carrefour and Waitrose, either as whole chicken or chicken portions.

Lamb

This is often a good choice because the animals are killed young and so hormones are not used and the meat does not have a chance to build up drug residues, the animals wander relatively freely and can exercise so, although it is a fatty meat, the chances are that it is free from some of the disadvantages of other meats.

> **My choice**
>
> When buying meat I choose organic or free-range produce. Of poultry, corn-fed chicken and Poulet Noir have more flavour. Liver is also a good buy, on occasion, and so are leaner cuts of lamb.

MILK

See also BABY FOOD.

When we looked at cheese we were rethinking our approach to it from a high-protein food to a high-fat food. Milk comes into very much the same category.

At one time it was regarded as essential for protein, as milk protein is ranked second to eggs in the scale of usability for the body, and in front of meat, but protein is something we do not go short of in the West and the quantity found in milk is small.

On the other hand fat is something we have too much of and because we use a lot of milk we are increasing our intake of saturated fats through drinking milk rather than increasing our intake of protein. Milk accounts for 19 per cent of the saturated fat in our diet and 14 per cent of all fats. In the UK we drink 12,000 million pints a year (as at July 1986) and of that only 20 per cent is skimmed and semi-skimmed, but this is a huge improvement on the 1 per cent skimmed and semi-skimmed drunk in 1980. Lower-fat milks really took off in 1984, when 1983's 4 per cent trebled to 12 per cent of all liquid milk. The reasons? Health consciousness, price and availability.

You will not lose out nutritionally with lower-fat milk because most of the vitamins and minerals and protein are in the watery part of the milk. All that is missing from these milks is the creamy layer, or top of the milk (and that is saturated fats) and the fat-soluble vitamins A and D, which are found in green and yellow fruit and vegetables or can, in the case of vitamin D, be made by the body when the skin is exposed to sunlight.

The doorstep pinta is unique to Britain and although delivery is convenient, milk in bottles left to sit on the doorstep will have a lower nutritional value than milk in a carton, because up to 80 per cent of the vitamin A and 9 per cent of the vitamin B (riboflavin) can be lost through light-sensitivity. Plastic bottles, though, can be even worse and milk in these containers left under fluorescent lighting in supermarkets may lose up to 14 per cent of its riboflavin in twenty-four hours. Cartons block out destructive light.

Processing milk

Pasteurization

In pasteurization the milk is heated to 72°C and held at that temperature for 15 seconds before being cooled to 5°C and bottled. The aim is to destroy natural spoilage bacteria and make the milk last longer. Pasteurization causes a 10 per cent loss of vitamins B_6, B_{12}, and folic acid (a B vitamin) and 25 per cent of vitamin C. It also alters the folate protein bonds, making folates (folic acid) less usable by the body.

Proteins are also altered or denatured by pasteurization of milk. There are two types of protein, casein and whey; the caseins are resiliant to heat treatment but the whey proteins, which are of a higher nutritional value, are denatured by 10 per cent. Many scientists say this denaturing is harmless to humans, but some people think that the altered milk proteins are more likely to cause allergies among those susceptible.

Bacteria are destroyed by pasteurization, but so are the enzymes and anti-microbial micro-organisms which regulate the bacteria in the milk. Raw milk (unpasteurized) proponents say that post-pasteurized contaminated milk goes off quicker than raw milk because the naturally present enzymes and micro-organisms actually slow down the process of spoilage.

They must alter the milk, because if raw milk is left to go off it will naturally sour into soured cream or cheese, but when pasteurized milk goes off it must be thrown away because it has been colonized purely by spoilage micro-organisms, not by natural bacteria and enzymes – these are destroyed by pasteurization.

Sterilization

Sterilized milk is homogenized, bottled and sealed, and then heated to above boiling point for 10–30 minutes. Sterilized milk has a lower nutritional value than pasteurized and has an un-

Milk

pleasant cooked flavour. Vitamins B_6 and B_{12}, folic acid and vitamin C are all lost in far greater quantities than in pasteurized milk. Because UHT milk and sterilized milk have long shelf-life, they are likely to be even lower in nutritional value, as vitamins are also lost during storage.

Homogenized milk

This process forces the milk (before pasteurization) through a fine aperture to break down the fat globules so that they remain evenly distributed throughout the milk, giving everybody equal shares of the cream from the top of the milk. As far as breakfast arguments go this might be good news, but as far as health goes it is bad news. At least with pasteurized milk you can pour off the top of the milk to lose the fatty layer (though this is not as effective as using skimmed or semi-skimmed milk).

Ultra Heat Treatment

This process heats the milk to 132°C before packing it into sterile containers, so the milk is of poorer quality nutritionally.

Bottle guide

Silver	Pasteurized	Silver top has 3.8 per cent fat and 380 calories per pint.
Red	Homogenized	Red top has 3.8 per cent fat but it has been evenly distributed throughout the milk so there is no creamy layer on top. It has 380 calories per pint.
Blue (Plastic bottle)	Sterilized	Blue top has 3.8 per cent fat and 380 calories per pint, but lower vitamin levels than silver or red top because it is heat treated.
Gold	Channel Island Pasteurized	Channel Island milk comes from Jersey and Guernsey cows and has 4.8 per cent fat and 445 calories per pint. It is very creamy.
Red/silver stripe	Semi-skimmed (may be	Semi-skimmed milk has 1.5–1.8 per cent fat and 263–280 calories per

Milk

	pasteurized, sterilized or UHT)	pint, but it retains all the protein and calcium of silver and red top. Vitamin-content depends on whether it is pasteurized, sterilized or UHT.
Blue/silver check	Skimmed (may be pasteurized, sterilized or UHT)	This has just 0.1 per cent fat (legally it has to be less than 0.3 per cent) and only 195 calories per pint, but retains the calcium and protein and vitamins of silver and red top if it has not been sterilized or ultra-heat treated.
Green top	Untreated/raw unpasteurized	Fat content will depend on the herd, i.e. if it is Jersey/Guernsey it will equal that of gold top, if Friesians or other non-Channel Island it will be the same as silver or red top; ditto calories.

Which is the best choice?

The blue/silver check of skimmed milk is the best choice for most people. The red/silver stripe of semi-skimmed comes next and in third place the green top untreated milk, if it is available. Unfortunately green top is only sold at the farm gate because of prevailing government agricultural preference. It must be from a brucellosis-accredited herd, retains all the natural vitamins and minerals and undergoes no protein-denaturing heat treatments. Fourth choice is silver top.

Forget the rest . . .

> **My choice**
> Skimmed or semi-skimmed fresh pasteurized

Milk in cartons

Milk in cartons generally follows the same colour coding as milk in bottles, but some supermarkets may use their own colours for cartons to designate skimmed and semi-skimmed. Usually

Milk

pasteurized is in blue cartons, skimmed in red and semi-skimmed in green or purple.

Evaporated milk

This has had about half the water evaporated. It is usually homogenized first, before being sterilized in the can, which destroys some of the vitamins, and normal strength evaporated milk usually has no added sugar.

Condensed milk

This is made in a similar way to evaporated, from either full cream or skimmed milk, but it has sugar added to it before being canned and sterilized.

Fermented milk

Yoghurt is the best known of these. See separate entry for YOGHURT, which also includes information about kefir, buttermilk and acidophilus milk.

Alternatives to cow's milk

Goat's milk

This is slightly different in composition to cow's milk and, for many people allergic to cow's milk, goat's is a good alternative. The fat does not rise to the top in a creamy layer because it is naturally homogenized; this makes it easier to digest, but it is higher in fat than cow's milk and the fat is saturated (as is cow's milk) so it has no health advantages in that way. Goat's milk is about 4.5 per cent fat compared with 3.8 per cent for whole cow's milk. Because the fat is homogenized, goat's milk can be frozen successfully and it is sold frozen in many supermarkets. It can also be bought dried and powdered.

If you cannot find goat's milk locally, the British Goat Society at

Rougham, Bury St Edmunds, Suffolk (telephone Beyton 70351), may be able to tell you your nearest stockist.

Sheep's milk
This is now becoming more widely available in health-food shops and supermarkets. Like goat's milk it is often tolerated where cow's milk is not, but it is high in fat, having nearly 6 per cent fat content.

Soya milk
See separate entry for SOYA MILK.

Slimmers' milk

Most of these products are long-life ultra heat treated or sterilized. Trimmilk, Balance and Slimcea are long-life skimmed milks, but Slimcea is also sold fresh. For comments on heat-treated milks, see p. 317.

Shape, from St Ivel, has less than half the fat of whole milk – 1 per cent fat – but more than skimmed milk, which has less than 0.3 per cent. Shape is a mixture of fresh pasteurized skimmed milk, whole milk and dried skimmed milk. It also contains a stabilizer to hold these extra solids in suspension. They are added to give the milk more body and make it taste more like regular milk. It has 45 calories per 100 ml.

Dried milk

Dried skimmed milk is a useful store-cupboard standby; it does not usually contain additives and sugars so it is better to use this, if you don't use fresh milk, in coffee and other hot drinks, than a coffee whitener or creamer, which usually does contain additives and sugar.

There are, however, straight dried skimmed milks and ones that contain additives, so you should read the small print on the plastic bottle or tub. The examples below illustrate the point:

Milk

St Ivel Five Pints: as well as dried skimmed milk, it contains vegetable fat, dried glucose syrup, E471, anti-caking silica, lecithin and vitamins A and D, which all adds up to 270 calories per reconstituted pint.

Marvel is a dried skimmed milk powder which is simply made from skimmed milk with added vitamins A and D, vitamins which are lost when the fat is removed from the milk.

Milquik from St Ivel is another widely available dried skimmed milk powder without any additives.

Dried skimmed milk with vegetable fat

A new category of dried milk, which replaces the old dried skimmed milk with non-milk fat, is labelled 'with vegetable fat'; it is in effect a 'fat-filled' milk which is higher in calories and fat than regular dried skimmed milk powder. Although the fat is not saturated animal fat, it is still fat and is not really a necessary addition to dried milk. Its fat content is about 13 g per reconstituted pint compared with about 1 g in dried skimmed milk. The calories are about 260 per pint compared with 200.

Dried goat's milk

Getting fresh supplies of goat's milk is often difficult and a store-cupboard standby of dried goat's milk is useful. There are several varieties available.

Healtheries is imported from New Zealand. It is checked by the NZ Milk Marketing Board and packed in tins with resealable vacuum lids which keep it fresh for ten weeks after opening.

Dietary Specialities do another spray-dried goat's milk powder which is available in tubs.

Tregaron Foods is a powdered spray-dried goat's milk powder produced from goat herds in Wales and the south-west. It is available in five-sachet cartons; each sachet makes 1 pint.

All these are sold in health-food shops.

Antibiotics in milk

Antibiotics are routinely used on the farm in the treatment of mastitis and they often find their way into the milk we drink. The Milk Marketing Board tests for antibiotics when the milk is delivered, but the tests take so long that the results are received after the milk has been bottled and has gone out to your doorstep. Farmers are paid less for milk which contains antibiotics; greater deductions are made for persistent offences.

The MMB says that the effect of antibiotics will be diluted by the milk being mixed with milk from other farms, but the opposite could also be the case! However, the MMB reports that the average levels in milk are now far lower than they were twenty years ago and the number of farmers failing the test is fewer.

Consumers' associations and committees have recommended that farmers who fail the test should get nothing for their milk, but the MMB has no plans to implement this (which is hardly surprising as they are a body designed to look after the farmers' interests!).

At the moment there are no plans for penalizing farmers who submit milk contaminated with pesticides, and testing for these is done on a far more random basis than for antibiotics. The tests are also much slower and more complicated. The MMB says levels of pesticides in milk are lower than the amounts 'permitted' by the World Health Organization – but they *are* there.

Other contaminants in milk, are radioactive fallout, which is higher in milk from cows near nuclear power stations and re-processing plants, and aflatoxin moulds from mouldy animal foodstuffs (see p. 340).

MINCEMEAT

This is traditionally a dried-fruit and nut preserve made with suet and sugar to give it a long shelf-life, but new versions are now available which are free from saturated animal fats and are also additive-free.

Mincemeat

Prewett's range, sold in health-food shops, is free from artificial additives, but the recipe does contain some fat and sugar. The sugar is raw cane and the other ingredients are: vine fruit, apple, vegetable fat, citrus peel, malt vinegar, nutmeg and cinnamon.

Down to Earth Apricot and Brandy Mincemeat is free from added sugar and salt, and from animal fat and additives. The ingredients are: apricots, organic dates, apple, vine fruits, apple juice, brandy, almonds, mixed peel, spices, natural essences (i.e. lime oil), acetic acid. Because it is free from added sugar and fat it must be stored, after opening, in a fridge. Unlike standard mincemeat it is suitable for vegetarians and vegans and those on a fat-free, kosher or halal diet.

De L'Ora Exotic Mincemeat is free from additives and added sugar, but it does contain honey. The fat used is vegetable and the fruits include a surprising range of exotic fruits. The ingredients are: grape juice and honey, chopped dates, apple and banana, guavas, vegetable fat, lime oil, mixed spices, sultanas, currants and citrus peel.

> **My choice**
>
> De L'Ora is delicious. It's less like mincemeat, but very tasty. Down to Earth is also good, but I find Prewett's too sweet.

NUTS
See SNACK FOODS.

OILS

Oils are produced from a wide range of ingredients – animal and vegetable – which are naturally rich in fat. They must state on the label whether they are of animal or vegetable origin, accompanied by the word 'hydrogenated' if the oil has been hardened. The type of processing ranges from the simple cold pressing of oils to methods employing chemical solvents to liberate the oils.

Cold pressing squeezes the oil from the plant mechanically – unlike the majority of oil-processing methods it does not use heat or chemicals, thus ensuring that little of the oil's natural content of vitamins and minerals is destroyed. Look out for the words 'Cold Pressed' or 'Unrefined' on the label of the bottle. Unless the oil is labelled as such it will have undergone numerous processes such as degumming, neutralizing, washing and drying, bleaching and deodorizing.

Oils with the highest levels of polyunsaturated fatty acids are safflower, sunflower, corn and soya oils. At the other extreme are palm oils and coconut oils, which are highly saturated and go to make up the cheaper blends of oil where the oil used is unspecified.

Between the two extremes is olive oil, which is 'neutral', by which we mean it is composed mainly of monounsaturated fatty acids which, as far as we know, are neither good nor bad for health – they do not seem to contribute to, or help prevent, heart disease. It has been suggested that the use of olive oil in place of animal fats is connected with the relatively low incidence of heart disease in some Mediterranean countries. Olive oil is about 70 per cent monounsaturated fats and 10–15 per cent polyunsaturates, most of which are the beneficial linoleic acids.

It is important to buy a good-quality oil for salad dressings and for cooking, especially if you are aiming to change the ratio of saturated to unsaturated fats in your diet.

For cooking, choose corn, soya, olive, or sesame oil – cold-pressed if possible. These oils are more stable at a high temperature because they have more saturated chemical bonds (i.e. they are lower in polyunsaturated fats). Oils which are less stable may break down when heated to produce free radicals – they may have only a temporary existence, but they have been linked with carcinogenicity. If the oil you use is more stable, it will taste better and last longer, and so will save you money in the long run. If you cook with oil, keep it to a minimum (see Chapter 4 for ways to cut down) and do not be tempted to reuse it. Always discard any oil that has darkened or froths.

For salads, use an oil that is high in polyunsaturates, or olive oil for flavour.

Oils

Unrefined oils (cold-pressed-oils)

These are usually sold at health-food shops and delicatessens; some of the more widely available, and wider ranges, are from:

Sunwheel, who have a range of five natural cold-pressed oils sold in glass bottles, including safflower, corn, sesame, olive and sunflower.

Western Isles oils are also sold in health-food shops. It is a range of unrefined oils which are produced without heat or chemical solvents, including corn, peanut, safflower, sunflower, sesame and soya.

Prewett's have an organic olive oil and *Vitaquell* have an unrefined walnut oil.

There are other brands, too, so look around shops in your area and make use also of supermarket own brands; they are often cheaper for oils such as olive oils.

Olive oil

This is produced in several 'grades' or qualities. The highest grade is 'Virgin Olive Oil', which is the result of the first pressing of the best-quality olives. It is extracted by cold pressing and the oil is dark green or golden; it is not refined. There are several grades of virgin olive oil – 'Superfine' is the best, followed by 'Extra' and then just plain 'Virgin Olive Oil'.

The second pressing uses heat and pressure; the oil obtained from this pressing, and from the third pressing, is mixed with some virgin olive oil to improve it.

Two other terms used are 'Pure Olive Oil', which means the oil is produced from pressing the fruit only, and 'Olive Oil', which can be extracted from the fruit and/or the seed.

Oils high in polyunsaturates

We have mentioned the type of oils that are highest in polyunsaturates (safflower, sunflower, soya, corn) but it is also useful to know some brand names:

Flora sunflower oil is pure sunflower oil and is 66 per cent polyunsaturate, 23 per cent monounsaturated, and 11 per cent saturated.

Spry Crisp'n Dry is a refined vegetable oil made from soya and rapeseed oil: 57 per cent polyunsaturated, 31 per cent monounsaturated and 12 per cent saturated.

Prewett's pure corn oil has added vitamin E which acts as an antioxidant. The oil is 51.6 per cent polyunsaturated, 30.7 per cent monounsaturated and 17.2 per cent saturated. Prewett's sunflower oil is similar, but with a higher polyunsaturate content at 65 per cent; the safflower oil in the range has 75.5 per cent polyunsaturates and the soya oil 59.4 per cent.

Dufrais Pure Grapeseed Oil has a polyunsaturate content that compares well with safflower and sunflower oils at around 70 per cent. It also has a high linoleic acid content. *Martlet* do a grape-seed oil which they blend with 10 per cent olive oil for added flavour and colour.

Blended oils

These are often labelled 'cooking oil', 'salad oil', or 'vegetable oil', and the type of oil used will depend, probably, on what is cheap for the manufacturer at the time of making, which is why specific oils are not mentioned on the label. The oils will be highly refined to ensure consistency between one batch and another, especially as different raw materials may have been used each time. It may be that the polyunsaturate level will be quite respectable if the oil used is high in polyunsaturates, but there is no way of telling. It is probably best to assume that they do not have a high polyunsaturate content or the manufacturer would be shouting about it and

Oils

putting the price up! Better to pay more for a higher-quality oil and to use less of it.

> **My choice**
> I'm hooked on organic olive oil for most culinary jobs.

ORGANIC FOODS

Organic food, either fruit and vegetables, or animal produce, is produced without the use of chemical fertilizers or pesticides, or hormones and antibiotics in the case of animals. But it is not always easy to tell if what you are buying is organically produced and not just labelled 'organic' by an unscrupulous grower or retailer. However, the organizations that set the standards in Britain are in discussion with the Ministry of Agriculture and Trading Standards officials to try to produce a legal definition that can be enforced under the Trades Descriptions Act.

Traditionally the concept of 'organic' encompasses a whole system of agriculture, and when food is described as organic it usually implies that it has been grown using a special system of agriculture. The problem is that Trading Standards officers require something they can check and measure when taking organic food off the shelves in shops. They would like to see a definition based on the absence of all chemical residues such as pesticides, for example, but the Soil Association puts the point that the world is so polluted that it is not possible to guarantee that food is entirely free from chemicals, pesticides, radioactive fall-out, etc. They can only guarantee the method of agriculture.

Who sets the standards?

The overall regulatory body in the UK is the British Organic Standards Committee, (BOSB), which was formed in 1980 with members from the Soil Association and other groups of organic growers and experts. Each of the organizations involved in organics puts its standards before BOSB for approval, which means there are several different symbols and slightly different systems in operation. Below is a guide to the ones to look out for.

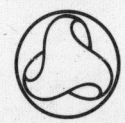

The Soil Association symbol is awarded to farmers, growers and processors of organic foods who conform to the Association's organic standards. These do not allow the use of synthetic fertilizers, pesticides, growth regulators, antibiotics and hormone growth stimulants or intensive livestock systems. They rely on rotation of crops, natural nitrogen fixation, recycled farm manures, manure, biological pest control and ethical livestock systems. A two-year transition period has to elapse from the last chemical crop before Soil Association status can be conferred. The standards is internationally accepted and farms are inspected by the Soil Association.

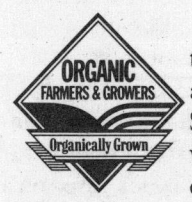

Organic Farmers and Growers is a cooperative set up by former Soil Association member and editor of the Soil Association journal David Stickland. The reason for the new organization was that Mr Stickland felt more needed to be done on the marketing and promotion side of organic food, so he formed the OFG as a cooperative where farmers and growers are on contract to grow for OFG, which markets and sells their produce, OFG sets its own standards, which are virtually the same as the Soil Association. They also organize annual inspection and certification of members. They have a second symbol for farms in the process of changing from chemical to organic growing.

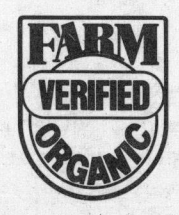

Farm Verified Organic (FVO) was set up in 1979 in America to verify international bulk trade of organic foods between Europe and the USA. In 1986 it was launched at shoppers' level in the UK as a seal to guarantee organic quality food. It does not set organic standards but far-

Organic Foods

mers, growers or processors who become members can use the seal which is licensed to them. They are inspected annually to make sure they are growing to organic standards set by the Soil Association or OFG. A system of lot numbers means the individual ingredients in each bag of muesli, for example, can be traced back (i.e. verified) to the farm on which they were grown, irrespective of country of origin.

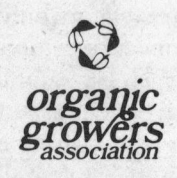

You may see the symbol of the Organic Growers Association on paper bags and biodegradable plastic bags in health-food shops selling fresh organic fruit and veg. It is the symbol of a groups of growers, a trade organization to provide advice on growing methods, marketing, research, etc. They encourage members to grow to Soil Association standards and to apply to become symbol holders.

Members of the Guild of Conservation Food Producers grow to Conservation Grade. The difference between this and organic is that the Guild will allow fertilizer compounds containing ground rock phosphate and rock potash, for example, whereas organic fertilizer is based on a self-sustaining system of mixed farming and crop rotation. Conservation Guild is particularly useful for cereal producers who don't operate a system of rotation or mixed farming which would provide them with manures. For this reason they are allowed to use bought-in manure. Many growers using the system supply W. Jordon Cereals, (makers of Original Crunchy Bars and cereals and flour millers), but dairy produce, meat and poultry are also produced to the standards laid down by the guild, which authorizes the use of its symbol under supervision and inspection.

On some products in health-food shops you may see the Demeter symbol, the symbol of the foods grown by biodynamic methods of agriculture. The symbol is a registered trademark and may be used only by farmers and growers licensed by the Biodynamic Agriculture Association. The method is based on the teachings of Rudolf Steiner, founder of Steiner Schools, and the system applies standards similar to organic standards; they disallow any chemical farming but do allow certain natural composts and biological methods to encourage compost breakdown and fertility. In addition, the system takes into account planetary movements to time planting and harvesting, and claims to be in tune with the universe and satisfy all aspects of human nutrition for body, soul and spirit. There are about ten British symbol holders but most Demeter food is imported.

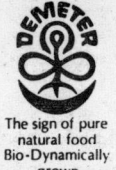

The sign of pure natural food Bio-Dynamically grown

Fruit and veg

Most organic fruit and vegetables is sold through health-food and wholefood shops. Some can be found in supermarkets (see SUPERMARKETS, table).

Organic stockists are listed in *The New Organic Food Guide*, edited by Alan Gear of the Henry Doubleday Research Association and published by J. M. Dent. A copy of the Soil Association's list of approved suppliers can be obtained, on receipt of 50p, from the Soil Association, 86 Colstone Street, Bristol BS1 5BR (telephone 0272 290661).

Frozen vegetables

A pack of mixed frozen organic vegetables produced by *Sunrise* is sold in health-food shops with freezer sections. The mix of vegetables in the 10 oz pack varies according to what is seasonal at the time of freezing – should be called 'surprise', not sunrise!

Organic meat

Organic meat can be found in some local farm shops and butchers'. For addresses, see MEAT.

Organic Foods

Specialist stockists

There are few shops that specialize in organic produce; major ones are:

Wholefood, 24 Paddington Street, London W1M 4DR; this is a wholefood shop with an organic greengrocer and an organic butcher in the same street.

Infinity Foods Cooperative, 25 North Row, Brighton BN1 17A, stocks a complete range of organic foods and is also an organic wholesaler and distributor with a cash-and-carry at 67 Norway Street, Portslade, East Sussex BN1 1YA.

Neal's Yard, Covent Garden, London WC1, where you will find organic fruit and vegetables, plus general produce.

Beehive Restaurant and Shop at 11a Beehive Place, Brixton, London SW9, where fruit and vegetables are sold, plus bread, dairy produce and baby food.

Real Foods, 37 Broughton Street, Edinburgh, stock a wide range of organic foods, but not fresh fruit and veg.

Another source of supply is the Organic Farm Foods cash-and-carry and wholesale-distribution warehouse at Unit C, Hanworth Trading Estate, Hampton Road, West Feltham, Middlesex PW13 6DH.

Your local health-food or wholefood shop will have some organic products.

Why organic?

Organic food exists because many people prefer to eat food that does not contain chemical and drug residues from modern farming techniques. They may prefer the taste, they may think it contains more vitamins and minerals and they may think it more wholesome. They may feel there is an unnecessary risk to health from the methods of modern farming.

The Soil Association originally polarized the aims of organic food production in Britain in the 1940s. Its philosophy was based on the concept that our health depends on the quality of the plant and animal products we eat and the quality of that food depends on the health of the soil.

Organic soil is soil that has no chemical-fertilizer or pesticide residues. Soil that is sprayed with chemicals and nitrogenous fertilizers to the extent that it cannot support life without yet more chemicals being added to it is unhealthy. The plants grown on such soil need chemicals to make them resilient against pests, etc. As the pests become resistant to the chemicals even stronger ones need to be used ... and so that vicious circle goes on, creating pollution and ill health.

The Soil Association, recognizing that the relationship of our health to the soil and the plants growing on it is irrevocably bound up with the future of life on earth, set up experimental growing areas in Suffolk to research sustainable, non-polluting, long-term methods of agriculture. Today they have moved to Bristol to new headquarters shared with the British Organic Farmers and the Organic Growers Association, both created in the 1980s, in order to coordinate their efforts to promote organic growing.

Not only does this method of agriculture hold out hope of a healthier diet, but it also gives protection to wildlife, being non-polluting; protection to the countryside; protection against soil erosion; protection for conservation; and many other advantages too, better explained by experts like Lawrence D. Hills in *Organic Gardening* (Penguin Books).

PASTA

For years pasta has been regarded as fattening, but the high-fibre revolution has now put pasta back where it belongs, as a good food for energy so long as it is a wholemeal pasta that releases the energy slowly, giving us fibre, vitamins and minerals at the same time. A wide range of different pasta shapes and sizes is now available in wholemeal pasta, so it is not difficult to make the switch from white to brown. Green pasta is also a good bet when it is made from spinach to give it the colour rather than just food colouring.

Most health-food chains have their own-label wholemeal pastas, as do the large supermarket chains like Sainsbury's and Waitrose; some of the specialist brands are listed below.

Record Pasta is the big name in wholemeal pasta. To prove the value of slow-release nutrition Record have fed London marathon runners on a meal of wholemeal pasta before the big event (not *just* before they set off, of course). As well as their range of dried spaghetti, macaroni, spirals, shells, etc., made from stoneground flour, they have a convenient, partially cooked wholemeal pasta called Fasta Pasta which cuts down cooking time, particularly for dishes like lasagne. Their Tomato Spaghetti is coloured and flavoured with natural tomato powder and the Verdi Pasta with spinach powder. Natural ingredients are also used in their Natural Spirals, pasta twists in red, green and white.

Euvita is a range of organic wholemeal pasta imported from Holland where it is made from Italian-grown organic durum wheat. Euvita have a complete range of dried pasta, including spaghetti, macaroni, tagliatelle, etc.

Buitoni, the brand leader in the UK dry pasta market, has launched the *Country Harvest* range of pasta made from durum wheat, semolina and added bran. It is not wholemeal, but has the same fibre content and is free from additives.

Wheat pasta is the basis of virtually all the pasta sold in the UK; it is made from durum wheat because it is high in protein, which makes it elastic and easy to work. Buckwheat pasta is more popular in the East (see 'Noodles' below) – one buckwheat range is available from *Sunwheel*, made from 40 per cent or 100 per cent extraction flour.

Fresh pasta

Fresh pasta shops are few and far between but fresh pasta is becoming more easily available through supermarkets, delicatessens and specialist shops. The two main suppliers of fresh pasta are *Pasta Reale* and *Spaghetti House* who pre-pack their fresh pasta in see-through plastic trays. Some varieties are plain, such as tagliatelle; others, like ravioli and tortellini, contain meat or cheese fillings. The cheese fillings are usually ricotta cheese and spinach and some of the fresh pastas are pasta verde (green pasta) made with spinach. They are free from preservatives and most are free from colourings. At the time of writing, Spaghetti House were phasing out all colourings in their pastas.

Pasta Reale are free from additives; they also do three fresh chilled sauces – tomato, mushroom and bolognese.

Try also *Signor Rossi's* fresh pasta products, sold in supermarkets.

Canned pasta

Spaghetti in tomato sauce has now been joined in the *Crosse & Blackwell* range by wholewheat spaghetti, wholewheat rings and wholewheat spirals in tomato sauce. All three are free from additives and have, on average, a 1.4 per cent fibre content. The sauce is based on 30 per cent tomato solids with water, starch, flour, herbs, spices, salt and sugar.

Buitoni have also brought out a wholewheat ravioli canned in a tomato, ham and pepper sauce (not quite wholefood).

The *Heinz Weight Watchers* range is free from added sugar, artificial colour and preservatives, but the pasta is not wholemeal.

For other spaghetti dishes see READY MEALS.

A Note on Quantities

The amount of dry-weight pasta you need for an average serving is only 2 oz (55 g) because it absorbs a lot of water. Fresh pasta packs state the number of servings.

Pasta

Noodles

Noodles were originally made in the Orient where, the story goes, Marco Polo discovered them and took them back to Italy, now the home of pasta. Anyone lucky enough to visit Hong Kong, China or Japan will have seen the noodle-market stalls where a fantastic range of fresh and dry noodles is on sale. They make an excellent snack lunch and a very nutritious one; in a noodle bar they are served with lots of fresh vegetables or some meat. This basic meal has been turned into a British convenience-food version – pot noodles.

A look at the contents of a Golden Wonder Spicy Curry Flavour Pot Noodle will show you what it contains: wheat flour, vegetable oil with antioxidants E320, E321, spicy curry flavour, acidity regulator 262, colourings E102, E110, E124, 154, flavour enhancer 621, artificial sweetener (saccharin), citric acid, maltodextrin, processed soya pieces, salt, peas, carrots ('real' food at last, a hint of the original dish), preservative E220; and a sachet containing curry sauce.

Japanese noodles, called *ramen*, are like a thick twist of noodles or a skein of spaghetti rolled up and folded on itself; they are available in Japanese shops or health-food shops. They are made from wholemeal buckwheat or wheat and are very quick and easy to cook – just like pasta. Chinese egg noodles are also sold in specialist shops and supermarkets, but watch out for additives in these. *Sunwheel* sell some noodles with sauces; these are free from additives and based on Japanese savoury sauces.

> **My choice**
>
> Fresh pasta, with or without sauces, from Pasta Reale and Spaghetti House are very good; for dry pasta, Euvita and Record are also excellent. Japanese buckwheat noodles make a pleasant change. Otherwise, try own brands such as Holland & Barrett's; your supermarket's own brand is often a good buy.

PASTRY

There are now some ready-made frozen wholemeal pastries available.

Loseley, best known for its yoghurts and ice-creams, has a 100 per cent wholemeal frozen shortcrust pastry made with stoneground flour which is organically produced. The pastry is made with vegetable fat and is free from additives.

Jus-rol, the pastry specialists, produce a frozen wholemeal shortcrust pastry made with all-vegetable margarine. It has no additives as such, but the vegetable margarine used in the pastry does contain natural colours and emulsifier E471, plus an antioxidant E321.

Sooner Foods produce an all-vegetable white-flour puff pastry and a white-flour shortcrust pastry, which may be useful for vegetarians. They also produce a ready-made frozen wholemeal pastry.

Viota Bran Pastry Mix is made from white flour with added bran. It is a dry sachet product needing water to mix, and contains vegetable fat, plus the emulsifier E471.

Greenose Frozen Foods supply health-food chain Holland & Barrett with frozen wholemeal puff pastry. The ingredients are wholemeal flour, margarine (containing 'natural' emulsifiers E322, E471), water and salt. It comes in a 13 oz (370 g) pack which makes about twenty vol-au-vent cases or two pie crusts.

Down to Earth produce a frozen wholemeal puff pastry made from 100 per cent wholemeal organic flour, vegetable fat and salt, and on sale in health-food shops.

> **My choice**
>
> I'm lucky enough to be able to make my own wholemeal pastry, but if I broke my arm I would choose Loseley's.

PÂTÉ

The majority of meat pâtés are very high in fat, virtually all of which is saturated fat. They are made from the fattier and lower-quality meats. Pâté is the sort of product that contains reconstituted or mechanically recovered meats; to give them flavour and extend their self-life, flavourings and preservatives such as nitrites are added.

The Meat Regulations state that pâté should have a 70 per cent minimum meat content, but of that 70 per cent only half needs to be lean meat. The result is that more than 65 per cent of the product is fat. No wonder non-meat alternatives are being produced . . . vegetable pâtés have another advantage over meat pâtés – they contain some fibre and most are also free from colours and preservatives. They are available through the health-food trade and from delicatessens.

Cauldron Foods produce two varieties of vegetable pâté, vegetable and mushroom, which are 9 per cent vegetable protein and 12 per cent fat.

Tartex is a Swiss vegetable pâté in cans and tubes, in either Plain or Herb flavours. It is free from additives and is made entirely from vegetable ingredients. *Snack Packs* of vegetable pâté (Mushrooms, Herb, or Pâté with Peppers are the three varieties) are packed in individual portions with wholemeal crackers and a spatula for spreading the pâté. A handy vegetarian snack food.

Leisure Vegetarian Pâté imported by Leisure Drinks – there are three varieties available in ring-pull cans. They are Golden Harvest, Mushroom and Tropical; all are free from additives and animal products.

Spring Hill Vegetable Pâté is made almost entirely from organically produced vegetables and is flavoured with herbs. The pâté is made with cold-pressed vegetable oils, vegetables and yeasts. It is also low in salt.

Devon Country Foods Vegetable Pâté is available in three flavours, Waldorf, Mushroom and Orange and Tomato, made from the main ingredients plus vegetable oil, vegetables, bouillon, nuts, soya protein, modified starch, herbs, spices, flavourings – and the dreaded sodium nitrite E250; shame about that! Available from Waitrose and other stores.

Euvita Olive Pâté is made from organically produced olives and cold-pressed olive oil, plus herbs. Suitable for toast, crackers, canapés, pizzas. Sold by Wholefood of Paddington Street, London.

Other imported varieties are sometimes to be found in delicatessens and food halls . . .

> **My choice**
>
> I love olives, so Euvita Olive Pâté is a favourite of mine. Of the regular pâtés, I like the texture and flavour of the Spring Hill pâté best.

PEANUT BUTTER

Peanut butter is another savoury food that has been 'invaded' by sugar. Most of the larger manufacturers add sugar and also emulsifiers, to prevent the natural oil separating out from the bulk of the product. (In natural peanut butters, which contain just peanuts and salt, this oil can be stirred back into the butter before use without any alteration to the flavour or texture.)

Peanut butter is made by crushing roasted, shelled and skinned peanuts to a smooth crunchy paste, and adding salt (and sugar and other ingredients if they are used). There are no laws governing the composition of peanut butter, but all of them contain more than 90 per cent peanuts.

Peanut butter is a high-protein spread – it is about 25 per cent protein – but remember that it is also high in fat (40–50 per cent) from the naturally occurring oils in their nuts (and any extra oil the manufacturer may add). Most, however, are high in monoun-

Peanut Butter

saturates, and peanut butter is also a good source of B vitamins and fibre. If you eat it on wholemeal bread it will give you extra protein because this is a good combination of two different sorts of vegetable protein (see BAKED BEANS for a fuller explanation).

Aflatoxins

Aflatoxins are toxins produced by moulds that live on the peanuts' skin (and on other nuts and foods), and the government is considering introducing legal limits for levels in peanut butters since food analyses have shown up high residues in some peanut butters. Aflatoxins are carcinogenic, but the government is not naming the offending brands. See also 'Blue Cheese', p. 208, and 'Antibiotics in milk', p. 323.

Buying peanut butter

Before you buy, remember to read the label carefully:

- Is there added sugar?
- Are there added vegetable oils, and if so are they hydrogenated?
- Does it contain additives? E471 is the most commonly used emulsifier in peanut butter and this is a mono- or di-glyceride derived from fatty acids, which may be of either animal or vegetable origin, so unless the label states which, vegetarians and vegans will not know if the product is 'animal-free'.

Natural peanut butters

The following is a selection of the peanut butters which use just peanuts and salt, or have no-added-salt versions.

Whole Earth make Old Fashioned Peanut Butter, which comes either crunchy or fine, and with or without added sea salt. Also available is American Style, with no added sugar, in either Smooth or Crunchy, with added apple juice and palm oil.

Boots Second Nature is free from additives, etc. It has just peanuts and sea salt and is sold in either crunchy or smooth versions.

Peanut Butter

Granose sell a smooth peanut butter and Granose Peanut Crumble, which is a crunchy peanut butter.

Prewett's have a crunchy natural peanut butter.

Sunwheel sell both smooth or crunchy, with or without added sea salt.

> **My choice**
>
> I like the crunchy, no-salt peanut butters from Sunwheel and Whole Earth, and the texture of Granose Peanut Crumble.

Other peanut butters

Gales, smoother or crunchy, is one of the most widely available. It is free from additives, the ingredients being roasted peanuts, hydrogenated vegetable oil, sugar, salt. The hydrogenated vegetable oil acts as emulsifier to stop the ingredients separating out.

Sun-Pat is also widely available, either smooth or crunchy. The ingredients are 90 per cent skinned peanuts, less than 2½ per cent added sugar and less than 1½ per cent salt. The stabilizer used is E471, but Sun-Pat (i.e. Rowntree Mackintosh) are planning to switch to a vegetable-based stabilizer to make their product suitable for vegetarians and vegans – the E471 they use at present is of animal origin.

The *Co-op* have smooth or crunchy peanut butters which use E471 of vegetable origin as an emulsifier. The other ingredients are roasted peanuts, sugar and salt.

Tahini

This is listed with peanut butter because it is a similar savoury spread. It is a paste made by crushing sesame seeds to a thick greyish-brown paste. Some varieties have added salt. Tahini is used to mix with crushed cooked chick peas to make the Middle Eastern hummus. Two good brands, *Harmony* and *Sunwheel*, are

Peanut Butter

available in health-food shops; the *Cypressa* brand is available in supermarkets and delicatessens.

Sunflower spread

This is similar to tahini, but is made from crushed sunflower seeds. It is made by *Sunwheel*, with or without added salt, and sold in health-food shops.

POPCORN
See under SNACK FOODS.

POULTRY
See under MEAT.

PORK PIES
You may have seen claims for 'healthy' pork pies from *Pork Farms*, who produce Floracrust Pork Pie (nothing to do with Flora margarine, but they do use a fat high in PUFAs). This non-additive pork pie contains pork (minimum 30 per cent), wheat flour, sunflower-seed oil, vegetable oil and hydrogenated vegetable oil, water, rusk, salt, gelatine, wheat starch, pepper, pork stock, egg. It's up to you...

PULSES
See also BAKED BEANS.

Pulses are an excellent source of vegetable protein; they are high in fibre and low in fat. I have not listed all the brands because there are too many of them. Virtually all supermarkets have their own brand and so do health-food shops, delicatessens, etc. They do not undergo any unnatural processing – they are just dried pulses.

However, there are organically grown pulses available and two impressive pre-packed ranges come from *Springhill Farm* and from *Real Foods*. Your local health- or wholefood shop will probably also have loose pulses available and these are often cheaper. They also have the benefit of allowing you to buy any quantity.

> **Save Your Teeth . . .**
>
> Remember always to pick them over and wash them well. You do not want to break your teeth, or those of your friends, on any grit and stones which find their way into your dishes. Wash as for rice (see RICE).

Most pulses have to be soaked for some time before cooking, and then cooked for quite a long time. Don't add salt until the cooking is completed. If you have a pressure cooker, this reduces the cooking time considerably; split peas and lentils take less time than most, and lentils need no soaking.

READY MEALS

With two out of three women under sixty working and an increasing number of single-parent families, there is a growing demand for quick and easy convenience meals. Birds Eye estimate that the frozen-meal market is now worth £225 m. Other estimates define ready meals as those which need nothing adding (Birds Eye products usually need vegetables adding) and put the value nearer £75 m.

So we are spending a lot of money on these meals, but are they all good news? *The Egon Ronay Guide Lucas 1986* is ecstatic about 'the revolutionary trend', 'their excellence and convenience may put a growing number of people off cooking, except as a hobby'. After tasting 300 meals from nine supermarket chains they gave *Marks & Spencer* top marks, followed by *Sainsbury's* and *Waitrose*, then *Tesco* and *Safeway*.

Marks & Spencer pioneered the first 'recipe dishes', as they prefer to call them, in the 1960s and since then have built up a

Ready Meals

range of about forty dishes which changes quite regularly. The sophisticated chilled production and transport system means that food can be delivered fresh rather than frozen, so M & S do not have to use as many additives as other food manufacturers, which is good news for the health shopper. It has always been M & S policy to use their chilled distribution system, rather than over-reliance on additives, as a means of controlling food safety.

The M & S fresh chilled range now also includes vegetarian dishes which were developed when they discovered that people were using their vegetable accompaniments as main meals.

The other most likely place to find additive-free meals is in health-food shops, and more and more are now going into fresh and frozen foods, stocking vegetarian, wholefood and 'healthy' convenience meals.

Frozen meals can now be prepared by cooking, followed by immediate blast freezing, which cuts nutritional losses to a minimum. Specialist 'health-food' companies have gone into this market to fill the needs of the estimated three million vegetarians in Britain and the seventeen million who, market research tells us, are cutting down on their meat consumption and looking for ready-to-eat vegetarian meals for one or two meals each week.

The growth of *Vegetarian Feast* frozen meals, from a range of five launched in 1984 to a total of thirteen in 1986, shows the uptake of the products, with supermarkets stocking them as well as health-food shops with freezers and the ninety branches of the Iceland Freezer Centres. *Realeat* is another company supplying this demand, with its frozen *Vegeburgers* and vegetarian meals – these too are found in supermarkets as well as health-food shops.

At the other end of the scale *Findus* have put £3½ million worth of advertising behind its *Lean Cuisine* range of twelve recipe dishes 'imported' from America and aimed at slimmers and the 'health conscious'. Sadly, only one is free from additives.

Marks & Spencer have *Calorie Counted* range of menu meals, aimed at a similar market; and these are more useful, being free from preservatives and colours and containing only 300 calories per meal.

The following is a round-up of the ready meals that might find their way into your shopping basket. They are all free from additives (unless stated otherwise) and wholefood dishes have been included in preference to non-wholefood lines.

Vegetarian meals – fresh chilled

Marks & Spencer's range of dishes 'suitable for vegetarians' are a generous portion for one and they are all additive-free. They include Vegetable Lasagne, Vegetable Chilli, Fresh Vegetable Bake, Broccoli in Cream Sauce, Filled Green Pepper and Ratatouille. Where cheese is used it is vegetarian cheese. Other dishes that are suitable, but not specifically marked as meals for vegetarians, are Aubergine Gratin, Cauliflower Cheese, Crispy Mushrooms and Cauliflower and Sweetcorn Pie, which contains vegetarian cheese. Other dishes, such as baked potatoes and salads, may also be suitable. None are wholefood.

Waitrose has a wide range of fresh ready meals and several are suitable for main-course meals for vegetarians; among them are Cauliflower Cheese and Légumes Mornay. Again, not wholefood.

Since 1984, *Spaghetti House*, a well-known chain of Italian restaurants, have been selling fresh chilled packed versions of the meals served in their restaurants, through the supermarket chains Waitrose and Sainsbury, as well as smaller London chains. The range is not wholefood, but they are additive- and colouring-free and include meat and vegetarian dishes. Green pasta gets its colour from spinach, not dye.

Vegetarian meals – frozen

Vegetarian Feasts offer a range of thirteen meals, from everyday dishes such as Wholewheat Macaroni Cheese and Beans à la Greque, to a more exotic gourmet range of dishes including Sweet and Sour Almonds with peppers and pineapple and Spinach and Walnut Lasagne. Available from many supermarkets and health-food stores.

Ready Meals

Realeat is best known for the Vegeburger, but they also produce a range of four meals which are excellent for everyday eating, three pasta-based and one veg cottage pie. Available from supermarkets and health-food shops.

St Nicholas Wholefoods offer a Nutty Vegetable Pie, with hazelnut and wholewheat pastry, and a Leek and Lentil Cobbler that are almost meals in themselves; other products in the range, such as flan, samosa, potato and sweetcorn cakes, need accompaniments. Their products are made from stoneground wholemeal flour which has been milled at the Thanet village of St Nicholas-at-Wade for 250 years, and by the Tapp family, who produce the range, for fifty years. Available from supermarkets and freezer centres.

Capricorn Meals started as a home-production unit before moving to special premises and producing about 2,000 meals a week; they do vegetarian dishes with an international flavour, as well as Cottage Pie and Lasagne, Pizza and puds such as Apple and Sultana Charlotte. Available from Leeds area health-food shops and some London and Bristol distribution centres.

Vege-Dine offer a range of twelve vegetarian dishes including pasta dishes, pies, curries and casseroles. They also make more unusual bakes, nut roasts and crumbles, straight vegetable dishes and terrines. Some with printed outer cardboard containers, others simply in foil containers with a printed label on the lid. Available in the Bournemouth area and in Bristol and London health-food shops.

Wholefayre offer four dishes, three of which are vegan: Vegetable Seed Crumble, Vegetable and Nut Curry and Chilli con Carne. Nut Lasagne contains a vegetarian cheese sauce and so is not for vegans. Available in health-food shops in Bristol and the southeast.

Haddington's kosher dishes, such as stuffed aubergines or peppers, and nut lasagne, are available in health-food stores in the south of Britain.

Mr Chef offers rare 'continental cuisine' for vegans. The dishes are based on tofu, and include exotic oriental ingredients like seaweed. Mostly in single-size servings. Available in the Midlands in health-food shops. Some, such as their Nut Roast, are frozen in foil containers; others, such as the Vegetable Curry come in two separate bags which they are boiled in, one bag containing the curry and one the brown rice. Others include Vegetarian Sausage and Mash with Peas, Pancakes, and Cottage Pie.

Nature's Harvest is another company based in the south-west producing ten complete convenience meals in individual servings.

One of the twelve dishes in the *Findus Lean Cuisine* range, Zucchini Lasagne, is suitable for vegetarians who eat cheese. It is free from additives.

Country Cooks ready meals are made by Cordon Bleu cook Jenny Allday. There are three gourmet frozen vegetarian meals and one made with wholefood vegetarian ingredients; they include Mixed Vegetable Crumble, Blackeye Bean Bake and Peanut Lasagne. Relatively cheap and available in Bath, Bristol and London area health-food shops.

French Chef is a range of vegetarian meals – Vegetarian Gratin, Vegetarian Biriani and Vegetarian Lasagne. It is carried in a third of the Waitrose stores.

Birds Eye Menu Master range now contains four vegetarian meals, Vegetable Curry with Pilau Rice, Cauliflower Cheese, using low-fat vegetarian rennet cheese, Vegetable Lasagne, which Birds Eye says is 'lower fat' and Mushroom and Pasta Italienne. All single serving packs which can be microwaved or boiled in the bag. All are free of colour and preservatives, but not wholefood.

Vegetarian meals – Alutrays

Alutrays involve a similar process to canning. Food is prepared and put into the shallow trays, the lids are sealed in place and then the Alutrays are heated until the food is sterilized. These can sit on

Ready Meals

a shelf in a shop in the same way as cans, without refrigeration. They are supposed to be cooked at a lower temperature and for a shorter time than with canning, but Alutray meals taste to me the same as canned products.

Because the food is cooked in the container, any vitamins leaching into the cooking liquid remain part of the dish, as the sauce is eaten with the main ingredients. Although the trays are aluminium they have a polypropylene lining which prevents the food being burnt and also means that the food is not in direct contact with the aluminium, which might of concern to some health-conscious people – aluminium contact is something to be avoided. The effect of the lining is a 'boil in the bag' one.

Boots has launched a range of vegetarian ready meals. They are not wholefood – the rice is white, as is the pasta and flour used. Some of the meals also contain additives such as phosphates which, although 'safe', may be too frequent in our diet. An interesting collection of dishes including Risotto, Lasagne, Country Casserole, Vegetable Curry and Ratatouille. Available at Boots Food Centres.

Prewett's range offers four pasta dishes – Wholemeal Ravioli, Wholemeal Canneloni, Lasagne and Tortellini, made with TVP fillings – and other ready meals, Vegetable Curry, Vegetable Goulash, and Lentil Stew. There is also a Bolognese Sauce for use with spaghetti, etc.

Eden soya-based vegetarian meals are imported from Germany by Leisure Drinks. There are four varieties: Soya Fricassé, Soya Ragoût, Goulash and Rondules. The dishes include vegetables and soya in a thick sauce. They are unusual in that the sophisticated sauces are made using alcohol-free white wine and natural flavourings. The fat used is vegetable but milk and milk protein is used, so the range is not suitable for vegans. Makes a generous single serving, or might serve two people with smaller appetites.

Vegetarian – dry mix meals

Prewett's a range of meatless meals for the lone diner is called *Just for One*. Each pack contains two sachets, one of brown rice or pasta and the other of the vegetable or bean mix: Vegetable Curry with Brown Rice, Vegetable Provençal with Brown Rice, Savoury Vegetables with Wholemeal Spaghetti, Neapolitan Vegetables with Wholemeal Spaghetti.

Holly Mill Singles is the name of a range which includes Spicy Mexican Mix, a vegetable chilli with kidney beans, herbs and spices, Hungarian Mix, Vegetable Goulash and Tasty Italian.

Granose dry mixes for Nut Roast and Lentil Roast come in a foil tray to which water is added before baking. Each serves four people.

Vegetarian – canned

Whole Earth Brown Rice and Vegetables can be heated and served within one minute. The rice is organically grown and the other ingredients are of the unusually high standard demanded by all Whole Earth products. No added sugar or artificial ingredients of any kind. From health-food shops and speciality stores.

A conventional can has a tin-plate lining and it will probably be soldered at the joins. Whole Earth use a superior method of electrical welding with the special inert lining of non-migratory plastic which acts as a barrier between the tin and the food and makes a lead-free seam. It is a little more expensive, but avoids any possible risk from metal contamination.

The *Granose* range of vegetable protein foods includes many canned products from vegetable pâté to Sausalatas; they also include some canned ready meals such as Chicken-style Curry, Country Vegetable Pudding, Savoury Pudding, Goulash, Mexican Bean Stew, and Lentil and Vegetable Casserole. Soya protein, vegetable protein vegetables and wholefood ingredients make up this well-established range. Available from health-food shops.

Ready Meals

Hofels is another name that has been around on the health-food scene for some time. They offer three canned vegetarian meals – Vegetable Curry, Savoury-style Curry (with TVP) and Cheese Hot Pot. All ingredients such as pasta are wholemeal. Available from health-food shops.

Itona is a company specializing in TVP; it has developed a new method of making it which it has called B-Tex, standing for Biologically Textured vegetable protein. Made from soya beans (like other TVP) it is produced by a biologically live process similar to that used in cheese making, rather than spinning or extruding – the usual methods. Itona's method is unique and it means the soya beans do not have to be exposed to such high temperatures or be processed so much. The range, which is available from health-food shops, includes Soya Pieces in Gravy and Sweet and Sour.

Hotcan's Curried Vegetables with Fruit is in a container that actually heats the food. The food can sits inside a larger can; by puncturing the outer rim of the can water is released on to a lime mixture below, which causes a chemical reaction to produce heat and so heat the contents of the inner can. The food is stirred for time to time during the 12–15 minute heating period and is then ready to eat. The product does contain MSG, but no other additives. Included for novelty value!

> **My choice (vegetarian)**
>
> I think the M & S vegetarian dishes are well presented and appetizing, though rather too salty for my taste. Spaghetti House pasta dishes are also good. Personally I do not like the canned or Alutray products – not only do they taste overcooked, but they also look unappetizing. However, there is one exception – Whole Earth canned brown rice, which is versatile and tasty.

Ready Meals

Non-vegetarian – fresh chilled

Marks & Spencer have an extensive range of fresh chilled meals, many of which do not contain additives, but because their range changes so frequently it is not possible to list named recipe dishes. Watch their shelves and read the labels! The current *Calorie Counted Menu* range includes seven dishes of single-portion size, six of which have no preservatives or colouring. The rice and pasta in the range are not wholefood. Each meal is less than 300 calories.

Waitrose have twenty fresh ready meals and all are free from colouring, preservatives and flavouring. They include several vegetarian dishes (see above) as well as Spicy Meat Balls, Lamb Curry, Chilli con Carne, Lamb Boulangère, Cod and Broccoli Mornay and Plaice and Prawn Véronique. The ingredients are not wholefood.

Spaghetti House have a range of fresh chilled meat-based pasta dishes which are made to the recipes used in their restaurants and frozen. They are sold through supermarkets and delicatessens, and are free from preservatives and colour, but they are not wholefood.

Today's Table from *Wall's* is a range of meat-based fresh chilled meals such as Chilli con Carne, Beef Casserole, Lancashire Hotpot and Sausage and Mash. Not particularly 'healthy', but they are free from artificial colourings and preservatives, although they do contain modified starch and some caramel.

Non-vegetarian – frozen

Marks & Spencer have a smaller range of frozen foods, since they concentrate mainly on the fresh-chilled sector; many of their fish dishes are free from additives – check the labels.

Waitrose have recently reintroduced their range of Indian dishes which are prepared with natural ingredients to authentic Indian recipes. Main dishes are either lamb, beef or chicken, with

Ready Meals

vegetable dishes of rice, lentils or samosa, which can be eaten as snacks or accompaniments to the ready meals.

Country Cooks, run by Jenny Allday, who also prepares frozen vegetarian foods (see the vegetarian section, above) has a range of gourmet dishes such as Boeuf Bourguignon, Chicken Marengo and Navarin of Lamb, and some more everyday dishes; Chilli con Carne, Moussaka, Lasagne, Fish Pie and Seafood Crumble. The range is not wholefood, but it is free from artificial additives.

They are available from Harrods and other Sloane shopping haunts, and up-market regional stores.

Co-op Stir Fry Meals are completely additive-free, but water is top of the ingredients list. Chinese Chicken contains a minimum of 14 per cent chicken, plus water, cooked rice, peas, onions, bean sprouts, sweetcorn, mushrooms, water chestnuts and bamboo shoots. Indian Chicken contains a minimum of 16 per cent chicken, plus water, cooked rice, beans, onions, sweetcorn, sweet red pepper, apple, spice, seasoning mix, sultanas.

Non-vegetarian – Alutrays

Healthline is a range of six recipe dishes based on international recipes. Launched by John Capito, they claim to use only lean meat 'more than the usual number of vegetables and other natural ingredients'. Dishes include Lamb à la Grecque, Elizabethan Spiced Beef, Turkey Marengo, Chicken Cacciatore, and Liver Mexicaine. Available from major Boots Food Centres, delicatessens, department stores and independent chemists. The ingredients are not wholefood.

Kitchen Classics are the own-brand range by Swissco, the importers of Alutray and manufacturers and packers of meals for other companies. The range includes Cannelloni with beef filling, Chicken Curry with Rice, Lasagne and Sweet and Sour Pork with Noodles. The ingredients are not wholefood.

Ready Meals

Lockwoods are also packing conventional meals in Alutrays and so doing without preservatives and artificial additives. The range includes Beef Casserole, Lamb Casserole and Chicken Casserole. The ingredients are not wholefood.

Non-vegetarian – canned

Newforge Foods has now dropped the MSG from its canned meat meals, such as Irish Stew, and uses spices instead to achieve flavour. Sold under an *All-Natural* sub-brand, the range includes Beef Casserole, Chicken Casserole and Hot Pot. The additive-free range is aimed to increase Newforge's 25 per cent share of the canned casserole market.

Vegetarian or non-vegetarian – packet

Casa Fiesta is an American product that has crossed the Atlantic to bring us the increasingly popular flavour of Mexican food. The range is free from artificial additives; it includes taco shells and sauces as well as green chillies. The vegetarian filling is Refried Beans and the non-vegetarian filling canned Beef Taco Filling (minced beef with onions), or you could use fresh minced beef and flavour it with the beef spice sachet which is part of the range. Colourfully packaged, they offer a nice change from other ready meals. The taco shells are made with stoneground corn (maize) and the sauces are made from vegetables 'processed within twenty-four hours of picking to retain their freshness', say the makers.

> **My choice (non-vegetarian)**
>
> M & S fish recipe dishes come out on top for me, followed by the Waitrose Indian range. The M & S Calorie Counted recipes are also good, but too salty for my taste.

RICE

Rice is an ideal food to form part of a healthy eating plan. Like wholemeal bread, brown rice is a complex-carbohydrate food that produces slow-release energy combined with the value of high-fibre food. Like bread, potatoes and pasta (wholemeal), it is a 'healthy food' and is no longer regarded as 'fattening'. Although the raw-weight calorie count is around 105 per ounce this is equal to only 35 calories per cooked ounce of rice.

	Fibre per ounce (g)
Brown rice, raw	1.25
Brown rice, cooked	0.4
White rice raw	0.75
White rice, cooked	0.25

White rice has had the husk, bran and germ removed, leaving only a refined white starch. Cooks in about 15 minutes.

Parboiled, pre-fluffed or easy-cook rice. Whatever the colour, this has been steam-pressure processed before being milled, which increases the nutritional value a little because it drives the vitamins and minerals from the husk into the grain as it hardens the grain (so that it does not overcook). It gives white rice a slightly yellow appearance. The rice takes slightly longer to cook than standard white or brown rice.

Brown rice has had only the husk removed, leaving the bran and the germ intact, so it has more fibre and higher nutritional value than white rice. Cooks in 35–45 minutes.

Wild rice is a luxury food; it is really the seed of an aquatic grass, not a rice. The grains are longer than rice and dark brown in colour, but when it cooks, it splits to reveal its white centre. It is produced in North America, mainly Minnesota, where it is hand-harvested by Chippenewa Reservation Indians. It is organically produced and cooks in 30–40 minutes.

> **Washing Rice**
>
> Always wash rice thoroughly before cooking, especially brown rice. Place in a container and cover with water to a good hand's depth above the rice. Stir gently to free the husks, dirt and dust these will float to the top and can be poured off. Repeat until the water is clean. Then cook in plenty of boiling water. It is not necessary to pre-soak rice; this will leach out the valuable vitamins and minerals and they will be lost in the water.

Jordans Country Rice and Grains
This is a blend of six whole grains, including brown rice. The advantage of mixing several grains is the enhanced protein value. The product is also high in fibre and low in fat, with a good flavour and nice chewy texture. The grains are brown rice (25 per cent), oats, barley, wheat, rye, buckwheat and sesame seeds.

Whole Earth Brown Rice and Vegetables
See p. 349.

> **My choice**
>
> For special occasions my choice is wild rice. It will go further if you mix it with brown rice and both have similar cooking times. Of the brown rices I prefer Basmati long-grain brown rice as a vegetable rice, and Italian medium or short grain rice for Risottos – it is often organic – plus American easy-cook brown rice if people are going to be late!

SALAD DRESSING/CREAM
See under MAYONNAISE.

SANDWICH SPREADS

These are often rather tart and acidic, and use unspecified oils and vinegars. They also, usually, contain additives, but products from the health-food trade, based on tofu, are lower in fat and the fats that are used are high in polyunsaturates.

Sandwich Spreads

Duchesse All-Natural Sandwich Spread is a dill pickle in a cholesterol-free dressing; 50 per cent of the oil used is polyunsaturated. It is low in sodium, with only 0.7 per cent being added and has 2 per cent added sugar. It is suitable for vegans and vegetarians.

Tofu Tomato and Garlic Spread and *Soychiz* are spreads based on tofu and are free from additives. They are also free from dairy products and could be used as a thick salad dressing as well as a sandwich spread.

Tofu Spread made by *Living Foods*, is an organic product based on tofu and free from additives. It is available as a Sandwich Spread, or in Natural, Celery or Garlic varieties. Typical ingredients of the 220 g jars are: tofu, safflower oil, apple cider vinegar, apple juice concentrate, celery, carrots, onion, sea salt and guar vegetable binder.

> **My choice**
>
> I hadn't used sandwich spread for years until I discovered Duchesse...

SAUCES

See also MAYONNAISE, SALAD DRESSINGS and STOCK, 'GRAVY'.

Say ketchup and you think of tomato sauce, right? But there are other ketchups too – brown sauces and other spicy sauces. Salt is often a major ingredient and most contain around 1,500 mg of sodium per 100 g. Not only that, most ketchups are high on added sugar, too – around 20 per cent in some cases. If you can't (or don't want to) kick the ketchup habit, here are some that are lower in salt and sugar than the two most popular brands, Heinz and Daddies. They *are* expensive, but they have to use more expensive ingredients to achieve a good flavour.

Tomato ketchup

The two most popular brands:

Heinz tomato ketchup contains tomatoes, sugar, spirit vinegar, salt and spices.
Sodium: 1,450 mg/100 g.

Daddies tomato ketchup contains tomatoes, sugar, spirit, vinegar, salt, modified starch, citric acid, spices and flavouring.
Sodium: 3,200 mg/100 g.

These are both free from additives and are included by way of comparison with the following varieties.

*

Whole Earth Tomato Ketchup is free from added sugar and salt, and from additives. It is made using a high-quality vinegar and the ingredients are: tomato purée, apple juice, barley malt vinegar, onion powder, kelp, garlic powder, cinnamon, cayenne, nutmeg, cloves.
Sodium: 1,040 mg/100 ml.

Life Low Sodium Tomato Ketchup: the emphasis is on keeping the sodium content lower than most ketchups and it contains about fifty times less than the average. It is free from additives and is made from: sieved tomatoes, cider vinegar, apple juice concentrate, honey, onion, garlic, whole spices, cornflour, guar and xanthan gums and natural flavourings.
Sodium: 35 mg/100 g.

Prewett's Low Sodium Tomato Ketchup is another additive-free product, although it is thickened with modified starch. The ingredients are: tomato purée, cider vinegar, water, apple juice concentrate, modified maize starch, onion powder, garlic powder, spices, autolysed yeast.
Sodium: 45 mg/100 g.

Sauces

Brown sauce

The brand leader in the brown sauce stakes is HP Sauce which has a pretty respectable list of ingredients. Others are not so good. The alternatives listed are lower-sodium versions.

HP contains: vinegar, tomatoes, sugar, dates, molasses, salt, rye flour, raisins, onions, starch, tamarinds, spices, soy sauce, modified starch, colour (caramel), defatted soya flour, garlic, mustard, flavours.
Sodium: 3,200 mg/100 g.

*

Life Low Sodium Fruity brown sauce has about 1.1 per cent of the sodium content of regular brown sauce and it is also free from artificial additives. It contains: apples, cider vinegar, water, dates, blackstrap cane molasses, cornstarch, whole ground spices, onions, natural xanthan gum and natural flavours.
Sodium: 40 mg/100 g.

Prewett's Low-Sodium Spicy brown sauce is another all-natural product containing: cider vinegar, apple juice concentrate, molasses, onion powder, garlic powder, modified maize starch, spices and vegetable gum stabilizer. (Well, perhaps the modified starch is not so natural!)
Sodium: 45 mg/100 g.

Whole Earth Kensington Sauce is a brown sauce which is free from added sugar, and artificial additives. It contains: barley malt vinegar, apple juice, apple purée, date juice, water, tamari soy sauce (soya beans, sea salt, well water), onion powder, sea salt, spices, apple pomace, rye flour, *miso* soya purée (soya beans, sea salt, water), guar gum.

> **My choice**
> I prefer the Whole Earth products in both tomato ketchup and brown sauce.

Worcestershire sauce

The best known of these is *Lea & Perrins*, which is free from artificial additives, but cannot be used by vegetarians and vegans because it contains anchovies. The ingredients are: vinegar, molasses, sugar, salt, anchovies, tamarinds, shallots, garlic, spices and flavourings. The sodium content is 1.5 per cent, so it is not a low sodium product; the sugar content is 16 g/100 g.

Life Worcestershire Sauce is probably the only non-animal Worcestershire Sauce – it is free from anchovies. It is also free from additives and added salt and sugar.

Fruit sauce

Wendy Brandon do a range of unusual and upmarket sauces including Spiced Apple, to an American recipe, Plum, Cranberry, and Cranberry and Orange. All are free from additives and are based on pure fruit sweetened with apple juice.

Tartare sauce

Usually a no-no for those wishing to avoid all additives but *Life* Tartare Sauce is free from additives and 50 per cent of the 25 per cent oil in the product is high in polyunsaturates. It is also egg and dairy-product free, probably making it a unique experience for vegetarians and vegans, who will obviously not use it with fish, but who could use it for other dishes. Also useful for fish eaters on an egg-and-milk-free diet.

Horseradish sauce

Many horseradish sauces are suspect because they contain additives.

Life Horseradish Sauce is free from additives, added salt and sugar, and is also suitable for vegetarians, but not vegans.

Burgess Hot Horseradish Sauce does contain salt and sugar, but no additives, and the colouring used is natural.

Sauces

Anchovy essence

For those of you who are into these gentlemanly relishes, the *Burgess Anchovy Essence* uses 'natural' colours and stabilizer, but it is high in sodium. The ingredients are: anchovies, water, salt, stabilizer E413 (tragacanth gum) and colour E172 (a natural iron oxide).

Soy sauce

With the increase in popularity of Chinese foods, the soy sauce bottle is becoming as common in British homes as the brown sauce bottle, both for use as a condiment with Chinese food and for use in cooking. Most of it is imported from Japan and China and British food laws have no compositional requirements for it.

Soy sauce is really a cheap version of the 'real' thing which is shoyu sauce (see below). A good-quality soy sauce will be made by fermentation of soya beans, wheat and added salt. Poor-quality soy sauce will contain monosodium glutamate, caramel colouring, defatted or hydrolysed soya beans, glycerine, ethyl alcohol, hydrochloric acid and/or caustic soda. These are all used to speed the process or produce the flavour that comes naturally through the long, slow, traditional fermentation. In particular, good-quality soy sauce does not need MSG, because the fermentation produces glutamic acid naturally.

Shoyu sauce

This is made from equal parts of soya beans and wheat, plus salt. It is fermented slowly, without the use of chemical additives or processes, and is the 'real' soy sauce. When buying, to test a good shoyu sauce, shake the bottle; if the natural froth that is formed remains for a minute it is a good-quality sauce. Soy sauce will not do this.

Tamari

This consists of soya beans fermented with *koji*, a starter (*Aspergillus oryzae*) and salt. It has a longer fermentation and lower salt level than shoyu and soy sauce. It is free from wheat grain and so suitable for coeliacs who want to use a soya-flavoured sauce. It tastes as good as shoyu, but a little stronger.

Spaghetti sauces

These are for heating and pouring over spaghetti (they are also useful for pizza toppings and in other dishes . . .), and are usually meat-based – bolognese – or tomato-based. They generally contain sugar and salt, although not always additives. There is one spaghetti sauce that is free from all these things:

Whole Earth Italiano! is a spaghetti sauce in which the water used is filtered, and the oil is olive oil and soya, which is high in polyunsaturates. The ingredients are: tomato, onion, filtered water, celery, tomato purée, barley malt vinegar, apple juice, soya oil, carrots, virgin olive oil, garlic, dried yeast, kelp, bay, lovage, cinnamon.

SAUSAGES

'Plenty of butchers make their own sausages, but you will have to hunt. It is worth the trouble because most of the pink, pasty sausages produced these days are not worth eating,' says David Mabey in *In Search of Food*, Macdonald & Jane's, 1978.

Other writers have been more forthright and called the sausage the equivalent of the food industry's dustbin. TV documentaries have also had their prod at the sausage and meat-product manufacturers. As a result, in 1984 sausage sales suffered a 9 per cent decline. TV revelations in 1985 resulted in a further 15 per cent drop in sausage sales, which manufacturers estimate would take a couple of months to recover from. (What short memories we shoppers must have!)

By law pork sausages have to be at least 65 per cent meat and other sausages 50 per cent meat, but only half the meat needs to be lean meat and the definition of meat can include many parts of the animal that we do not traditionally regard as meat, such as gristle,

Sausages

and rind, lips and meat slurry – mechanically recovered 'meat' forced from the carcass. We are not told whether these are in any particular meat product, so we are denied freedom of choice over whether or not we buy sausages that use these meats.

Because of the poor quality of the ingredients used in sausages they need a lot of colouring, flavouring and texturing agents to restructure them, as well as emulsifiers and preservatives, etc.

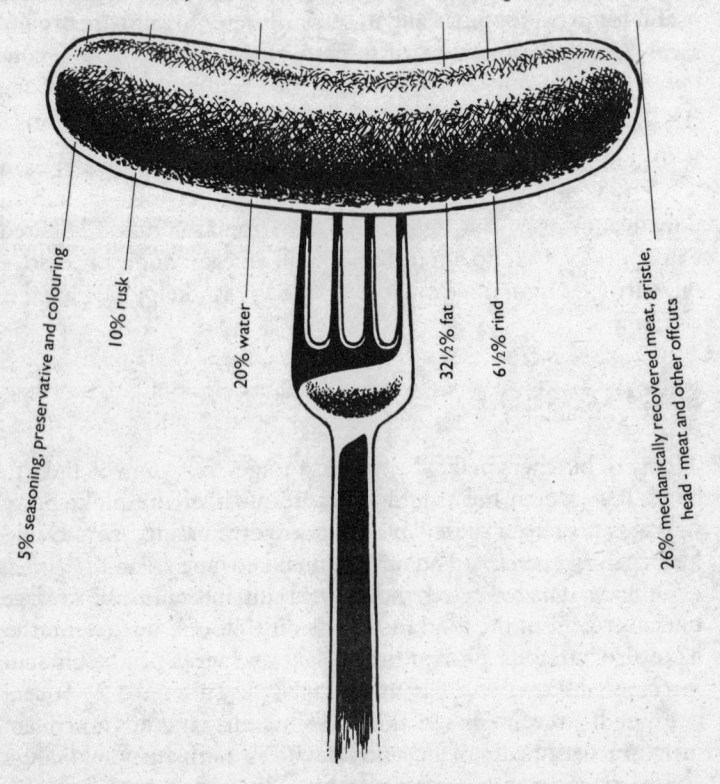

- 5% seasoning, preservative and colouring
- 10% rusk
- 20% water
- 32½% fat
- 6½% rind
- 26% mechanically recovered meat, gristle, head - meat and other offcuts

Source: From an illustration in the *Sunday Times Supplement*, 1984, by Bob Garrard.

The Law-abiding Sausage

This is what you pay for when you buy the typical supermarket pork sausage. According to the legal definition, it contains its due quota of 65 per cent meat (50 per cent for beef sausages).

Sausages are also bulked with binders and up to 20 per cent is allowed to be binder material such as cereal rusk and cheap fillers like skimmed milk. Even sugar goes into the sausage and water can be added – up to 5 per cent water can go in without the label having to state that it contains added water.

Even sausage skins are not what they used to be... The natural skins are made from cleaned and salted intestines, man-made ones are from collagen and they do not need pricking, as they don't burst like natural ones.

How to buy sausages
(if you must!)

Look out for the low-fat versions if you are a sausage addict, but do try to cut down sausages, because they give you lots of fat and fillers without much nutritional value. If you fry sausages, this adds even more fat, so grill them if you can.

Bowyer's Low Fat Sausages are pork sausages with half the fat of standard sausages. Available fresh in packets of eight and frozen in packs of twenty. They may be lower in fat, but they still contain additives.

Wall's Light and Lean sausages contain half the fat of standard sausages and 99 calories per sausage. Analysis figures from Wall's claim 10 g fat for 100 g English Recipe sausage, compared with 24 g fat in the same weight of ordinary pork and beef sausages. Other flavours are Country Recipe and Turkey Recipe. Fat content for Country Recipe is the same as English Recipe; the Turkey Recipe fat content is lower, at 8 g per 100 g.

Ingredients are pork, water, rusk, starch, salt, and less than 1 per cent soya protein concentrate, spices, herbs, tri-phosphates, antioxidant (ascorbyl palmitate, alpha tocopherol – vitamin E), preservative (sodium metabisulphate) and natural colour (cochineal); they contain a minimum of 50 per cent pork (minimum lean 40 per cent, maximum fat 10 per cent. Country Recipe is similar, but with 55 per cent pork (minimum lean 44 per cent, maximum fat 11 per cent) and Turkey Recipe has a minimum of

Sausages

50 per cent turkey (minimum lean 41 per cent, maximum fat 9 per cent). Turkey Recipe also includes starch and lactose. There are eight sausages to a 400 g pack; English Recipe is also available in 284 g packs of ten chipolatas.

Another sausage in their range is the 'high lean meat' Wall's Original Pork sausage, which has 66 per cent meat content, more than 75 per cent of which is lean meat. Salt content has been reduced in this recipe; it contains no sugar or artificial flavours. However, despite the lower fat levels, there are still some ingredients that might not attract all shoppers. As well as pork, they contain water, rusk, salt, and less than 1 per cent herbs, dextrose, sodium polyphosphate, antioxidant E304, E307, preservative E223, colour.

Sainsbury's Low Fat Premium Pork Sausages contain 53 per cent pork, 13 per cent fat and 34 per cent water, with rusk and seasoning (plus the usual additives).

Iceland Frozen Food Centre's Low Fat Pork Sausages contain 65 per cent pork, water, rusk, salt, pepper and vitamin C as an antioxidant.

Co-op Good Life Pork Sausages are 12.5 per cent fat, less than half that of standard sausages. They contain pork, water, rusk, potato starch, salt, spices, preservative E221, antioxidant L-ascorbic acid, colouring cochineal.

Other brands of reduced-fat sausages are also appearing, but make sure you read the labels to see if the other ingredients are the kind you want to buy.

Here are some questions to ask before buying:

- Are they high in lean-meat content – 80 per cent?
- Are they low in fat – 11–13 per cent?
- Are they free from sugar?
- Do they have a large proportion of skimmed milk, cereal rusks and other fillers?
- Are they free from additives?

Additive-free sausages

Dorset Farms is a Somerset company producing sausages that are low in fat and free from preservatives, colourings and other artificial additives, as well as added sugar and water. Their range includes Pork, Pork and Herb, Cumberland, Chipolatas and the ingredients are, for example: pork (80 per cent, 11 per cent fat), water, rusk, salt, herbs, spices. They are available in London, Hampshire, Berkshire and the West Country.

Hockey's. Philip and Carol Hockey are organic farmers in the New Forest in Hampshire. They produce organic meat products, and also make home-made sausages, free from additives. The range includes: pork, pork with herbs, venison, lamb with fresh mint, beef and veal with mixed herbs. For your nearest stockists send s.a.e. for list to Philip and Carole Hockey, Newtown Farm, South Gorley, Fordingbridge, Ringwood, Hampshire (telephone Fordingbridge 52542).

Other sausages

Turkey, venison and game sausages are available from specialist butchers and delicatessens; they are usually lower in fat than conventional pork and beef sausages. Look around for them in your area and ask about the ingredients if they are not shown.

A full list is beyond the scope of this book because, as the British Sausage Information Bureau point out, there are more than 15,000 butchers in Britain and many of them make their own sausages; there are also 150 specialist sausage-making companies. Don't forget to check the contents before buying – see opposite.

Cooking Sausages

Sausages are fatty enough without frying them in more fat – especially saturated animal fat. Grill them to drain off the excess fat. The average 2 oz (55 g) sausage, uncooked, contains around 150 calories. Grilling it will reduce this to 130 calories; frying it will add to the calories and fats. There is no need to prick sausages these days, because the skins are man-made and they do not burst like natural skins.

Sausages

F. A. and J. Jones, farmers and butchers, have been producing organic meat in Lincoln for many years. Their Farmhouse Meaty Sausages are made with traditionally fed pork (no antibiotics, hormones, etc.) and contain no artificial flavourings or preservatives. They have recently reduced the fat content and came in the Top Ten British sausages in a 1985 national sausage contest organized by the *Daily Express*.

> **My choice**
>
> When buying sausages I choose the additive-free versions, preferably made with organic meat. I can buy Hockey's in my area, but would like to try F. A. and J. Jones's if I lived in Lincolnshire. Otherwise I prefer my home-made sausages!

Home-made sausages

You can always make your own sausages at home and be in complete control of what sort of meat goes into them. Natural sausage casings are sold by Gysin and Hanson Ltd, 96 Trundleys Road, Deptford, London SE8 5JE (telephone 01-692 8217) for sausages, chipolatas, black puddings, salamis, etc. The casings are made from hog, sheep or ox and Gysin and Hanson supply a recipe leaflet and instructions. Sausage-making machines are available from Catermasters, West Street, Dunster, Somerset TA24 6SN, price £8.75 post paid (1986), which includes natural skins, seasonings, recipes and instructions.

Continental sausages

These include salami, cervelat, bologna, bierwurst and frankfurter sausages, and all the thousands of other varieties available in France, Germany, Spain, Poland, Italy ... Some are smoked and some are peppery, some are dried and some are fresh and need cooking; most are ready to eat.

One thing they all have in common – yes, you have guessed it – they are all high in fat and they are all likely to contain preserv-

Sausages

atives such as nitrates and nitrites. Check when you buy. Ask to see the print on the wrapper if it is not visible – but generally speaking you can tell by the bright pink colour many of them contain nitrites, and you can see the large lumps of white fat in them.

Average Fat Content

	(%)
Frankfurter	27
Liver sausage	27
Salami	45
Bologna	27
Cervelat	37
Polish sausage	30

(The British black pudding has around 37 per cent fat.)

Non-meat sausages

Vegebanger is a follow-up to Vegeburger (see BURGERS) by *Real Eat*. It is free from additives and sugar, and contains 4–5 per cent fibre and 8–12 per cent fat, depending on the method of cooking. The fibre is from the sesame-seed, oats, wholemeal-rusk and dried-vegetable content of the banger; it can be reconstituted from the dry packet mix with water, egg and/or oil. Also available as a frozen skinless ready-made sausage.

Haddington's sausages are kosher, and are based on soya protein and are free from additives. They have a 6 per cent fibre content and are flavoured with spices, herbs and yeast extract. The range includes Savoury Sausages, Tomato Sausages and Sausage Rolls in wholemeal pastry. They are frozen.

Hera produce a Vegetable Soysage mix made from soya protein, cereal brans, herbs and spices; it is reconstituted with water. It contains 9 per cent fibre and some dairy products, so is unsuitable for vegans.

Boots have a Vegetarian Sausage Mix in their vegetarian range; it is free from additives (except a natural cellulose stabilizer) and

Sausages

needs only water to reconstitute. The fat content may be vegetable, but it is very high at 33 g per 100 g – and frying would add extra fat and calories.

Mr Chef vegetable and soya sausages are fresh chilled. They are made from potato, carrot, wholemeal flour, soya mince, oil, water, breadcrumbs, rolled oats, pearl barley, soya protein, milk protein, onions, peppers, herbs and spices. One wonders how it all fits in these long thin sausages which are vacuum packed and wrapped in a plastic skin (which must be taken off before cooking). Shelf life is three weeks. No nutritional breakdown available.

Nutribanger is a frozen sausage that is free from additives and can be grilled, fried or barbecued straight from the freezer. Details unavailable.

Sausage rolls

Pork Farms have a Natural Recipe sausage roll which contains wheat flour, margarine, water, pork (minimum 15 per cent), soya protein concentrate, rusk, salt, pepper, herbs, pork stock, egg. There are no additives, but it's up to you to decide how natural is natural; it is not wholemeal.

> **My choice**
>
> Useful though these are, I am not too keen on this type of food; Haddington's tomato sausages and Mr Chef's are the tastiest, but try them for yourself.

SEEDS
See under SNACK FOODS.

SNACK FOODS
See also CEREAL BARS and FRUIT BARS.

Snack Foods

Crisps

Potatoes are an excellent food. Baked in their jackets they are a wholefood, high in fibre and low in fat (provided you go easy on the butter) and sugar. The carbohydrates in them are unrefined and not disruptive to the blood-sugar levels when digested. They are a cheap source of vitamin C and minerals. Like most vegetables they are high in potassium and low in sodium – the right balance for health.

Potatoes are also a cheap raw ingredient for food manufacturers who turn them into items like potato crisps and, as we saw on p. 64, this means lots of profit. But sadly, making them into crisps turns them from a healthy food to one that is high in fat, having been deep fried, often in animal or hydrogenated vegetable oils, and high in salt (or more exotic flavourings). They also usually contain antioxidants to stop all the fat going rancid, often the noxious BHT and BHA.

Contrary to the 1986 SNACMA (Snack, Nut and Crisp Manufacturers Association) report compiled by scientists at King's College, London, crisps are not in line with COMA recommendations for healthier eating, and they are certainly not a better snack than an apple – the report claimed that they are in line with the COMA Report on Diet and Cardiovascular Disease recommendations because they contain 36.8 per cent fat, the COMA recommended percentage of calories in the diet from fat. As has been pointed out, crisps are 36.8 per cent fat by weight, which means that 60 per cent of the calories they contain are from fat.

Potatoes, once an everyday food in their own right, have now become an everyday food in this new highly processed version. They form the basis, together with sweets, of schoolchildren's lunches and snacks, and with their addictive, salty taste, they are difficult to give up. Perhaps the right approach with children is to make crisps an occasional treat food, not a daily food.

The trouble is children like them because they have been given a taste for salty and artificial flavours early on. If you feel you have

Snack Foods

to provide crisps here are some of the better bets and options to start the weaning process . . .

Tesco has an own-label plain potato crisp with reduced fat and salt content – about four fifths of the fat of standard crisps and three quarters of the salt. The crisps are also free from artificial additives and are wrapped in foil.

Smiths are one of the most widely available brands and their Square Crisps contain 25 per cent less fat than standard crisps. Their Salt 'n' Shake crisps have a separate little blue bag of salt and so enable less (or no) salt to be added. Smiths Crisps and their Tudor Crisps are now free from preservatives, and the flavoured crisps are also free from colouring.

Sooner Foods have crisps which are free from antioxidants and the plain and salted versions are free from additives; however, the flavoured ones do contain additives.

Hedgehog brand crisps use only natural flavourings and their crisps, which claim to be 30 per cent lower in fat than standard crisps, and lower in salt, are cooked in vegetable oil and are free from additives.

Warburtons Traditional Potato Crisps are thick cut (which means more crisp, less fat) and they are free from additives, including antioxidants. To stop them going off they are packed in a thick foil bag which protects them from oxidation, rather than using chemicals. The crisps are cooked in vegetable oil and sea salt is used on them. Warburtons use either cottonseed oil or groundnut oil.

Zweifel Pomy is a leading brand of Swiss 'natural' crisps, cooked in groundnut oil and free from preservatives. They are in a double bag to prevent them going rancid and are flavoured with 'natural' flavourings.

KP Lower-Fat Crisps claim 30 per cent less fat than standard crisps and are available as Lightly Salted and Cheese and Onion and Beef. Vegetable oil is used to fry the crisps but the oil does contain antioxidants and some oil is hydrogenated. Lactose (milk sugar) is also added making them unsuitable for vegans (who wouldn't like the Beef flavour anyway!).

The *Co-op* has also removed antioxidants from its crisps. Ready Salted are free from additives; others contain some additives and flavourings. All are cooked in vegetable oil.

> **Just How Much Fat?**
>
> Independent research by the Consumers' Association has shown that supposed lower fat or low fat crisps are not always what they appear to be. For example the Hedgehog crisps were shown to contain the same amount of oil as standard crisps. Smiths Square, labelled 25 per cent less fat than regular crisps, contained 28 per cent fat compared with 35–39 per cent fat of standard crisps. KP Lower Fat and St Michael Lower Fat contained 23 per cent and 22 per cent respectively.
> *Source: Which?*, August 1986.

Tortilla and Corn Chips

These are often a better bet than potato crisps because they are free from additives and flavoured with natural spices, but they are more expensive. They are also packed in foil bags to protect them against oxidation. There are several good brands from *Marks & Spencer* and *Phileas Fogg*, who started the trend towards these 'snacks' for adults. Phileas Fogg brand uses stoneground maize as the basis for their Tortilla Chips and their Corn Chips, which are fried in vegetable oil. Another brand is *Meximan* sold in Holland & Barrett health-food shops.

Twiglets are old favourites that have been around for fifty years. Made with 80 per cent wholemeal flour, no 'nasties', and a yeast extract flavour.

Phileas Fogg have also removed the additives from their Natural range, including Cheesey Curls, Crunchy Sticks and Potato Rackets.

Snack Foods

> **My choice**
>
> Corn Chips or Tortilla Chips from M & S or Phileas Fogg, but don't forget, either, good old Twiglets.

Alternative crisps

Benson's Natural Choice Bran Snacks are 'crisps' made from 30 per cent bran and maize. They are free from additives and the flavours are of natural origin. They are cooked in polyunsaturated oils and seasoned with sea salt; they are free from sugar. (Even the bags are biodegradable.)

The Great Taste Company produces *Wheat Sticks* which are free from additives and available in several flavours: Italian Tomato, Mexican Chilli and American Bar-B-Q. They are based on wheat and rice and cooked in groundnut oil. They have added salt and sugar, whey powder and sodium bicarbonate, so low-salters beware!

Ready Salted Wholewheat Crisps, as the name suggests, are made from wholewheat dough which is deep fried in groundnut oil and sold under the *Natural Snacks* brand. Each packet contains 100 calories, which is a lower calorie-count than standard crisps.

Sainsbury's Wholewheat Crisps are similar, being made from stoneground wholemeal flour, vegetable oil, sea salt and flavouring as appropriate to the variety – 210 calories per 80 g bag.

Allinson's Wheat Eats are also made from wholemeal flour, baked instead of fried, so they contain less fat and half the calories of standard potato crisps. They are free from additives and available in Natural, Cheese, Onion, Pizza and Peanut Butter flavours.

Crispy Soybits are made by another health-food company, *Hofels*, who produce these snacks from soya protein with rice. The product is 20 per cent vegetable protein and 10 per cent fibre; it is flavoured with natural spices and herbs. It is also very low in fat – 0.5 per cent and only 53 calories a bag.

> **My choice**
>
> Wheat Eats, both for flavour and for lack of calories!

Nuts

Peanuts are another popular snack food, mostly salted and roasted. Nuts are already high in calories because of the natural oils in them, but they are made even more calorific if oil is added to roast them.

Dry-roasted nuts may have the benefit of lower oil content but they usually contain sugar and a mixture of artificial flavours and flavour enhancers like the ubiquitous MSG (monosodium glutamate), which is renowned for its ability to provoke allergic reactions. Some packaged nuts are free from additives. Generally the mixtures of nuts and raisins are not salted and are a better bet than the salted versions.

Marks & Spencer produce naturally roasted peanuts, which are roasted without added oil and are not salted.

Sooner Foods' peanuts are free from additives.

KP Roasted Salted Peanuts, Mixed Nuts and Raisins, and Raisins and Cashews are all free from additives.

Macadamia nuts are very expensive luxury nuts roasted in their own oil with added sea salt. They are free from additives and are usually sold in foil bags to prevent them going rancid.

> **My choice**
>
> M & S roasted peanuts without salt and oil are jolly good; for very rare occasions, macadamia nuts (but remember they are high in saturated fats and often cooked in coconut oil, another source of saturated fats, so choose the version which is roasted without added oil).

Snack Foods

Seeds

If you thought these were only for the birds or for planting then think again. Sunflower and Pumpkin seeds make a nutritious snack food and an alternative to nuts and crisps. However, like nuts, they are high in oils and so should be eaten in moderation, but they are also high in protein (around 30 per cent). They are available from health-food shops and supermarkets either plain or roasted and flavoured with soy/tamari sauce. Pumpkin seeds are often sold salted. Sunnies are made by *Hofels*, a health-food company; they are roasted sunflower seeds with sea salt.

Popcorn

Popcorn can be great fun to make at home. Popping corn can be bought from the health-food shop and some delicatessens. It makes an instant 'sweet' or savoury snack that is high in fibre and the only additives will be the ones you put in.

To make it, place 1–2 tablespoonfuls of oil in the bottom of a heavy-based pan with a well-fitting lid and heat the oil until hot but not smoking; throw in about 4 oz (115 g) popping corn and place the lid on firmly. Shake the pan from time to time and don't let it get too hot. After a minute or two you will hear the corn beginning to pop. Don't take the lid off until the popping has stopped or you will have a kitchen full of corn. Melt a little carob in another pan and stir it into the corn for a sweet treat, or use a little honey. Use herbs, seasoning, salt or yeast extract for a savoury treat.

Poppola is a ready-made popcorn sold in bags similar to large crisp bags; it has no added salt or sugar. It is a savoury popcorn made with vegetable oil and flavoured with mature Cheddar cheese powder, onion powder and dried yeast to give a cheese and onion flavour. From health-food shops and selected stores.

Pop 'a' Lot is the brand of popping corn sold by *Green Giant*. It has a sachet of corn and a sachet of sauce with which to flavour it. The Barbecue and Toffee flavours contain sugars and artificial flavours, but the Original variety has a sachet of reduced-sodium mineral salt with which to flavour the corn.

Mixes

Bombay mixes and Indian spicy mixtures of roasted seeds, grains and wheat products are sold prepacked or loose and are often free from additives, although some might be rather oily. They can be a less salty snack than crisps and salted nuts.

Fruit and nut mixtures are also available either prepacked or sold loose; they consist of dried fruits, nuts, baked or deep-fried banana chips, etc. Some may be quite high in sugar, but they are low compared with much chocolate confectionery and sweets, and they also offer fibre and other nutrients from the fruit which are not available in sweets.

Carob

Carob bars look like chocolate bars and they are the 'healthy alternative to chocolate'. They are sold in health-foods shops and are made from roasted, ground pods of the carob tree instead of the roasted and ground cocoa bean.

The carob pod is naturally sweet, whereas cocoa is bitter, so carob is lower in added sugar and some carob bars are free from added sugar. They are also available with mixed nuts and fruits and flavoured like chocolate.

The main advantage over chocolate is that they are free from caffeine, theobromine and phenylethylamine, which are stimulants and migraine triggers in some people. Carob is also free from oxalic acid, so it is less likely to cause spots. Oxalic acid in chocolate blocks the absorption of calcium and zinc, which is needed for a healthy skin and clear complexion.

Kalibu carob bars are available in Plain, Peanut, Orange, Peppermint and Krunchy (with bran and raisins) varieties either with raw cane sugar or in no-added sugar varieties. They are free from additives and are sold in 60 g bars.

Snack Foods

Plamil make a carob bar with non-dairy produce, based on vegetable fat and soya flour, called Non-dairy Carob. It contains raw sugar. Plamil also make Plain Chocolate with Soya, which is a non-dairy chocolate made using soya; it is suitable for vegans and those who cannot take dairy products. Both bars weigh 100 g.

Carob- and yoghurt-coated nuts and raisins

There is quite a large range of carob confectionery available which offers a 'natural' alternative to chocolate-coated confectionery; it is sold in specialist shops such as the Happy Nuthouse and in health-food shops.

Nearly all confectionery is high in sugar and fats and really we should not eat much; if you are swapping from a regular type of confectionery to the alternatives, do also try to cut down on quantity in the process and reserve sweets and confectionery for special occasions only.

> **My choice**
>
> Don't forget dried fruit and fresh fruit – they are the best snacks.

SORBET

Sorbet is often lower in calories than ice-cream, and may be free of dairy products, making it a possible treat for vegans.

Loseley, who also make yoghurt and ice-cream, make delicious sorbets. Ingredients include real fruits, such as lemon, orange and black cherry, and brown sugar, water, glucose solids, skimmed milk powder, Jersey double cream, citric acid and a vegetable gum as a stabilizer.

Wall's Alpine range includes real fruit lemon and orange sorbets, which contain water, sugar, glucose syrup, lemon or orange, natural gums as stabilizers, citric acid (vitamin C), natural flavourings – the lemon also contains natural colouring. Additive free.

Prospero is a brand found in health-food shops and delicatessen in the London area. The sorbets are made from real fruit, sweetened with grape juice and set with a natural pectin, so they are sugar-free. The range includes flavours such as Peach, Blackberry, Passion Fruit and Guava, Strawberry.

SOUP

Home-made soup may be an excellent and nutritious food, rich in fibre from the vegetables it is made with. Many people associate canned soups, too, with healthy eating (possibly subconsciously relating it to the image the advertisements portray for it), but a glance at the ingredients panels will show the wide use of additives, including flavour enhancers, stabilizers, antioxidants, etc. It will also reveal the addition of sugar in its many forms and the use of salt. Dried packet soups may also contain sugar, but canned soups seem to contain more.

There are strict controls over the composition of soups, and looking at them reveals that you probably get less of the main ingredient than you might expect from the pictures on the labels. For example, the following soups can have as little as 6 per cent meat content: meat soups, oxtail soup, mock turtle, kidney, mulligatawny (poultry), and game. Tomato soup need contain only 3 per cent tomato solids and for meat consommé there is no fixed amount; the proviso is that the named ingredient must be the predominant ingredient (which actually means you probably do get more of it!).

If you are comforted by the idea of a can of soup or a packet of dried soup mix being in the cupboard, then here are a few of the more acceptable products . . .

Additive-free soups

Of the leading brands of soup only a few are free from the ubiquitous MSG, and most contain sugar, salt and modified starch.

Soup

Baxters
Soups in the Baxter range which do not contain MSG, or other additives apart from modified starch, are

Tartan Range – Highlander's Broth, Pea and Ham, Scotch vegetable, Poacher's Broth, Cream of Tomato, Minestrone, Lentil, Cock a Leekie, Scotch Broth, Chicken Broth, French Onion.
Special Occasion – Lobster Bisque, Cream of Pheasant, Game Consommé, Cream of Scampi.
Size: 425 g cans.

Crosse & Blackwell
Currently reformulating their soups and removing some additives. *Healthy Balance* claims '25 per cent less salt and no added sugar' (Garden Vegetable contains saccharin) for three of its four flavours and 'less added sugar' in the Creamed Tomato. The soups are also free from added preservative, artificial flavour and colour. Sunflower oil is used in the manufacture.
Size: 15 oz/425 g cans.

Crosse & Blackwell have also introduced a range of soups in cartons under the *Four Seasons* brand with blue labels for everyday soups and gold labels for special-occasion soups. There may be an advantage over canned soups where some metal will be released into the food, but the soups are still heat-treated for long life (nine months). They also contain MSG and other additives, although they are free from artificial colours and preservatives.
Size: 400 ml (serves two) cartons.

Campbells
The vast majority of Campbells soups contain MSG, added sugar and salt. There are a few from their four ranges that do not. They are

Condensed – Tomato, Tomato Rice.
Size: 10.6 oz/300 g.

Granny's (made for Scotland – semi-condensed) – Mushroom, Tomato.

Size: 15 oz/425 g.
Main Course – Beef and Vegetable.
Size: 15 oz/425 g.

Boots
Boots do a range of vegetarian canned soups which are free from additives, but do contain added sugar and salt; their *Second Nature* brand dried packet soups are also vegetable-based. Both ranges are suitable for vegans with the exception of Mixed Vegetable with Spices, which contains dried skimmed milk.

Canned Vegetarian – Country Vegetable, Bean and Pepper, Red Lentil, Potato and Leek.
Size: 15 oz/425 g.

Second Nature (dried) – Mixed Vegetables with Spices, Thick Potato, Thick Green Bean.
Size: 70 g (serves four).

Prewett's
Prewett's have a range of six dried packet soups, all of which are vegetarian, but not vegan because they contain skimmed milk. They are described as 'high fibre' and free from added salt, although raw cane sugar is added.

Easy to Cook – Tomato, Lincoln Pea, Mushroom.
Size: 50 g (serves two).

Soup in Seconds – Mushroom, Tomato, Lentil.
Size: two-sachet packs, each 40 g (one serving).

Hugli
This is another 'health-food brand' available through health-food shops and imported from Switzerland. All are dried and in packets which make four servings. They are free from artificial additives and modified starches, using instead natural gums such as carob to thicken and hold the vegetable pieces in suspension. Some contain dried skimmed milk – Potato and Five Herbs, Carrot,

Soup

Asparagus, 5 Cereal, Mushroom, Vegetable – so are not suitable for vegans. Tomato contains added raw cane sugar.
Size: 80 g (serves four).

Smedleys
This is a small range of soups in five popular flavours, available in two sizes of can. Each variety contains modified starches, and added sugar and salt; only Tomato is free from MSG.
Range: Tomato, Mushroom, Oxtail, Chicken, Vegetable.
Size: 15 oz/429 g and 1.75 lb/793 g cans.

Heinz
One of the first ranges of canned soups, available in four types: *Original* (red label), with twenty varieties, soon to carry the flash 'free from artificial colourings and preservatives' on the cans (unfortunately most contain MSG, and Cream of Chicken and Golden Chicken and Mushroom also contain polyphosphates – see below for soups free from MSG); the *Big Soup* range of four also contains MSG, as does the *Classic* range of five (surprising when the label flashes 'finest ingredients'; *Invader* soup for children, which contains strange spaghetti shapes, *is* free from MSG. Nutrition panels are soon to appear on all Heinz soup labels. *Original* (red label) – Beef Broth, Mulligatawny and Oxtail are all free from MSG.
Size: 300 g/10 oz, 425 g/15 oz and 800 g/28 oz cans.
Invader – Cream of Tomato with Pasta (free from MSG).
Size: 435 g cans.

Heinz Weight Watchers look tempting, with only 60–75 calories a serving according to the label, but all contain MSG, polyphosphates, modified starch and saccharin.

Miso cup

There are several varieties of instant *miso* soup in single serving sachets, based on Japanese soup made from the condiment *miso*. This is a fermented and matured soya-bean paste which comes in several flavours and colours. These vegetarian and vegan soups are sold in health-food shops and Japanese specialist stores.

Vegetable bouillon/stock

These make a good basis for home-made soups. See separate entry, under STOCK.

> **My choice**
>
> I don't often use packet soup, but I was pleasantly surprised when I tried the Hera and Hugli soups.

SOYA MILK

Soya milk sales are booming; they are now around £3 m a year and estimates are that they will reach £20m in the next three years. Why? Because more people are catching on to the low-fat, non-animal fat health benefits of soya.

It is the alternative milk for those who are cutting down on dairy products and milk in particular and, as more information comes to light about the relationship between cow's milk and all kinds of health problems, from skin complaints and catarrh to arthritis, asthma and migraines, more people are trying soya milk.

In large areas of the world the population cannot tolerate cow's milk because of lactose (milk sugar) intolerance. Virtually all peoples of non-European descent lack the enzyme lactase, which is needed to digest lactose. Although lactose is in human breast milk, many races – and about 20 per cent of white Europeans – lose the ability to produce lactase after weaning. (This is not a 'milk allergy', however.)

In China and Japan and other oriental countries, the milk of the soya bean has been used for centuries and dairy produce has not been used at all. Soya milk is curdled into a curd called tofu (p. 186) in the same way that we make cheese from cow's milk; the health advantage is its high protein content and low fat content.

Soya Milk

Soya milk is high in protein and low in fat, and can be used hot or cold at the table or for cooking; it can also make ice-creams and home-made yoghurts. It is mainly imported from Japan, but there are now firms making it in Britain. It is made by boiling and crushing soya beans and taking off the resultant liquid. Most varieties are UHT and packed in cartons, so they are long-life products; others are canned.

Buying soya milk

There are several things to look out for when buying:

- Remember some varieties have added sugar, so check that the brand is sugar-free.
- Read the ingredients panel for additives (although soya milk is usually free from them, being sold mainly though health-food stores at the moment).
- Some soya milks are concentrated, so decide if you want ready-to-use or concentrated and check on the pack.
- There are several flavoured soya milks on the market – check to see if they have added sugar and colours, etc. (most are of 'natural' origin).
- Watch out for claims about being sugar-free or free from added sugar. While this may be true, the product may contain added malt, honey or sugar in another disguise.

Storing soya milk

If you haven't used it before here are some tips on keeping soya milk:

- Do not dilute concentrated soya milk until the moment of use; leave the rest undiluted.
- Do not cover the carton or can once opened – excluding the air 'incubates' the milk and reduces keeping time; allow it to breathe.
- Do not store opened milk in a can – pour it into a non-metallic container.

Soya Milk

- Once opened, keep it in the fridge – soya milk keeps fresh there for about five days.

What to buy

Cereal Mate is the most widely available and it is being cleverly marketed to give it a specific use – for the breakfast table along with the cereal. To purists it's not the real McCoy, as it contains sugars, but people who don't find soya milk palatable like this one... Difficult. The ingredients are water, dehulled soya beans, raw cane sugar, barley, malt, sea salt and natural vanilla. It is made by Alpro, who have been making Provamel (see below) for many years for the health-food trade.

Provamel is a range of soya drinks made by *Granose*, who also produce Granose Soya Milk and Granose Sugar-free Soya Milk. The drinks are sold in cartons and have a shelf-life of eight months, unopened. Sizes are 1 litre and 500 ml.

Soya milk: green label – sugar-free soya milk.
Soya drink: green carton – soya drink sweetened with honey and malt
    red carton – soya drink with no added sugar
    brown carton – soya drink flavoured with carob.

They also do strawberry-flavoured soya milk.
Plamil made the first British soya milk in 1965. The products are all free from animal fats and animal ingredients and contain no additives. Plamil concentrated soya milk is available in 500 ml long-life cartons and in 420 ml cans of concentrated soya milk.

Cartons: green and red label – concentrated soya milk with raw sugar
        blue and mauve label – concentrated sugar-free soya milk
        light blue and dark blue – ready-to-use sugar-free soya milk.
Cans: green – with raw sugar
    blue – sugar free.

Sunrise is a British-produced soya milk made from Canadian soya beans and Welsh mountain water. Sunrise products are free from animal produce, lactose, cholesterol and salt. The soya milk is

Soya Milk

UHT and long-life, lasting six months unopened. It is available in cartons and will keep for seven days in the fridge after opening.

No colour code. The upright 500 ml carton is sweetened with raw cane sugar and the squat 500 ml brick carton has no added sugar.

Sojal is a 'nutty' flavoured soya milk under the *Hera* label. Available in 1 litre cartons and free from added sugar and salt. One variety – dark blue carton.

Prewett's is another health-food company producing soya milk. It is sweetened with honey and packed in 500 ml cartons with a shelf-life of six months. One variety – dark blue and red carton.

Itona was one of the first British producers of soya milk. It is sold in cans (15 fl oz) under the *Golden Archer* brand name, and is sweetened with unrefined sugar.

Eden and Bonsoy are two products imported from Japan. They are packed in sachet/pouches in individual servings and are available as plain or flavoured soya milks. They have no added sugar.

> **My choice**
>
> I don't use much soya milk, which is one reason why I choose the small sachets of Eden and Bonsoy – I also think they taste better. The carob versions are good.

Dried soya milk

Like cow's milk and goat's milk, soya is also available in dried and powdered form. Several of the above producers also produce dried soya milk:

Soyagen Powdered Soya milk is made by *Granose*, who also make *Granolac* powder soya milk for infants.

Soyvita is an instant soya milk made from spray-dried powdered soya milk by *Healtheries*. It is sweetened with corn-syrup solids and has added vitamins and minerals.

Rice pudding and custard

No, I am not suggesting you eat them together, but pointing out that rice pudding and custard made with soya milk are also available and made by *Itona* under the *Granny Ann* brand – the rice pud is made using brown rice – and *Plamil*.

SQUASH

See 'Fruit Squash', under FRUIT JUICE.

STOCK

Most stock cubes contain flavour enhancers such as monosodium glutamate, and the majority are meat based. For a more delicate flavour and for use in non-meat dishes there are several high-quality vegetable bouillon stocks available without additives. Some are also salt-free.

Stock cubes

Hugli – regular and low sodium
Sold in packs of two stock cubes, each makes up to 1 litre (1¾ pints) when mixed with boiling water. The ingredients are hydrolysed vegetable protein, sea salt (not in the low-salt version), vegetable fat, lactose, starch, dehydrated vegetables and spices.
Suitable for vegetarians.

Morga – regular and low sodium
Sold in packs of two, each stock cube makes up to 1 litre (1¾ pints) when mixed with boiling water. The ingredients are sea salt (not in the low-sodium version), hydrolysed soya and wheat proteins, hydrogenated peanut and coconut oils, salt, dried vegetables and spices.
Suitable for vegetarians and vegans.

Plantaforce – no added salt
Sold in packs of two, each cube makes up to 1 litre (1¾ pints)

Stock

when mixed with boiling water. The cube is free from salt but contains lactose.
Suitable for vegetarians.

Friggs
Friggs stock cubes from *Kallo Foods* come in three varieties, Vegetable, Tomato, and Onion. All are free from additives and from lactose. Sea salt is included – there are plans for a salt-free version.
Suitable for vegetarians.

Stock concentrates

Vecon contains seaweed to boost its mineral content and can be used in sandwiches as a spread. It looks like a yeast extract and is free from additives, added salt and animal ingredients. The contents are: hydrolysed vegetable protein, yeast extract, dried yeast powder, seaweed powder, dried vegetables and celery seed. Available in three sizes: 4 oz (100 g), 8 oz (225 g), 1 kg.

Lotus Brown Stock is a small pot of concentrate (2.8 oz/80 g) which is free from additives and animal products, but it does contain added salt. The ingredients are: hydrolysed vegetable protein, salt, starch, fructose, dried onion and spices.

Marinating paste

Rechard Instant Marinating Paste is a concentrated purée free from additives, fats, salts and sugars. So what's in it? The paste is simply made from stone ground chilli peppers, vinegar, garlic, ginger, shallots, tamarind, cumin, cinnamon, cloves, cardamon, saffron and mustard. Rechard is the name of an authentic Indian Goa paste which has been used for thousands of years and until now has been limited to imports for ethnic communities. Now it is made by D'Silva foods of Manchester and adds flavour without additives and calories. As well as marinating, it can be used, well diluted, in stock and in many dishes.

Gravy

This is usually made from meat stock but one product may be useful for vegetarians. It is a meatless Gravy Mix under the *Pantry Stock* brand name and can give flavour to all sorts of dishes. The ingredients are: wholemeal flour, cornflour, yeast extract, sea salt, caramel powder, onion powder, herbs and spices. It thickens too, like gravy browning.

A Low Salt Gravy Mix made by *Applefords* uses herbs and spices for flavour; it is available from health-food shops.

> **My choice**
>
> First choice is the no-added-salt stock cubes from Hugli, but all of these are worth a place in the kitchen.

STUFFING

The usual poultry stuffing mixes are complete with a whole range of artificial additives to give them flavour but there is one range that is not only free from additives, but also has no added fats and sugar or salt and is based on wholemeal breadcrumbs with bran. *Mr Harvey's Original* range of stuffing mixes are reconstituted with boiling water and 1 tablespoonful of oil and come in 3 oz (85 g) packs. Varieties include: Chestnut, Parsley and Thyme, Roasted Hazelnut, Sage and Onion, Stuffing Mix with Bran.

SUGAR

Thoughout this book I have emphasized that we are eating too much sugar – too much sugar from the sugar bowl and too much hidden sugar in the 80 per cent of our diet that is processed. There is still a feeling in some quarters that unrefined brown sugar is to white sugar what wholemeal bread is to white bread, yet current research suggests that *all* sugar is equally likely to promote disease – from dental caries to cancer.

Sugar

Nevertheless, you will probably want to bake a cake occasionally, and not necessarily a sugarless one, so it is probably useful to look at the differences between sugars. There are more nutrients in unrefined sugar than there are in white – minerals in particular – but they are present in very small quantities. We would have to eat a lot of unrefined sugar for the vitamins and minerals in it to make a meaningful contribution to our diet – and that is something we do not want to do.

Brown sugar

From an aesthetic point of view unrefined sugars are much more pleasing than white sugar. They have some character, colour and flavour, and the real unrefined ones have a definite aroma. But all brown sugars are not the same. Most brown and some golden granulated sugars are simply refined white sugars with colour and flavour added.

The real unrefined sugar has been made from raw cane sugar, not beet sugar, and is refined in the country of origin. Billingtons, the producers of this type of quality sugar, have devised a symbol to identify genuine unrefined sugars from the refined alternatives that are in fact white sugars with dye added (see opposite).

Some people would say this is just a marketing ploy, an attempt to get sugar a 'good press', and strictly from a health point of view it might be seen as such, but from the point of view of the cook who wants to use sugar, it is useful to be able to identify a better-quality product. The symbol has now been adopted by *Prewett*'s, *British Home Stores*, *Budgen*, the *Co-op*, *Fine Fare* and, of course, *Billingtons*.

Unrefined sugars

Demerara has the lightest, clear crystals of a large consistent size and a rich aroma. It is named after Demerara, in Guyana, where it is produced.

Muscovado is from Barbados; it is a fine-grained, soft, sticky and dark brown sugar. It is rich in molasses and is tackier

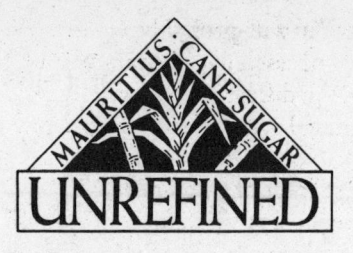

The Billingtons Symbol

than demerara because of this. *Light Muscovado* contains less molasses.

Molasses sugar is also called *Black Barbados* or *Demerara Molasses*; it is stronger in taste than muscovado due to its higher molasses content.

Refined sugars

London demerara is large crystals of white sugar or washed cane sugar, with molasses or syrup added to 'dye' them brown.

Soft, light, golden or dark brown sugar is in fact white or washed cane sugar tossed in molasses, treacle or syrup to replace lost flavour or colour.

Brown coffee crystals are larger white crystals tossed in molasses or in bright synthetic dyes.

Granulated is standard white refined sugar.

Golden granulated has had most of its molasses coating removed, leaving it pale and free flowing.

Caster (or castor) is smaller crystals of granulated sugar.

Icing sugar is powdered granulated sugar with calcium or phosphate added to keep it free flowing.

Cubes are granulated sugar mixed with water and compressed.

Brown cubes are coloured white sugar treated in the same way.

Quick dissolving cubes are less compressed than ordinary cubes.

Preserving sugar is larger crystals of granulated, but with no special benefit over granulated for preserving.

Vanilla sugar is white sugar flavoured with vanilla flavouring.

Sugar

Naturally occurring sugars

These are other names under which sugar often appears on the ingredients panel of foods.

Fructose or fruit sugar is one and a half times sweeter than sucrose (table sugar), so less can be used. It occurs widely in nature, especially in honey, and is metabolized slowly (compared with sucrose), so it is used in diabetic products because it is less disruptive to blood sugar levels.

Glucose is found also in honey, but not in many foods. It is less sweet than sucrose and appears in most foods as glucose syrup.

Sucrose is table sugar manufactured from sugar-cane or beet.

Lactose is milk sugar and only one sixth as sweet as table sugar; it is used in many foods and in some sweeteners.

Maltose is a product of malting barley in beer-making and other processes such as malting grains for bread and flour. It is one third as sweet as sucrose.

Honey – see below.

Syrups

Syrups can be either the by-products of sugar-refining or they can be made from sugars such as glucose.

Cane syrup is made from concentrated cane juice before the sugar is extracted.

Corn syrup is made by treating corn or maize starch with acid, which produces glucose and fructose. It is more used in America in the manufacture of foods.

Golden syrup is a light treacle, being a mixture of refined sugar syrup and invert sugar (produced by splitting sucrose, and used in brewing and food processing).

Glucose syrup can be bought from chemists; it is used to make sweets and in royal icing.

Maple syrup is made from the sap of the maple tree and is a distinctive amber in colour. 'Maple-flavoured syrup' is an imitation of the real thing.

Molasses is a dark black syrupy liquid, in its strongest form in

Sugar

blackstrap molasses, which is the richest in nutrients of refined sugars. Molasses is made from the leftovers of the cane once all the other products have been extracted; it should be treated as other sugars, but stored in a cool place because it is liable to ferment.

Treacle is partially refined syrup with molasses in it which gives it the dark look and liquorice flavour that characterizes gingerbreads.

Malt

This is a by-product of malting barley and is sold in products like *Cookie Malt* in health-food shops as a sweetener for baking. It is free from additives and less sweet than sugar. *Sunwheel* also produce a Barley Malt Syrup.

Honey

Honey is mainly glucose and fructose, both of which are less disruptive to blood sugar levels than sucrose because they are metabolized comparatively slowly, yet they are still sugars. Honey contains about 20 per cent water; it also contains about 180 other substances and some pretty outrageous health claims have been made for it.

There may be minerals and vitamins present, but they are in minute amounts, not large enough to contribute to the nutrients in our food. (Honey should not be eaten in such large amounts that these nutrients contribute significantly to our diet!) Other powers attributed to honey have centred on its pollen content, which is used as a dietary supplement, but although there is an average of four million pollen grains in each one-pound jar, they weigh only one thousandth of an ounce, not enough to be medicinally useful. Similarly, the enzymes contained in honey are present only in very small amounts.

Buying honey
Honey is usually sold as clear (often called liquid) or as set (which is also called crystallized or granulated). If clear honey is dull or

Sugar

cloudy crystallization has begun. This process occurs naturally after the honey is taken from the hive. It is perfectly harmless and to bring the honey back simply stand the jar in hot water. (Commercially produced honey is heat treated to retard crystallization.) Conversely clear honey can be made to crystallize by adding a small amount of crystallized honey to it to 'seed' it.

Honey can replace sugar in baking; it is 20 per cent water, so where a recipe says 8 oz sugar you might want to add 10 oz honey, but for the sake of cutting down on sugar it is better to add only the 8 oz and 'save' yourself 2 oz.

Natural set honey should have a relatively fine grain, but not be too rough, and should be uniform in colour. Liquid on the surface is a sign of fermentation, as is a moist bubbly surface; frosting at the top and sides of the jar occurs where air has been trapped between honey and jar.

Soft-set honey is natural set honey that has been softened, stirred and reset. It should have the characteristics of natural set honey, but with a softer set so that it is always spreadable.

Instead of sugar

You might like to put these items on your shopping list instead of sugar – they give sweetness without the calories and other effects of sugars and honey:

cinnamon, cloves or mixed spices add sweetness to cooked apples
cinnamon sweetens rhubarb
chopped nuts and dried fruits sweeten cooked fruits and baked foods
grated orange rinds
no-added-sugar jams, marmalades and fruit purées, – especially purées of dried fruits – can be used as sweeteners
some herbs, for example, lemon thyme, angelica, cicely
vanilla pods
date sugar, made from ground cooked dates
orange and lemon oils and vanilla essence.

Artificial sweeteners

Having read all about the disadvantages of sugar in Chapter 1, you may be looking for other ways of adding sweetness, and you may be tempted by sweetening tablets (used in hot drinks) and powders (for sprinkling on cereals, etc.).

Before you add them to the shopping list, however, do have a think about the fact that they do nothing to re-educate our taste away from sweet things. They just encourage the British sweet tooth. If the reason for using them is to lose weight, then there is even more incentive to change your eating habits rather then switching to another method of satisfying the desire for sweet things.

So let's now take a look at artificial sweeteners and see if they do have anything to offer.

Saccharin

This is the most established of the sweeteners. It is a coal-tar derivative and has had a stormy past. It was given the 'all clear' for food use in America before their stringent testing procedures for food additives came into force, and since then it has been subject of much controversy. The current position in Britain is that the Food Additives and Contaminants Committee began to study all sweeteners five years ago and produced a report in 1982 which permitted saccharin, pending completion of new studies.

Cyclamate

This is an artificial additive that was banned in Britain in the 1970s after it had been banned in the US. The ban has been challenged but upheld.

Aspartame

This is the newest sweetener, permitted in Britain in 1983 after extensive testing. It is 200 times sweeter than sucrose and tastes similar. It is virtually calorie-free and has been described as a 'natural' sweetener because it is a compound of two amino acids (aspartic acid and phenylalanine). *Canderel*, the commercial aspartame product, does, however, contain additives: an anti-caking agent called silicon dioxide and lactose (milk sugar), plus leucine (another amino acid) and cruscarmellose sodium A, a thickening agent. It is not suitable for baking.

Controversy surrounded the launch of Canderel (available as tablets and powder) because high doses are dangerous for people with phetylketonuria, which means they cannot metabolize the amino acid phenylalanine, and build-up in the brain results in mental retardation. About a million people in Britain have this problem.

Aspartame is also used commercially in soft drinks and other manufactured good under the name of *Nutrasweet*.

Acesulfame K
This is a non-nutritive artificial sweetener made by Hoechst and approved for use in the UK in 1983, at the same time as Aspartame. It is chemically similar to saccharin and its main use is in manufactured food and drink; it also appears in some table-top sweeteners. It is 200 times sweeter than sugar.

Thaumatin
This is a naturally occurring protein found in the West African katemfe fruit; it is said to be 2,000–3,000 times sweeter than sugar. The trade name is Talin. At the moment it is used only in manufactured foods.

So far I have seen no adverse reports of either acesulfame K or Talin.

What's What in Sugar Substitutes

Bisks Slim Sweet	saccharin
Boots Shapers	saccharin
Canderel	aspartame
Diamin	acesulfame K
Hermesetas	saccharin
Hermesetas Gold	acesulfame K
Natrena	saccharin with flavour enhancers
Saxin	saccharin

Sucron	saccharin
Sweet 'n Low	saccharin and sugar
Sweetex	saccharin
Sweetex Plus	saccharin plus acesulfame K

> **My choice**
>
> I don't add sugar or sweeteners to drinks or fruit or breakfast cereal – I have found it easy to adapt to taking these without sugar. In cooking I use a good-quality unrefined sugar, where necessary, in small amounts, or I use clear honey. Whichever you choose, you need less than when using regular sugar.

SUPERMARKETS AND HIGH-STREET STORES

The following is a brief guide to the ways in which the various supermarkets and high-street chains may be helpful to you when you are shopping for health.

It is impossible to make direct comparisons because they differ considerably. For example, Boots has taken an interest in healthy eating but is primarily a chemist, and although Marks & Spencer is an especially useful port of call for the shopper who wants really fresh produce, it is not exclusively a food store. Similarly, it is very difficult to generalize about the Co-op because it varies regionally.

It is interesting to note that supermarkets have for a long time kept the cost of food down by the use of food additives, which make cheaper ingredients possible, and now, under pressure from shoppers, they are having to reverse the trend – remove the additives and go for higher-quality ingredients.

Some of the stores do not have own-label products, e.g. ASDA, so they cannot be included in the table on p. 397, and there are brands which are sold in a wide variety of independent shops, such as Mace, Spar and VG.

Supermarkets and High-street Stores

How fresh?

The Egon Ronay Lucas Guide 1986 put supermarkets to the test over the freshness of their produce and concluded, after visiting representative stores from each chain in different parts of the country, that more information on freshness should be given to the shopper, through better datestamping and by telling shoppers which of the apparently fresh foods had been frozen beforehand. Only *Sainsbury's* and *Safeway* marked their goods 'Do not freeze – previously frozen' where appropriate. Improvements were also needed in the presentation of fresh fish.

The store to come out top for freshest food was *Marks & Spencer*. Egon Ronay's findings, not surprisingly, coincided with those of this book – that *Marks & Spencer* has created a range of fresh foods that reflect the current trend towards healthier eating and help the shopper attain this, especially in the area of fresh, ready-prepared salads and recipe dishes.

In another survey by the *Sunday Express Magazine*, headed by Robert Carrier, more than 500 items were tasted in twenty-two food categories from the major food chains and here *Waitrose* came out top for value for money, but *Marks & Spencer* were top for quality.

The Carrier team also points to the supermarkets' and *M & S* filled sandwiches and packaged lunch salads, which offer office workers a healthy alternative to most of the instant meals and snacks available.

Bejam

Bejam Freezer Food Centres have their own 'Healthy Eating' campaign running through 1986 and has analysed the diets of 4,000 customers, giving them advice on healthy eating.

Areas of special interest are:

Bejam poultry is free from polyphosphates
their Golden Baked range is free from colourings
Bejam Premium Pork sausages are additive-free
a growing number of Bejam ready meals including Chilli con Carne,

Supermarket Guide	Boots	Fine Fare	Gateway (International)	Harrods	Marks & Spencer	Safeway	Sainsbury's	Superquinn (Ireland)	Tesco	Waitrose
(These products are not necessarily available at all branches.)										
Free-range eggs				✓	✓	✓	✓	✓	✓	✓
Organically grown fruit/veg				✓		✓	✓	✓		✓
Fresh fruit juicing facilities				✓ juice bar			✓	✓		
Wet fish		✓	✓	✓		✓	✓	✓	✓	✓
Additive-free fresh pasta						✓				✓
Own Label										
Additive-free ready meals				✓	✓	✓				✓
Vegetarian ready meals	✓			not own label	✓	✓	✓		✓ not own brand	✓
Additive-free frozen meals					✓	✓				
Fresh pre-washed salads					✓	✓				✓
Vegetarian cheese					✓	✓	✓		✓	✓
Reduced-sugar jams	✓									
No-added-sugar jams					✓					
Low-fat cheese							✓			
Fruit canned in natural juice		✓				✓	✓			
Vegetables canned without salt						✓	✓			
Additive-free wholemeal bakery products	✓				✓	✓	✓	✓	✓	✓
Health-food sections	✓					✓			✓	
Additive-free (etc.) foods lists					✓					
Additive-free fish-fingers						✓	✓		✓	✓
Additive-free wholemeal pizzas						✓	✓			✓

* Organic (hormone-free) meat will probably soon be available in some high-street shops, with Boots Food Centres rumoured to be among the first to take it.

Supermarkets and High-street Stores

Meat Lasagne, Beef Stew and Dumplings, Fish Lasagne and Fish Pie are additive-free

their smoked trout and mackerel fillets are free from artificial colouring.

Boots

Boots was one of the first high-street chains to launch its own-label high-fibre range of products (under the *Second Nature* label). The most recent additions have been additive-free wholemeal bakery goods in the Boots shops with Food Centres – the range even includes an excellent wholemeal doughnut!

Areas of special interest are:

Boots wholemeal bakery range

Boots own-label range of long-life vegetarian ready meals

Boots range of cereal mixes and soya vegetarian mixes for convenience vegetarian meals

Boots canned bean and pulse range

health-food sections in many Boots stores which also sell a selection of non-Boots brands

health-education leaflets with advice on diet and free computerized diet analysis for a limited period, both in store and by use of postal leaflets

more than 65 per cent of their 450 lines are additive-free; Boots aims to remove additives from many of the remainder and avoid them in new products.

Co-op

Although there are regional variations, the Co-operative Wholesale Society has produced an *Eat Right, Eat Well* healthy-eating campaign and taken initiatives in nutrition labelling and food additives. There is an advice centre for customers and in-store information leaflets:

nutrition labelling has been introduced in conjunction with a Consumer Care logo and the aim is that this will be on all 1,500 own-brand foods by the end of 1987

high, medium and low statements on products for fat, protein, carbohydrate and fibre content have been introduced with high = over 10 g per 100 g, medium = 3–10 g/100 g, low = up to 3 g/100 g

all additives in own-label products are under review with a view to minimizing or removing them
low-fat sausages, cheese and other own-label foods
the intention is to introduce more high-fibre, low-fat, low-sugar foods.

Fine Fare

Fine Fare are trying out free-range eggs and fresh juicing facilities in their stores. They have fifty-seven stores with wet-fish counters and in-store bakeries producing loaves made from Allinson's stoneground flour.

Harrods

Harrods has an extensive range of healthy-eating accoutrements in its basement Pantry, with a wide range of brands.

Areas of special interest are:

the Pantry, with its range of 'health-food' goods
the bakery section, with an extensive range of wholemeal and wholegrain breads and baked goods, including organic unwrapped wholemeal bread
own-brand range of cereals, dried fruits, seeds and nuts
large selection of 'real' additive-free cheeses
free-range eggs, both poultry and game
a wide range of low-fat game and lean-meat cuts in Food Halls
fresh-fish hall where farmed fish sold have not been fed with dye-containing food
additive-free vegetarian ready meals from the frosted-food department.

Iceland frozen food centres

Like many other stores, Iceland now has a policy of removing additives from own-label products 'wherever possible', and has a free booklet, 'An Iceland Guide to Additives', that gives a brief explanation of additives and a guide to Iceland's additive-free products.

Areas of special interest are:

Supermarkets and High-street Stores

'Family Favourites' such as fish-fingers, pizzas and beefburgers that are free from artificial preservatives, colourings and flavourings

additive-free ice lollies

special symbols on pack fronts for at-a-glance identification of additive-free items.

Marks & Spencer

Marks & Spencer are unique in selling only own-label foods. It has always been their policy to avoid food additives and promote fresh foods by use of a highly controlled chilled chain of supply. By controlling strictly areas such as preparation and chilled distribution M & S are enabled to avoid additives in foods where other stores might use them. Listing products is difficult because they change on a regular basis, especially their ready meals and chilled recipe dishes. However, lists of foods for special requirements – e.g. additive-free or sugar-free meals – are drawn up each three months by the Customer Service Department and given, on request, to customers to enable them to shop for their special dietary needs.

Areas of special interest are:

the *Lite* range of low-fat dairy produce which uses the 'natural' sweetener aspartame instead of sugar

free-range eggs

free-range poultry

strict pesticide and residue analysis of all fruit and vegetables is carried out by M & S on a regular basis

all sources of supply are visited, be they Birmingham or Brazil, and strict specifications are laid down

free-range poultry are available; the feedstuff is specified by M & S and has been hormone-free for twenty years; other drugs are not allowed, except against coccidiosis

a wide range of wholemeal bread and bakery products – but none is entirely free from additives

vegetarian recipe dishes available, as well as special additive-free vegetable recipe dishes

Calorie Counted Recipe Dishes are additive-free, and some are vegetarian

Supermarkets and High-street Stores

vegetarian rennet cheese is used in vegetarian dishes
wide range of ready-prepared salads which are free from additives
ready-prepared salad meals: ready-washed vegetables together with dips and cold meats/fish
freshly squeezed orange juice also sold, not made from concentrates.

Safeway

Safeway has, in some branches, a Natural Foods section which offers 'health-food' branded products. They also regularly sell organic vegetables and have a programme of customer health education through free booklets on subjects such as food additives. Safeway was the first supermarket chain to come out with a 'hit list' of fifty-one additives which it is removing from its products (see Chapter 2).

Areas of special interest are:

organically grown fruit and vegetables
Safeway's own range of canned fruits in natural juices and vegetables canned without added salt
own-label wholemeal flours, brown rice, pasta, etc.
wide range of pulses and cereals, as well as ethnic foods from Mexico, China, the Middle East, etc.
special low-fat foods for children, i.e. fat-reduced crisps and low-fat sausages
vegetarian cheese
a range of additive-free delicatessen items, including Indian savouries such as samosas and *bhajis*
a gluten-free symbol is being used on their own-label products
first supermarket chain with their own range of no-added-sugar jam and marmalade.

Sainsbury's

Sainsbury's is another chain of supermarkets working on the reduction of use of food additives in its products and has given priority to food items frequently used by children; they have introduced *Mr Men* 100 per cent natural yoghurts (some have sugar) and tartrazine-free ice-cream, as well as a fruit squash with a high juice content. They also offer, on request, extensive listings of food free of MSG, artificial colouring, preservatives, and foods needed for special diets – gluten-free, lactose-free, etc. They are currently investigating organic vegetables. Additives in 3,000 own-label products are under review.

Areas of special interest are:

comprehensive nutritional labelling
a range of low-fat dairy produce, such as cheeses, yoghurt and cream. They were the first with the low-fat skimmed milk, Vita Pint, with added solids to enhance the flavour
free-range eggs
free-range poultry
wide range of wholemeal breads
own-label wholemeal pizzas and flans
about to launch new exotic additions to fruits canned in their own juice, also vegetables canned without salt
a microprotein pie – made by the action of micro-organisms
in some stores, facilities for the fresh juicing of oranges
Mr Men range of additive-free yoghurts for children
tartrazine-free ice-cream
Hi-juice orange squash with 50 per cent orange-juice content (does contain sulphur dioxide)
fish-fingers with no additives
all breaded Sainsbury products are free from colouring
free information leaflet, 'A Healthy Look at Sainsbury's Labels', outlining the role of additives, and explaining nutritional terms and labelling
healthy-eating cookbooks.

Superquinn

(Ireland)

Superquinn have not introduced health items on their own label, Thrift, but there are other areas in the stores that are of interest:

free-range eggs in most branches, in the fruit-and-vegetable section
organically grown vegetables available, but supply varies seasonally
fresh juicing facilities in most fruit-and-vegetable departments – mainly orange juice

in-store bakeries producing a wide range of wholemeal and high-fibre, additive-free breads

wet-fish counters in all branches; the emphasis is on sea fish, but when farmed fish are used, they try to obtain those not fed flesh dyes.

Superdrug

This is mainly a chemist but they have entered the healthy snack market and stock health books. Superdrug usually stocks products like soya milk and juices, decaffeinated coffee, cereals, skimmed milk, cereal bars, wholewheat crisps, etc.

Tesco

Tesco was the first supermarket chain to launch their own comprehensive nutritional labelling. They have a range of free leaflets in a series on healthy eating which are linked with the nutritional labelling and give useful and sound information.

Areas of special interest are:

in-store bakeries producing wholemeal products with several new items planned

fish-fingers now free from additives

all but three own-label biscuits use only natural colouring; antioxidants are also being removed from own-label biscuits

vegetarian cheese available, loose or prepacked

vegetarian ready meals are stocked, but none of those under their own label is vegetarian or free from additives.

Waitrose

In common with other stores, Waitrose has been removing additives from its products and now has a hundred own-label additive-free lines – and more using only 'natural additives'. They have extensive lists of information on own-label products that are free from additives, lactose, suitable for vegetarians, suitable for vegans, etc., on request to the Customer Services Department, to help shoppers with special dietary needs with their shopping.

Supermarkets and High-street Stores

Areas of special interest are:

a wide range of additive-free wholemeal breads and bakery goods, including organically produced wholemeal bread

organically grown vegetables available in a pilot scheme in some branches

their fresh fish are not fed flesh dyes

virtually all ready meals, fresh and frozen, are free from additives

free-range eggs available

additive-free fish-fingers, jams, ketchups, soups, biscuits, etc., among their own-label lines.

> **My choice**
>
> There is no supermarket where you can do all your shopping – or at least that is what I find. For preference I shop for organic fruit and vegetables at a local supplier and then use either Marks & Spencer, Waitrose or Safeway, supplemented by a fishmongers and an organic butcher, plus a health-food shop for other items such as tofu, shoyu sauce, agar agar, some nuts, rice and pulses, and dried fruit without preservatives.
>
> There is an excellent range of fresh foods at M & S, but you would need to travel further afield for items such as olive oil, flour, etc., making Waitrose, Sainsbury's, etc., a better bet for all-round shopping.

TAHINI
See PEANUT BUTTER.

TAKEAWAYS

Nearly a quarter of all the money spent on food outside the home is spent on takeaway meals. Although as a nation the latest Gallup Poll shows we are actually eating out less often, we are 'eating out' at home *more* often.

According to Gallup, many people buy a takeaway meal once a week, often to eat while watching a video. If you are a takeaway buyer how can you make sure that you are getting good health

Takeaways

value for money, since it seems that takeaway meals are particularly high in salt and fat?

A lot, it seems, depends on where you buy your takeaways. Researchers at Leeds University have shown that there are differences in fat content in different parts of the country. In the south, the polyunsaturate content of meals is higher than in the north; portion size varies too, not just between areas, but also from season to season – you get more chips when you buy in June than you do in December!

Some studies have shown that the amount of fat in chips varies according to the method of cooking. Double frying (par-frying followed by finish-frying just before serving) results in fattier chips than those cooked just once. But the Leeds survey showed a negative relationship between the percentage of fat and the portion size; the fat only increased by 50 per cent when the portion size doubled. Chip fans will be glad to know that the least fat is found in thicker-cut chips.

There is also a difference between chips and fries. You not only get a lot more potato in a portion of chips as opposed to the slim, sophisticated fries, but you get a lot less fat, too. In the north, fries tend to be thicker than in London, but in London chip portions are bigger than in Leeds.

There is a higher ratio of polyunsaturated fats getting into our takeaways these days, but not because they are becoming more health conscious. It seems the salads served with burgers are raising the levels of polyunsaturated fat because of the salad dressings. Although this might sound good on paper the takeaway burger meal is still very high in fat.

For a lower-fat takeaway you might be better off with some ethnic dishes. Indian food in particular offers lower fat, especially if you choose the rice and bread dishes and some of the salads and fresh relishes. However, although you are getting *less* fat in Indian and Chinese food, Italian pizzas and Greek kebabs and pitta breads and salads, you are getting *more* salt.

Takeaways could be healthier if the sodium was reduced in ethnic meals in particular and if the batter on fish was reformulated so that it did not soak up so much fat.

Takeaways

The following analyses from the Leeds University research shows the fat content of typical takeaways. It also gives a polyunsaturated/saturated fat ratio for each meal.

Chinese Meals

Item	Source	Fat per portion (g)	Kcals (MJ) per portion	Energy from fat (%)	P/S ratio
Sweet and sour	Leeds	48.2	1,232 (5.15)	35	.37
pork with rice	London	59.1	1,456 (6.09)	37	.85
Beef chow mein	Leeds	29.5	646 (2.70)	41	.76
with noodles	London	24.9	570 (2.38)	39	1.45
Chicken and					
mushroom	Leeds	26.7	774 (3.24)	31	.66
with rice	London	27.2	876 (3.66)	28	1.18
Chicken fried	Leeds	30.4	866 (3.62)	32	.63
rice	London	22.8	751 (3.14)	27	.83
Prawn chop	Leeds	15.2	643 (2.69)	21	1.15
suey	London	16.4	769 (3.21)	19	1.35
Pancake roll	Leeds	14.8	249 (1.04)	53	.33
	London	11.4	208 (0.87)	49	1.57

Indian Meals

	Source	Fat per portion (g)	Kcals (MJ) per portion	Energy from fat (%)	P/S ratio
Lamb bhuna	London	46.5	1,000 (4.18)	42	1.05
Meat curry	Leeds	42.5	910 (3.80)	41	.53
Chicken biriani	London	41.4	973 (4.07)	37	.99
Chicken curry	Leeds	37.8	852 (3.56)	39	.54
Vegetable					
curry	London	34.1	834 (1.81)	36	1.85
Tandoori					
chicken	London	21.7	737 (3.08)	25	.63
Chicken tikka	London	17.0	686 (2.87)	22	.51

Note: Each meal includes a portion of rice.

Takeaways

Italian Meals

	Source	Fat per portion (%)	Kcals (MJ) per portion	Energy from fat (%)	P/S ratio
Lasagne	Leeds	33.4	679 (2.91)	43	.15
Spaghetti bolognese	Leeds	21.6	742 (3.10)	26	.34
Canneloni	Leeds	37.9	713 (2.98)	47	.27
Spaghetti supreme	Chain London	11.3	512 (2.14)	19	.63

Greek Meals

	Source	Fat per portion (%)	Kcals (MJ) per portion	Energy from fat (%)	P/S ratio
Doner kebab with salad and pitta bread	Leeds	21.2	442 (1.78)	42	.12
	London	50.1	790 (3.26)	57	.07
Kofte kebab with salad and pitta bread	Leeds	14.5	355 (1.42)	36	.16
	London	23.9	510 (2.08)	41	.16
Shish kebab with salad and pitta bread	Leeds	8.1	288 (1.14)	25	.26
	London	14.5	416 (1.68)	31	.22

Note: The data for these tables was collected in 1983–4; some chains, for example Wimpey, have since switched to the use of more unsaturated oils.
Source: J. Pascoe, J. Dockerty and J. Ryley, British Nutrition Foundation Annual Conference 1985.

Note on the tables
The COMA recommendation for the polyunsaturated/saturated fat ratio in the diet (not individual foods) is 0.45, so any foods with less than 0.45 in the last column of the tables will have a polyunsaturates/saturates ratio of less than 0.45:1 and so will not meet COMA requirements. If a large percentage of your daily food comes from takeaways, the rest of your diet would have to be very low in fat (particularly in saturated fat) to achieve the

Takeaways

COMA recommendations. Although COMA has set a target of 0.45:1 polyunsaturate/saturate ratio, some people believe that we should be aiming for a ratio of 1:1, in order to lower our blood levels of saturated fat, since by adulthood they are usually too high.

TEA

Tea is Britain's favourite drink. About half the liquid we drink is tea and most of it is drunk with milk and sugar, which that adds up to a hefty whack of fats and calories during the year. By switching to skimmed milk in hot drinks and by gradually cutting down and eliminating the sugar you can save lots of calories in the long-term, and reap the benefits of having less sugar and fat in the diet.

Like coffee, tea is a stimulant. An average six-ounce teacup will contain 50–60 mg of caffeine (compared with 100–120 mg in the same amount of coffee), and most of us drink tea by the mugful, not the cupful! Tea is also acidic and may cause indigestion in susceptible people because of its tannin content (in the form of tannic acid), although the Tea Council says that this acidity helps stimulate the digestive juices (which caffeine also tends to do). This may be acceptable, perhaps, after a meal, but if tea is drunk more frequently it will be a constant source of stimulation. (Impossibly large amounts would have to be drunk for the tannin content to be actually toxic.)

Tea has also been linked with constipation and it can inhibit the absorption of iron from our food, so it's not surprising that anaemia and constipation are common British health problems! That said, tea does have certain advantages over sugary or additive-laden soft drinks and over very milky sweet drinks. But it should be treated with respect!

Its strength will determine the level of caffeine and tannin it contains. There is a difference between the way caffeine in tea and caffeine in coffee acts: the release of caffeine in tea is gradual, giving a stimulating effect about 15 minutes after a cuppa, whereas the effect of coffee is almost instantaneous.

In Britain we drink mostly blends of black tea from India, Sri Lanka (which in the tea world is still referred to as Ceylon tea) and East Africa and these are higher in tannins than the green teas which are more popular in China and Japan. Green tea undergoes fewer treatments than black tea and is usually drunk very weak and without milk, so large amounts can be drunk without the same effect (or side-effects).

Twinings, one of the biggest speciality tea producers, give the following figures for the three types of leaf used in their teas:

Leaf type	Caffeine content of dry leaf (%)
Green (gunpowder)	1.9–2.2
Oolong	2.4–2.7
Black	3–4

When buying speciality teas, do read the description on the label beneath the name of the tea, because even though it might say, for example, Darjeeling, it could be a 'blend from various sources' and not genuine Darjeeling from the foot of the Himalayas – far more Darjeeling is sold each year than is produced there.

Green tea

This is packed at the beginning of the season. All tea is picked from the tips of the plant where two leaves and a bud form. The tea is steamed to kill enzymes (which are responsible for many of the chemical changes that turn green tea into black tea) and the leaves are then rolled and fired.

Oolong tea

This is mainly from south-east China and from Taiwan. The freshly plucked tea is withered and dried for some hours after being picked, and then rolled by machine to release the enzymes. Oxidation/fermentation then follows for a short period and the colour changes to copper; it is then fired. The taste is 'half-way' between that of green tea and black tea.

Tea

Black tea

This is plucked, withered and rolled like Oolong, but the fermentation is longer, after which the leaves are dried to stop the enzyme activity which is responsible for the production of a kind of varnish that coats the leaves, making them black and giving the tea its aroma.

Be ... BOP

When taking the wrappers off some packets of tea, you may have noticed the letters BOP printed on it, which refers to the quality or grade of tea. There are two basic grades: leaf grade and broken grade. The leaf grades are called:

    Orange Pekoe (OP)
    Pekoe (Pek)
    Flowery Pekoe (FP)

The broken grades are called:

    Broken Orange Pekoe (BOP)
    Broken Pekoe (BP)
    Fannings
    Dust

In the majority of tea we drink, the broken grades are mixed with leaf grades. The fannings and dust go into tea-bags to make instant tea and the top-quality leaf grades go to make speciality teas.

Decaffeinated tea

Two companies are now producing decaffeinated tea. The Health and Diet Food Company, Godalming, Surrey, are importers of Luaka Pure Ceylon Tea and they now have *Luaka Decaffeinated Tea* available in tea-bags. It has less than 0.2 per cent caffeine and is also low in tannin.

St James's Tea produces decaffeinated tea-bags in packs of eighty which have 15 per cent less caffeine than regular tea. They are available by mail order, minimum order two packs, from St James's Tea, Sir John Lynon House, Upper Thames Street, London EC4V 3PA (telephone 01-236 0611).

Alternatives

Rooibosch

Rooibosch tea is harvested in South Africa from a legume called *Aspalathus linearis*. It grows wild and is cultivated on the Cederberg mountains at the Cape. It is completely caffeine-free and has a very low tannin content, between 1 and 4 per cent, compared with around 12 per cent in Indian teas. It also contains vitamin C and, like tea, a wide range of minerals. It is sold in health-food shops.

Maté tea (or matte)

This has more caffeine than other herb teas and less than ordinary black tea, although some analyses fail to show any caffeine. The tannin content of maté is low (similar to Rooibosch). The tea is made from the dried, smoked and crushed leaves of a South American holly tree called *Ilex paraguayensis*. It is also high in minerals.

Herb tea

Herb teas are usually free from caffeine and tannin. There is controversy about just how much caffeine and tannin is in them, but the amounts will be small compared with regular tea and coffee. Some brands will be free from both and may state this on the label. It really depends on the plant or substance from which the tea is made.

There is a wide selection of herb tea available for everyday drinking and some of the most popular ones are: chamomile, peppermint, fennel, mixed fruits, rosehip and nettle. There are others that are used for specific problems such as migraine or circulation problems or during pregnancy; these include comfrey, feverfew, raspberry leaf, buckwheat and ginseng teas.

Blends of fruit teas are popular and they often go under names such as 'Goodnight', or 'After Meal', or 'Reviver', rather than the name of the ingredients. There are far too many herb teas and suppliers to list, but a visit to a health-food shop or wholefood shop, or even a herbalist if you live near one, will reveal a wide range. Give them a try to find one that you enjoy for everyday drinking, to make at least some of the drinks you take during the day of the non-stimulatory type!

> **My choice**
>
> The new decaffeinated teas from Luaka and St James's Tea are the ones I choose to drink during the day. For evening and after meals I prefer jasmine and Japanese green tea and China tea – all without milk.

TOFU

Tofu has been keeping the Japanese and Chinese healthy for centuries, and is an ingredient of many health-food substitutes for standard products. It is a high-protein and low-fat food, and can be used as a basis for savoury and sweet dishes, although in the East it is used exclusively as a savoury food.

It is made by coagulating soya milk into a curd and draining off the water, in the same way that we make cheese from dairy milk, and is sold in health-food shops in small blocks which are prepacked and can be used in oriental-style stir-fry dishes, or can be made into burgers, cheesecakes, etc. It has very little flavour, so it is versatile. It is also useful for making low-calorie salad dressings.

It is mostly sold as long-life product in vacuum packs or in cartons; fresh-chilled vacuum packs of plain and smoked tofu are also available from British manufacturers. Once open, tofu will keep in the fridge for about seven days if stored in chilled water which is changed daily.

Morinaga silken tofu is imported from Japan. It is a long-life product, sold in a carton, pasteurized, but free from preservatives.

Tofeata is available from *Hera*, and is vacuum-packed in a pouch inside a carton endorsed by the Chinese chef Ken Lo. The pack has several recipe ideas to get you started if tofu is new to you.

Cauldron Foods sell vacuum-packed tofu with a long shelf-life. It is packed in see-through pouches inside and is available plain or smoked.

Paul's Tofu is another chilled and vacuum-packed product in a see-through container.

> **My choice**
>
> I think Morinaga has a 'long-life' taste and I prefer Cauldron Foods tofu, but none of these products taste like freshly made tofu, which has a subtle and slightly sweet and nutty flavour. Much more interesting to Western tastebuds is smoked tofu.

VEGETABLE JUICE
See under FRUIT JUICE.

VEGETABLES
See CANNED FRUIT and VEGETABLES, FRESH FRUIT and VEGETABLES and FROZEN FOODS.

VINEGAR

In England the most popular form of vinegar is malt vinegar; the Scots prefer distilled malt vinegar and in the south-west of England cider vinegar predominates. In France and Italy wine vinegar is more popular.

Real vinegar is made in three stages. The first involves brewing and fermenting the malt barley (or cider or wine) the second is a controlled fermentation to turn it into vinegar and the third is a slow maturation to produce the characteristic flavours.

Real-vinegar brewers have recently started a campaign to alert us to the use of 'non-brewed condiment essence' which is a chemical by-product of refining crude oil. It is, they say, diluted and used in fish and chip shops as vinegar, but not labelled as such; simply put on the counters in unmarked dispensers. We are unlikely to come across this substance in the shops.

Vinegar

When buying vinegar, we need to know which is the right one for our particular requirements. Most of the malt and distilled malt vinegars are very harsh and acidic, and are a disaster in salad dressings. They are cheap, but they have no subtlety of flavour. For salad dressings it is better to buy wine vinegars, cider vinegars or speciality herb vinegars which are much more pleasant, though they still have to conform to the legal requirements that vinegar must have a level of 4 per cent acidity.

There is a wealth of speciality vinegars available, too many to list here, but one particularly useful range is from *Martlet*, part of the Merrydown Wine Company. It includes cider vinegar, red and white wine vinegar and a raspberry vinegar made from pure crushed raspberries and red wine vinegar. There are also other flavoured vinegars in the range – garlic and tarragon, and a high-strength cider vinegar, complete with a sachet of pickling spices, for home pickling. *Dufrais* is another company that offers a wide range of wine and cider vinegars, plus speciality herb and other vinegars.

WATER

To many people it seems a waste of money to buy bottled water when we have good drinking water 'on tap', but there are several reasons why some people prefer bottled water.

- One is to avoid fluoride if it is added to the water in the area in which you live. The safety of fluoride is a controversial subject and one beyond the scope of this book.
- Allergies to tap water are not as uncommon as might be thought.
- The taste of tap water in some areas can be quite unpleasant, and mineral water is usually a more pleasant drink. It has diffused slowly through the earth where it has been naturally filtered and can taste much better than tap water, especially if you live near the water works where the chlorine, etc., is added, because your water will taste stronger than that of someone at

the end of the chain of supply, where the chemicals will have had a chance to diffuse out.
- In old houses, lead piping may result in higher than acceptable lead levels in the drinking water.
- Bottled water also makes a better-tasting cup of tea or coffee, but this is an extravagance and a water filter is probably more economical here.

This list may seem a bit hypochondriacal to some readers, but water should be our main drink for quenching thirst, so it is important to be happy with it. If we like it we will drink more of it and less of the sugary or sweet soft drinks that we might otherwise be tempted by.

Bottled water

Bottled water is available either still or sparkling – for quenching thirst and everyday drinking the still versions are more useful.

Natural spa water is considered to be water from a well or spring 'acknowledged by the medical profession to have therapeutic properties'. It must be bottled without treatment other than filtration, it can be either still or sparkling.

New Natural Mineral Water Regulations came into force in February 1986, bringing bottled water in the UK under stricter control, in line with the rest of Europe. The following is an explanation of the terms used on the labels of bottled water.

Still waters

'Natural Mineral Water' is the best water, that has passed tests designed to standardize the composition of bottled waters. To have earned the 'Natural Mineral Water' label the company bottling the water has had to submit papers about the surrounding terrain and show how it is protecting the water from pollution. It will have had to give analyses of the chemical constituents of the water and microbiological analyses too, to comply with limits set down for metal contamination (which tap water also has to do). Filtering, decanting and bottling also come under close scrutiny under the regulations; sterilization of the water is not allowed.

Water

Criticism has been made of the absence of specific tests for pesticide levels in bottled waters and for the levels of nitrites and nitrates washed into the waterways from the chemical fertilizers used on farm land. These pollutants are finding their way into tap water, which is why some people are turning to bottled water, and it is therefore argued that the new legislation should have required specific tests for these chemicals to make sure that they do not find their way into bottled mineral water.

Sparkling water

'Naturally Carbonated Natural Mineral Water' is the phrase to look out for on the labels of sparkling mineral waters. This means that the water is naturally fizzy and has got its fizz underground – it has not been carbonated artificially. If the water has been 'enhanced' with added bubbles after being brought above ground it will bear the legend 'Natural Mineral Water Fortified with Gas from the Spring' – in this case the carbon dioxide used will have to come from the same source as the water. If the water is totally artificially carbonated it will be called 'Carbonated Natural Mineral Water'. In some cases the bottlers might want to remove some of the sparkle from the water and if they do this after it has been brought above ground the water will be described as 'Natural Mineral Water Partially Decarbonized', which means that some of the carbon dioxide has been removed.

Health claims

Claims about properties relating to the prevention, treatment or cure of health problems have now been outlawed; only strictly controlled clauses may be used, such as:

'low mineral content' – contains less than 500 mg/l inorganic residues
'very low mineral content' – contains less than 50 mg/l inorganic residues
'rich in mineral salts' – contains more than 1,500 mg/l
'contains bicarbonates' – more than 600 mg/l
'contains sulphate' – more than 200 mg/l
'contains chloride' – more than 200 mg/l
'contains calcium' – more than 150 mg/l

'contains magnesium' – more than 50 mg/l
'contains fluoride' – more than 1 mg/l
'contains iron' – more than 1 mg/l
'acidic' – contains 250 mg/l free carbon dioxide
'contains sodium' – more than 200 mg/l
'suitable for low-sodium diet' – contains less than 20 mg/l.

Which to buy

There are many brands of water available and choice will depend on your personal needs or taste (see above). Buying large 2 litre bottles (for still water) is cheaper, but only if you use it within two weeks of opening. Sparkling water will keep for about one week if the lid is tightly replaced.

A fascinating guide to the world's mineral waters is *The Good Water Guide* by Maureen and Timothy Green, published by Rosendale Press, 140 Rosendale Road, Dulwich SE21 8LG.

Water plus

Some new products are now appearing based on mineral water with a small amount of added fruit juice. One such is called *Piermont* – it is a sparkling mineral water with added apple juice; it is free from additives and is made by the Taunton Cider Co. Another is *Wells (Drinks) Cwm Dale* Sparkling Water with natural lemon flavour.

Perrier have introduced Perrier with a Twist, with natural essence of lime or lemon added to the naturally carbonated water. No sugar or additives are used.

> **My choice**
>
> For still water, I prefer Malvern, Evian and Volvic, and for sparkling occasions I choose Perrier, Spa or Badoit.

WINE

Wine labels can tell you a lot about the quality of the wine you are buying. They can tell you about the type of grape used, the area in which the wine was made, the amount of alcohol in the wine, the year it was made, whether it is a vintage wine, or has any other 'grading' ... What they don't tell you is whether there are any chemical additives, or whether any have been used in the making of the wine.

Wine is only covered by the general food and drink laws that say a manufacturer must not add to food anything which is harmful and no more than the specified amount of some of the additives that are used in the UK.

Additives in wine

Complex EEC regulations do regulate the additives used, but they do not make the wine producer state what has been used on the label. The wine you drink could contain any of twenty permitted additives. For example, sour grapes may be de-acidified with potassium tartrate, potassium bicarbonate or calcium carbonate – and there are lots of other additives

tartaric acid and citric acid may be used to improve flavours; citric acid is also used as a stabilizer
sugar may be used to increase alcoholic strength
sulphur can be added to kill bacteria and slow yeast activity
sorbic acid can be added to slow yeast
diammonium phosphate, ammonium sulphate and thiamin hydrochloride can be used to encourage yeast activity
potassium bitartrate and metatartaric acid are used to precipitate tartaric acid
tannins are used to preserve red wine
some sparkling wines are made by adding carbon dioxide to still wine.

Additives are also used during the processing of the wine. So if you don't know what's in the wine you are drinking and the makers or importers can't tell you, there is one way of avoiding them and that is to buy organically produced wine. This will also have the

Wine

advantage of being made from grapes that are grown to organic standards, because as well as the additives in the wine, other wines may carry over chemical residues from modern methods of viniculture.

France is the country that produces the most organic wines, products that have earned the legend *'Nature et Progrès'* these wines often carry a collar on the bottle to denote their organic origins along with the *'Nature et Progrès'* symbol. You are unlikely to find this wine in the supermarket or off-licence; specialist health shops do carry some, but most has to be ordered from suppliers.

Organic suppliers

The Organic Food Co. Ltd, PO Box 463, Portslade, Sussex BN4 1AJ (telephone 0273 424634.)

Bibendum, 113 Regents Park Road, London NW1 8UR (telephone 01-586 9761). Minimum order one case (twelve bottles), with discount for collection.

Infinity Foods Cooperative, 25 North Road, Brighton BN1 1YA (telephone 0273 424060). Minimum order one case. Can be bought by the bottle in the North Road shop.

Organic Farm Foods, Unit C, Hanworth Trading Estate, Hampton Road, West Feltham, Middlesex PW13 6DH.

West Heath Wines, West Heath, Pirbright, Surrey (telephone 04867 6464). Minimum order one case.

Wholefood, 24 Paddington Street, London (telephone 01-935 3924). Buy by the bottle in the shop.

Roy Cooke, Pine Ridge Vineyards, Staplecross, Robertsbridge, East Sussex (telephone 015 083 715). Britain's first organic-wine producer who supplies his wine.

The Lincolnshire Wine Company, Chapel Lane, Ludborough, near Grimsby (telephone 0472 840858), twenty-four-hour tele-

Wine

phone service and free delivery within thirty miles of Louth. German wines only.

The Organic Wine Company Ltd, PO Box 81, High Wycombe, Bucks. HP11 1LJ (telephone 0494 446557). Mainly French wines.

Merrydown wine and cider

In common with most wine and cider producers, *Merrydown* do use sulphur dioxide in their products as an antioxidant, but they are free from all other additives. They have none of the colours or flavourings used in similar products. Sugar is added at a final blending to adjust sweetness. The apples used in the cider and the soft fruit used in the *Country Wines* include a proportion of organic fruit.

Ciders include Vintage, Vintage Dry, Country, Traditional Draught.

Country Wines include 1066 Sparkling Elderflower, Mead, Apple, Gooseberry, Elderberry, Red Currant. The wines are made from fresh, local fruit and, following fermentation, they are matured for up to three years in oak vats.

Alcohol-free wine

The alcohol is removed by vacuum distillation at a low temperature and the resultant wine must have less than 0.05 per cent alcohol before it can be called alcohol-free. This is, in fact, less alcohol than in grape juice, in which the natural alcohol is 0.07 per cent and in sparkling grape juice a boozy 0.9 per cent. Alcohol-free wines are lower in calories and so are good for slimmers.

Jungs
These wines have until recently taken up around 90 per cent of the British market. The most popular is Schloss Boosenburg Sparkling which is carbonated after the alcohol has been removed.

There are also still table 'wines' Rotlak (red), Weisslak (white) and Roselak (yes, you've guessed it, rosé). They are available in full and half bottles from health-food shops, department stores, some off-licences – Bottoms Up and Peter Dominic list them – and hotel chains such as Trust House Forte. They are imported by Leisure Drinks.

Eisberg
This is a slightly sparkling white wine which starts life as a German hock from the Rheinpfaltz and is imported to the UK, where it is de-alcoholized; it is available in Bass pubs which specialize in food, and other Hedges and Butler outlets.

Motzel/Le Jacque
These two, the former from German and the latter from France, are imported by R.H.&M. Victuals. *Le Jacque* is a white and the *Motzel* range includes red, white and sparkling. Available from R.&G. Vinters, Price Busters in the Midlands, and Arctic Wine off-licences in London.

Paul Masson
An American wine made in the traditional manner from Chenin Blanc and Columbard grapes, dealcoholized by Masson's 'unique process' to remove 99.5 per cent of the alcohol. Light and fruity with a slight sparkle. Also contains grape juice, carbon dioxide and preservative sulphur dioxide, plus citric acid (vitamin C). Available from Oddbins, Gough Brothers, Budgen and some Sainsbury's.

> **My choice**
>
> Schloss Boosenburg Sparkling is a good choice and a nice fun wine, but for a still wine I prefer Masson Lite and Eisberg.

Wine

Aperitifs

Palermo is a 'vermouth'-flavour red or white aperitif from Leisure Drinks; they also produce a pastis called Blanca.

Katell Roc is a range of non-alcoholic aperitifs marketed by Brooke Bond. The range includes Americano, with a sweet flavour, Bacarat, a red vermouth, and a pastis called Anise. Each is made from a blend of herbs and spices and fruits and all, except Anise, contain sugar. They also contain E211, a preservative.

Cocktails (not alcohol-free)

A range of ready-mixed cocktails from Britvic called *Drivers*, is available through off-licences. They contain one tenth the alcohol of a normal drink and are ready mixed. The range includes whisky and ginger ale, rum and cola, gin and tonic. From the health viewpoint, although they are low in alcohol, they contain the usual additives.

> **My choice**
>
> Personally I don't like any of these, but friends who gave their opinions at tastings liked Americano and some opted for Palermo.

Low-alcohol beers

To be called 'alcohol-free', beer or lager has to be under 0.05 per cent alcohol. There is less alcohol to remove from beer than from wine, only 4–5 per cent compared with 12 per cent, but even this has an impact on the flavour and the 'fullness' of the beer.

Some manufacturers start with lager or beer and remove the alcohol. Others prefer to start with the wort (the mix of malt, hops, and so on that is fermented into beer) and then brew with a special yeast which makes a beer with very little alcohol.

Some of these special beers also have the advantage over real beer of being lower in additives, but not all of them are. More than eighty substances – including raw ingredients, additives, proces-

Wine

sing aids and adjuncts – are allowed in beer and these include some of the more troublesome additives such as the benzoates, nitrates and nitrites, as well as sulphates.

Clausthaler

This is the best-tasting low-alcohol beer. It is brewed by *Bindings Brauerei*, West Germany's second largest brewer, and is sold by Surfax and Leisure Drinks in this country. It is free from the additives found in similar products because of the strict German beer laws, the Reinheitsgebot, which allows only water, barley, malt, hops and brewers' yeast to go into beer (unlike the twenty-four or so additives allowed in British beers). Clausthaler is available in bottles from off-licences and from Waitrose.

Dansk LA

This is imported from Denmark, from Elsinore (home of Hamlet) by *Carlsberg* and is sold through some pubs, clubs and hotels. It is made by the traditional process, but the amount of sugar added keeps the alcohol content low. The ingredients are water, malt, maize, hops, carbon dioxide, antioxidants E300 and 330, colouring E150. The antioxidants are natural vitamin C products and the colouring is caramel. Dansk LA is available in 33 cl bottles.

Kaliber

This is brewed in Ireland by *Guinness*. It too contains only traditional ingredients, according to Guinness. It is de-alcoholized after brewing.

Panther

This is a French non-alcoholic beer imported by Leisure Drinks.

Barbican

The best known of the low-alcohol beers from *Bass*. Barbican contains water, malt, glucose, hops, yeast, carbon dioxide, enzymes, stabilizers, ascorbic acid and caramel.

Wine

St Christopher
Made by *Allied Breweries* (whose pubs include Ind Coope, Taylor Walker, Tetley and Ansells) this product contains water, malt, barley, glucose syrup, hops, brewers' yeast, carbon dioxide, flavourings, stabilizer and colours. Allied also import *Danish Lite*, another low-alcohol beer.

Birrell
This is *Watney Mann Truman*'s low-alcohol beer available through their pubs and off-licences.

Gerstel
Imported by *Courage* from the *Henniger-Brau* brewery in Frankfurt and available through their off-licences Arthur Cooper, Roberts, plus some motorway service areas.

> **My choice**
>
> I think Clausthaler is superb – the only problem is its limited availability.

Cider

A low-alcohol Belgian cider called *Cidre Stassen*, which contains less than 0.5 per cent alcohol, is now imported by Leisure Drinks from Stassen, the Belgian company. It is available from health-food shops.

YEAST EXTRACTS

Yeast extracts are very useful way for us to increase our vitamin B intake, especially for vegetarians and vegans who may be short of vitamin B_{12}, as many yeast extracts are fortified with it. Yeast extract can be spread on bread and toast and is a good starter for children to keep them away from sugary foods, but they should be used in moderation because they are high in salt.

Marmite is, I find, often confused with meat extracts, but Marmite is a vegetable product made with yeast extract, salt, vegetable extract and spices.

Bovril, however, does contain meat, or, to be precise, beef stock, yeast extract, hydrolysed beef protein, hydrolysed vegetable protein, beef extract, powdered dried lean beef, colour, carrots, starch, lactic acid, spices, flavour enhancers, ribonucleotide.

Natex is a low-salt extract with less than 1 per cent salt – most contain around 13 per cent. Natex is made from yeast extract, parsley flavouring, niacin (vitamin B_2) and vitamin B_{12}.

Barmene is a yeast extract suitable for vegetarians and vegans (as are the others, except Bovril). It is an entirely vegetable product made from yeast extract, hydrolysed vegetable protein, brown sugar, caramel, salt, natural flavouring, vitamins B_1, B_2, B_{12} and niacin.

Tastex is another vegetable yeast extract which has added vitamin B_{12}.

Vegemite, the Australian equivalent of Marmite, is made by Kraft Foods of Melbourne and is now available in Britain. The contents are yeast extract, salt, malt, caramel and spices.

Natex, Barmene and Tastex are available from health-food shops.

> **My choice**
>
> Marmite or Barmene are the ones I use on my 'soldiers' or for peanut-butter-and-yeast-extract sandwiches with wholemeal bread!

YOGHURT

About 3 million pots of yoghurt are sold in Britain every day; 1,000 million were sold in 1984, which added up to £165m worth of yoghurt, according to the *Review of the Fresh Chilled Dairy Products Market 1985* (Eden Vale). Most of this is fruit yoghurt

Yoghurt

and the projections are that we are going to continue to eat more.

Eden Vale attributes this success to the trend toward healthier eating, 'which means that people are looking for products that they know to be fresh, natural and nutritious, and are increasingly concerned over issues such as fat content and food preservatives'.

But just how natural and healthy are the mass-produced yoghurts? Certainly the majority of fruit yoghurt contains sugars, flavourings, colours, preservatives, thickeners, syrups and emulsifiers. They are far removed from the original sugar-free and additive-free health-food yoghurts made solely from milk and the bacteria needed to ferment the milk, which generated the 'health' image on which the sugary products are sold.

In fact, the growth in demand is for the sugar fruit yoghurts and the 'luxury' yoghurts which have added cream or are made from full cream milk. Do we think these yoghurts are healthy or do we simply dislike natural, sugar-free yoghurt?

What goes into yoghurt?

There are no laws about what is allowed in standard yoghurts. There is only a Code of Practice which indicates requirements for composition, added ingredients and labelling. A list of ingredients is not required by law on the pots if the yoghurt contains nothing other than the milk and the bacteria needed to ferment the milk sugars into acid, which produces yoghurt. Anything else in the yoghurt is listed on the pot under 'added ingredients'.

Additives

The Code suggests a maximum of 0.5 per cent stabilizers in flavoured and fruit yoghurts and up to 1 per cent of the more natural gels and pectins or starches. Emulsifiers may also be used. Thickeners are recommended only for yoghurt containing fruit or other particles, and preservatives are controlled by the general Preservatives in Food Regulations which allows them in fruit yoghurts or in the fruit used to make yoghurt. The fruit used in yoghurt can contain sulphur dioxide, the benzoate preservatives,

Yoghurt

and sorbic acid and other salts – these are used to prevent spoilage by yeast moulds on the fruit.

You can rest assured that there won't be any antibiotic residues in the yoghurt, as there might be in your milk, because the antibiotics kill the bacteria that are needed to make yoghurt. Dairies where yoghurt is made have to check very thoroughly to determine if there are any antibiotics in the milk delivered to them from the MMB and if there are they reject it.

Fat in yoghurt

The Code gives guidelines as to how much fat should be in yoghurts and suggests the amounts which should correspond to the various claims made on the pot:

	Fat content
low fat	0.5–2%
very low fat	less than 0.5%
skimmed milk yoghurt	less than 0.5%

It suggests all yoghurts should state the fat content in terms of 'not more than x per cent fat'. If it does not give a percentage, but just claims, for example, to be 'very low fat', it should comply with the categories given above.

'Live' yoghurt

There is often confusion about what the term 'live yoghurt' means. The word refers to the presence of the bacteria used to turn the milk sugar (lactose) into lactic acid. These bacteria are beneficial to health and they encourage a healthy gut flora. Often hospital patients who have been on antibiotics for some time are fed natural yoghurt to help recolonize their gut and regulate digestion problems. But even yoghurt that does not have the word 'live' on the pot will contain live bacteria so long as the yoghurt has not been pasteurized or heat treated *after* it has been made, which would kill the bacteria. Yoghurt which is made from

Yoghurt

pasteurized milk will still contain these bacteria – it seems they even survive the addition of food additives to yoghurt.

'Strawberry flavour' or 'strawberry flavoured'

It is not surprising that other confusions arise with yoghurt over the labelling of fruit varieties. Fruit yoghurt can only be labelled 'strawberry' or 'strawberry flavoured' or show pictures of real strawberries if all or most of the flavour has come from real fruit, fruit purée or syrup. If the flavour is from artificial flavourings or mostly from artificial flavourings, then the yoghurt must be labelled 'strawberry flavour'.

Skimmed milk solids

This is a term seen on many yoghurt pots and most commercial manufacturers use it. It means the addition of 'non-fat' milk solids to the yoghurt, i.e. the addition of skimmed milk powder, which gives the yoghurt body and thickness, as well as adding protein and calcium. (You can also add skimmed milk powder to home-made yoghurt to thicken it.)

Natural set

The words 'natural set' on the tub mean that the yoghurt was mixed and then cultured or incubated in the pot, which gives it more of a junket consistency. Most yoghurt in Britain, however, is stirred. All fruit yoghurt is made like this. It is incubated in a vat and then the fruit is stirred into it before it is put into the pot.

Homogenization

Most milk for making yoghurt is homogenized. It is forced through tiny holes at high pressure to break up the fat globules and distribute them evenly throughout the milk, to make the yoghurts smoother and creamier. It also helps stop 'wheying off' –

that is when the watery layer of whey separates out of the yoghurt when it is cut; this happens most often in natural-set yoghurt.

What to buy

Additive-free yoghurt is now becoming more widely available as manufacturers respond to the demand for products without additives. Here are a few of the ranges available.

St Ivel 'Real'
This range of eight fruit yoghurts is free from sugar, sweeteners and artificial additives. It is available in strawberry, black cherry, orange, pineapple, banana, Caribbean, raspberry and Fruits of the Forest. The range contains 1 per cent fat.

Co-op French Style Yoghurts
These come in a pack which contains four pots of yoghurt of different flavours: strawberry, lemon, vanilla and raspberry. They are free from additives and contain natural fruit juice as flavouring. There are no fruit pieces; they contain 0.9 per cent fat.

Chambourcy Nouvelle
These 'pure fruit yoghurts' do contain sugar, but the only other ingredient is fruit, fruit juice or purée, or natural fruit flavours. Chambourcy claim the *Nouvelle* range contains 30 per cent more fruit than standard yoghurts. Nouvelle are stirred yoghurts with 'not more than 1.5 per cent fat'. The range is pear and banana, raspberry, black cherry, apricot and apple, strawberry, peach and red currant, rhubarb. There is also a fruit and nut range: raisin and pistachio, melon and walnut, cherry and almond, apple and hazelnut.

Chambourcy Bonjour
This is a low-fat range, less than 1.5 per cent fat, of set yoghurts flavoured with natural fruit flavourings and containing sugar. Available in four and six packs the flavours include lemon, exotic fruits, strawberry, vanilla, raspberry, cherry, passion fruit, apricot, kiwi fruit, banana.

Yoghurt

Chambourcy Robot

This aims to attract children; although free from additives it does contain sugar. The yoghurt is flavoured with fruit purée and is free from fruit pieces, which they say some children do not like. Available in strawberry, banana, raspberry, black cherry.

Loseley

Describe their yoghurt range as very low fat, containing not more than 0.3 per cent fat. They are sweetened with raw brown sugar and are free from artificial additives. Made with real fruit, the fruit content and range is (percentages) apricot (11), raspberry (11), hazelnut (12), black cherry (15), blackcurrant (17), strawberry (20). Hazelnut does contain more fat, 2.5 per cent, because of the natural oils in the nuts.

Holland & Barrett

This health-food chain has two ranges of low-fat yoghurt, one without added sugar or sweetener in six flavours, and one with raw cane sugar in eight flavours, plus a goat's milk range in natural and six fruit flavours sweetened with raw cane sugar.

Eden Vale

Eden Vale has a Natural and Honey and a Natural and Grapefruit which are free from additives and contain only natural yoghurt with the named ingredients and vitamins A and D.

Ski

Ski blackcurrant is free from additives, but contains added sugar and modified starch.

Sainsbury's

Mr Men yoghurts for children are free from artificial additives and they are low fat, but they contain sugar; chocolate and fudge are included in the range.

Yoghurt drinks

These are a mixture of thin yoghurt and fruit juice. Sugar has been added in most cases and also flavourings and preservative. One typical ingredients panel reads: pasteurized skimmed milk (2 per cent fat), sugar, yoghurt culture, fruit pulp 4.7 per cent, flavouring, preservative E202. Some health-food shops have versions free from additives. There is a *Dan Mark* brand, imported from Denmark, which is additive-free and low-fat. The *Ambrosia* yoghurt drink contains synthetic colours but the *Prewett's* Yoghurt Drink with Honey is free from additives. It is made from low-fat yoghurt, honey, fructose and apple purée, so it's not sugar-free.

> **My choice**
>
> Personally I don't think you can better Loseley for fruit yoghurt, but when they are unavailable I choose Holland & Barrett's or St Ivel's Real fruit yoghurts.

Natural yoghurt

This is the healthiest of the yoghurts so long as it is low-fat and free from added sugar and additives – which it usually is. There are too many brands to list, but the natural yoghurt is a safe bet in most brands. Add your own fruit if you want to!

Strained yoghurt

There are several imported Greek yoghurts which are strained natural yoghurts and they are rapidly becoming more popular. They are higher in fat than most natural yoghurts and are creamy in consistency because they are strained to drain off the whey, or watery part of the yoghurt. The milk is homogenized to make the yoghurt creamier. They make an excellent substitute for cream and can be used in cooking. The only thing they lack is the tanginess of natural yoghurt, being rather bland.

Delta Greek Strained Yoghurt
Made from cow's milk, this natural yoghurt has a 10 per cent fat content and 135 calories per 100 g. Size: 250 g.

Yoghurt

Total Greek Strained Yoghurt
This is made from cow's milk; it has 10 per cent fat and 145 calories per 100 g. Sizes: 250 g and 500 g.

Loseley Greek-style Yoghurt
Described by Loseley as a 'concentrated' yoghurt, this one is especially creamy. It has a 9 per cent fat content and 143 calories per 100 g. Made from cow's milk. Size: 500 g and individual serving pots of 138 g.

St Michael Greek Style Yoghurt
This is unsweetened and free from additives; it is made from cow's milk and has a 9.3 per cent fat content and 130 calories per 100 g. Size: 150 g.

Greek and Pure
Another strained Greek yoghurt with 10 per cent fat content and 145 calories per 100 g. Made from cow's milk. Size: 240 g.

Velouté Natural Strained Yoghurt
This is made from cow's milk; it is imported from Cyprus. It has a lower fat content than its rivals at 7 per cent and 135 calories per 100 g. Also available in a Velouté Low Fat Natural Strained Yoghurt, which has a mere 1 per cent fat and only 80 calories per 100 g. This is also made from cow's milk. Both are homogenized to make them creamy. Size: 250 g and an individual 125 g pot.

Goat's milk yoghurt

Some people who have cow's milk allergies find goat's milk yoghurt tolerable. It is especially useful for those with eczema, asthma or hay fever who are on a cow's-milk-free diet. There are many varieties available and it is sold in supermarkets, delicatessens and health-food shops. Often local varieties can be found in both natural and fruit varieties; usually made for the health market and free from additives because they are not mass produced. Higher in fat than cow's milk yoghurt (see MILK).

> **Home-made Yoghurt Cream**
>
> You can make a thick 'double cream' from strained yoghurt, for use on desserts and for piping. It is much lower in calories than dairy creams.
>
> 8 oz (225 g) strained yoghurt
> ½ oz (15 g) gelatine
> 4 tablespoonfuls boiling water
> the white of 1 free-range egg
> flavouring, if liked – vanilla essence, lemon oil, etc.
>
> Place the yoghurt in a bowl. Sprinkle the gelatine on to the water and stir until dissolved. Fold thoroughly into the yoghurt. Whisk the egg white until stiff and fold in, with a couple of drops of flavouring, if used. Refrigerate until ready for use.

Sheep's milk yoghurt

This is often imported from Greece by the strained Greek yoghurt importers; it is higher in fat than cow's and goat's milk yoghurt. Two importers are Delta and Total; both ranges have 6 per cent fat and 100 calories per 100 g.

Soya-milk 'yoghurt'

For vegans and people with allergies to milk, yoghurt made with soya milk is quite useful. Because it is free from animal products (and is therefore low in cholesterol) it is not allowed to be sold as 'yoghurt', and producers have been told to call it something else. The argument that yoghurt is a generic name has not persuaded the trading standards officers, which means that until the law is made clear, or someone is taken to court, soya-milk yoghurt is being sold under some rather odd names, such as *Sojal Yoga*. This is made by *Haldane Foods* and is a natural 'yoghurt' made from soya milk. Yoga is available in two real-fruit varieties, strawberry and raspberry, and natural. It contains live bacteria as dairy yoghurt does, and is free from additives and sweetened with raw cane sugar. Another brand, which has not yet changed its name, is

Yoghurt

Sunrise Soya Milk Low Fat Yoghurt. Available from health-food shops.

> **My choice**
>
> Velouté's Low-fat Natural Strained Yoghurt combines the creamy texture of strained yoghurt with a lower calorie count; Total, Delta and M & S strained yoghurts are equally versatile for recipe dishes and when compared with creams, their fat content is still extremely low.

Other fermented milks

Smetana

This, like yoghurt, derives from Eastern Europe and, like yoghurt, it is widely used in Eastern cooking. Smetana is a cultured milk product, but it has a thicker, creamier texture than yoghurt and does not separate out into watery whey so easily. The difference between yoghurt and smetana is that a different bacterial culture is used. There are two types of smetana, ordinary and creamed; both are produced by the same bacteria.

Raines Dairies in Middlesex has been making smetana for twenty-five years and claims to be the only maker in Britain; they have national distribution through supermarkets and health-food shops. Creamed smetana has 132 calories per 100 g and a 10 per cent butterfat content, and standard smetana has 120 calories and 5 per cent butterfat.

Buttermilk

This is a byproduct of butter making; it can also be made by adding a culture to skimmed milk, in which case it is labelled 'cultured buttermilk'. Because most of the fat has gone into the butter, buttermilk is low in fat and calories. It has a tangy flavour like yoghurt and is sometimes flavoured with fruit to make a drink. Most drink products are imported from Germany, but *Raines* and *Churchills* both make buttermilk in this country. It is sold in health-food shops.

Kefir

This is another fermented milk drink, but not seen as commonly as the other two. It is sold in specialist ethnic outlets and the milk used to make kefir may be cow's or goat's. It is not heated to incubate bacteria like the other drinks; kefir starter, looking like gelatinous grains, sometimes in clumps like a cauliflower floret, is added to cold milk. The culture lasts for years and should be rinsed in cold water before starting each new batch.

Acidophilus

Acidophilus milk is used to recolonize normal bacteria in the gut after antibiotic use (as yoghurt is). To make acidophilus milk the milk is first homogenized and pasteurized and is then incubated with the bacteria in the same way as yoghurt. Acidophilus milk is often flavoured with fruit juice or vanilla.

There are many other cultured and fermented milk products made in the world but these are the only ones you are likely to come across in this country. They are valuable because of their bacteria content and because they are low in fat. They can replace creams and other rich toppings in the diet.

Further Reading

Barnes, Belinda, and Colquhoun, Irene, *The Hyperactive Child, What the Family Can do*, Thorsons.
Burkitt, Dennis, *Don't Forget Fibre in Your Diet*, Martin Dunitz.
Erlichman, James, *Gluttons for Punishment*, Penguin Books.
Eyton, Audrey, *The F-Plan*, Penguin Books.
Gear, Alan, *The New Organic Food Guide*, J. M. Dent. (A directory of names and addresses of suppliers.)
Gillie, Oliver, and Raby, Susana, *The A B C Diet and Body Plan*, Hutchinson.
Hanssen, Maurice, *E for Additives*, Thorsons.
Here's Health, *Health and Fitness Handbook*, Windward/Here's Health.
Manual of Nutrition, HMSO.
Mayes, Adrienne, *The Dictionary of Nutritional Health*, Thorsons.
Millstone, Eric, *Food Additives*, Penguin Books.
Robbins, Christopher, *Eating for Health*, Granada.
Tudge, Colin, *The Food Connection: the B B C Guide to Healthy Eating*, BBC.
Walker, C., and Cannon, G., *The Food Scandal*, Century.
Webb, T., and Lang, Dr T., *Food Irradiation: the Facts*, Thorsons.

References and Reports

NACNE (National Advisory Committee on Nutrition Education), *Proposals for Nutritional Guidelines for Health Education in Britain*, Health Education Council, September 1983.

COMA (Committee on Medical Aspects/Food Policy), *Report on Diet and Cardiovascular Disease*, July 1984, HMSO.

JACNE (Joint Advisory Committee on Nutrition Education), *Eating for a Healthier Heart*, Health Education Council/British Nutrition Foundation, September 1985.

Diet, Nutrition and Health: (Report of the Board of Science and Education), British Medical Association, March 1986.

Food Intolerance and Food Aversion, a joint report of the Royal College of Physicians and the British Nutrition Foundation, April 1984.

Look at the Label, free booklet from Ministry of Agriculture, Fisheries and Food, listing E numbers and common names (from MAFF Publications Unit, Lion House, Willowburn Trading Estate, Alnwich, Northumberland NE66 2PF).

Look Again at the Label, Soil Association – an interpretive version of the above (from the Soil Association, 86 Colstone Street, Bristol BS1 5BR).

Miller, Melanie, *Danger! Additives at Work*, a report on food additives, their use and control, London Food Commission, October 1985 (from the London Food Commission, PO Box 291, London N5 1DU, £5).

Food Additives, Description, Function and UK Legislation, British Food Manufacturing Industries Research Association (annual).

Consumer Attitudes to and Understanding of Nutrition Labelling, Consumers' Association/Ministry of Agriculture, Fisheries and Foods/National Consumer Council, June 1985.

Does the Consumer Really Care and *Who is Shaping the Nutrition Label?*, Food Research Policy Unit, Bradford University.

Guide to the Food Regulations UK, Leatherhead Food Research Association.

Index

acesulfame K, 394
acidophilus milk, 435
acids, 51, 94–5, 111–12
additives, 49–119
  'acceptable daily intake' (ADI) of, 58, 68
  allergies to, 70–73
  and academic success, 74
  and baby foods, 71; check list, 117
  and canned foods, 194–7
  and consumers' interests, 65–6
  and 'empty' foods, 63–4
  and hyperactivity in children, 70–71, 72, 141; checklist, 117–18
  and low-salt diets, checklist, 118–19
  and supermarkets, 76–81
  beneficiaries of, 64–5, 76
  'cocktail effect' of, 68
  consumer attitudes to, 61–2
  control of, 57–8
  definition of, 49
  functions of, 50–55
  harmful effects of, 69–74
  in bread, 163–4, 169, 174–5
  in cheese, 205–6
  in fish, 235, 238, 240–41
  in flour, 248
  in fruit juice, 259–60
  in margarine, 291–2, 300
  in meat, 309–11
  in milk, 60, 323
  in sausages, 365
  in soft drinks, 29
  in soups, 377–80
  in wine, 418–19
  in yoghurt, 426–7
  safety, checklist of, 83–100
  safety tests on, 66–8
  undeclared, 37–8, 59–61
  vegetarians and vegans, checklist for, 101–16
aflatoxins, 340
agricultural lobby, 19
alcohol/alcoholic drinks, 18, 19, 29, 39; *see also* beer; wine
allergies, 70–73
alkalis, *see* bases
aluminium, 85, 96, 122
Alutrays, 347–8, 352–3
amaranth, 75–6
American Institute of Biosocial Research, 74
amino acids, 12, 13
anchovy essence, 360
animal fats, 11, 21, 23, 301
animal protein, 13, 26
antibiotics, 59, 60, 82, 309, 323
anti-caking agents, 51, 95–7, 112–13
anti-foaming agents, 51
antioxidants, 51, 71, 73, 78, 88, 106
aperitifs, 422
aspartame, 393–4
Association of the British Pharmaceutical Industry, 72
azo dyes, 84; *see also* colours

Index

baby food, 41, 71, 117, 139–52
  and babies' needs, 145
  and salt, 140–41
  and sugar, 140–41
  and sweet tooth, development of, 142–3
  cereals, 143–4
  formula feeds, 139–40, 143
  juices, 152
  main meals, 146–52
  organic foods, 141–2
  rusks, 144–6
  weaning, 140
baked beans, 152–6
baked goods regulations, 39
Bakers' Union, 70
barley water, 265
bases (alkalis), 52, 94–5, 111–12
battery-hen system, 80
beans, 24, 26; *see also* baked beans
beefburgers, 129
beer, 39
  low-alcohol, 422–4
Bejam Freezer Food Centres, 80, 396, 398 and *passim*
benzoates, 70–71, 86
benzonic acid, 104
BHA/BHT, 60, 71, 89
Biodynamic Agriculture Association, 330–31
biscuits, 29, 157–62
bleaching/improving agents, 52, 98, 114
blood fat, 19; *see also* cholesterol
blood pressure, high, 16
blood sugar, 10, 15, 25
boiling, 130
Boots the Chemist, 79, 148–9, 398 and *passim*
botulism, 81–2
Bradford University Food Policy Unit, 47, 61–2
bran, 22, 24
bread, 162–77
  and nutrition, 173–7
  'brown', 164
  choosing, 165–8
  gluten-free, 168
  special, 168–71
  types of, 162–5, 166–71
  white, 164–5, 166
  wholemeal, 24, 163–4
breadcrumbs, 172
breakfast, 25
breakfast cereals, 177–84
  and salt, 179
  and sugar, 179–80
  nutritional analysis of, 185
British Food Manufacturers Industrial Association, 49
British Home Stores, 79 and *passim*
British Industrial Biological Research Association (BIBRA), 66
British Nutrition Foundation, 69, 71–2, 73
brown sauce, 358
buckwheat, 251
bulking aids, 52
burgers, 129, 184–90
butter, 20, 190–91
  fatty acids in, 293
buttermilk, 434

cake mixes, 191
cakes, 20, 29, 191–2
calories, 10, 11, 15, 16, 18, 28, 29, 41 and *passim*
CAMRIC, 271
cancer, 16; *see also* carcinogens
canned foods, 193–8, 242–4, 335
  additive-free, 194–7
  for vegetarians, 349–50
  ready meals, 353
  see also baked beans
caramel, 83–4
carbohydrates, 9–10, 12, 15
  see also sugar
carcinogens, 67, 71

Index

carob, 258, 375–6
cereal bars, 29, 199–203
cereals, breakfast, *see* breakfast cereals
cereals for babies, 143–4
cheese, 21, 26, 28, 203–10
   additives in, 205–6
   for vegetarians, 205, 207–8
   low-fat, 206–7
   types of, 206–10
Chinese food, 406
cholesterol, 11–12, 40–41
chutney, 211–12
cider, 424
citrus fruits, 131
clingfilm, 212
'cocktail effect' of additives, 68
cocktails, 422
coffee, 28, 213–19
colours, 52, 73, 76–8, 83–5, 101–3, 241
Committee on Food Additives and Contaminants, 75
Committee on the Medical Aspects of Food Policy (COMA), 17, 19, 42, 57
concentrates, additive, 52
constipation, 17
consumer attitudes
   to additives, 61–2
   to food labelling, 44–7
consumer education, 79
Consumers' Association, 44–5, 62, 66, 72
consumers' interests, 65–6
convenience foods, 16, 31
cooking, 120–33
   and flavour of food, 131–3
   and vitamins, 129–31
   equipment, 121–8
   hygiene in, 120
Co-op supermarkets, 79–80, 398–9 and *passim*
crabs, 239
crackers, 224–8

cream, 21, 219–24
   substitutes for, 220, 222–4, 433
   types of, 220–21
crispbread, 224–8
crisps, 369–71
crush, fruit, 265
custard powder, 228–9
cyanides, 95
cyclamate, 393

dairy foods, 13; *see also* butter; cheese; cream; eggs; milk; yoghurt
Dairy Trade Federation, 43–4
datemarks on foods, 32, 34–6
Davies, Dr Stephen, 72
desserts, 28
DHSS Committee on Toxicity of Chemicals in Food, 57
diabetes/diabetics, 15, 16, 285
   foods for, 41
diet, healthy, 9–30
   government recommendations, 17–19
diets, slimming, 12
drinks, 28–9; *see also* beer; coffee; fruit drinks; tea; water; wine
drugs in animal feed, 59–61, 82, 235, 238, 309–10

E numbers, 55–7, 75
EEC, 30, 58, 75
EEC, Scientific Commission for Food, 75
eggs, 26, 80, 230–33
'empty' foods, 63–4, 74
emulsifiers, 53, 89–91, 92–4, 106–8, 109–11
energy, *see* calories
excipients, 53

Farm Verified Organic (FVO), 329–30
farming, 59–61

441

Index

fats, 10–12, 15–16, 19, 37, 289–304
  cooking, 300
  cutting down on, 20–22
  hidden, 157
  hydrogenation, 11
  in cheese, 206–7, 210
  in cream, 219–20
  in crisps, 371
  in meat, 312
  in sausages, 363–4
  in yoghurt, 427
  labelling on, 42–4
  low-fat products, 206–7, 301–2 and *passim*
  monounsaturated, 11, 290; *see also* olive oil
  polyunsaturated, 11, 40–41, 290, 327
  saturated, 11, 290
  see also animal fats; butter; margarine; oil; vegetable fats
fatty acids, 10–11
Feingold diet, 72
fibre, 9, 10, 17, 153–4, 178, 180, 252
  increasing intake of, 22, 24
Fine Fare supermarkets, 399
firming/crisping agents, 53
fish, 80, 233–44
  additives in, 235, 238, 240–41
  buying, 234–5, 236–7
  canned, 242–4
  cooking, 132
  smoked, 240–41
fish oils, 12
fish pastes, 244
fish-fingers, 129, 244–5
flans, 245–6
flavour enhancers, 53, 77–8, 97, 113–14
flavour, cooking for, 131–3
flavourings, 33–4, 53, 73
  lack of controls on, 74–5
flour, 246–53
  additives in, 248

'brown', 249
extraction rate, 247
fibre in, 252
nutrients in, 253
special-purpose, 250–51
types of, 248–50
white, 250
wholemeal, 24, 249
fluoride, 261
Food Act (1984), 57
Food Additives and Contaminants Committee, 57
Food Additives Campaign Team (FACT), 66
Food Advisory Committee, 55, 57, 66, 75
Food and Agriculture Organization (FAO), 58
Food and Drugs Act (1955), 49, 57, 67
food industry/manufacturers, 19, 34, 41, 62, 64–5, 66
  and additives, 76, 81–2
Food Labelling Regulations (1984), 37, 41, 42, 57
food processors, 127
Food Safety Research Committee, 57–8
Food Standards Committee, 57
food workers, 69–70
France, 76
freezants, 54
French beans, 131–2
freshness of food, 34, 396
frozen foods, 256
  for vegetarians, 345–7
  ready meals, 351–2
  see also Bejam Freezer Food Centres; Iceland frozen food centres
fruit, 28, 29, 253–6
  canned, 193–8
  dried, 29, 38, 229–30
  exotic, 255–6

Index

frozen, 256
organic, 256, 331, 332
purées, 130–31
see also dried fruit
fruit bars, 257–8
fruit 'drinks', 262–3
fruit juice, 28–9, 258–69
   additives in, 259–60
   and fluoride, 261
   and labelling, 260, 262–3
   and vitamin C, 261–2
   choosing, 265–8
   concentrates, 267–8
   organic, 265–6
   sparkling, 266–7
fruit sauce, 359
frying, 132

gallates, 88
gallstones, 15, 16
glacé cherries, 230
glazing agents, 54, 97–8, 114
glutamates, 97; *see also* monosodium glutamate
goat's milk products, 320–21, 322, 432–3
government, British, 66, 75–6
   on diet, 17–19
grains, 26
granola products, 182
gravy, 387
Greek food, 407
Griggs, Barbara, 73
Guild of Conservation Food Producers, 330

haemorrhoids, 17
Harrods, 80, 399 and *passim*
health claims on foods, 32, 40–41, 416–17
'health drinks', 265
health-food industry, 40 and *passim*
heart disease, 11–12, 15–16, 19, 42
homogenization, 318, 428–9

honey, 391–2
hormones, 59, 60, 235, 310–11
horseradish sauce, 359
humectants, 54
hygiene, 120
Hyperactive Children's Support Group (HACSG), 70, 72
hyperactivity in children, 70–71, 72, 117–18, 141

ice lollies, 274–5
ice-cream, 269–75
   CAMRIC, 271–2
   dairy, 270–71
   'healthier', 272–3
   luxury, 274
   non-dairy, 271
Iceland frozen food centres, 399–400
Indian food, 26, 406
instructions for use (packaged foods), 32, 36
irradiation, 275–9
   advisory committee's findings, 277–9
Italian food, 407

jam, 279–83
   'extra', 282–3
   no-added-sugar, 281–2, 286–8
   reduced-sugar, 281, 288–9
JECFA, 58
jelly (spread), 284–5
Joint Advisory Committee on Nutrition Education (JACNE), 17, 43
junk food, 63; *see also* 'empty' foods

kefir, 435
kidney stones, 15
kitchen equipment, 121–6

Labelling Regulations (1980), 49

443

Index

labels, food, 31–48
  and 'flavour', 33–4, 428
  and fruit juice, 260, 262–3
  consumer attitudes to, 44–7
  ideal, 47–8
  ingredients list, 32, 37–40
  nutritional, 42–8
  on fats, 42–4
lamb, 315
legal definition of foods, 33
linoleic acid, 291
lipoproteins, 11–12
London Food Commission, 64, 69–70
lunch, 26

main meals, 25–7, 146–52
malt, 391
manufacturers, *see* food industry/manufacturers
margarine, 20, 289–304
marinating paste, 386
Marks & Spencer, 80–81, 400–401 and *passim*
marmalade, 283–4
marzipan, 304–5
matzos, 228
mayonnaise, 305–6
meat, 21, 23, 59–60, 309–15
  additives in, 59–60, 309–11
  antibiotics in, 309
  hormones in, 310–11
  leaner, 312
  mechanically recovered, 64–5
  organic, 311–12, 313
menus, planning, 30
Merrydown products, 420
microwave ovens, 128
milk, 21, 178, 316–23
  additives in, 60, 323
  alternatives to cow's milk, 320–21, 322
  bottle guide for, 318–19
  dried, 321–2
  fermented, 434–5; *see also* yoghurt
  processing, 317–18
  types of, 317–22
Millstone, Dr Erik, 66–7
mincemeat, 323–4
minerals, 14, 18
Ministry of Agriculture, Fisheries and Food, 21, 44, 57 and *passim*
miso cup, 380–81
monosodium glutamate, 53
muesli, 181–2
mussels, 238
mycotoxins (moulds), 82

NACNE, 17, 18, 19, 42
names of foods, 32
  misleading, 33–4
National Advisory Committee on Nutrition Education (NACNE), 17, 18, 19, 42
National Consumer Council, 44
National Food Survey, 21
'nectars', fruit, 263
net quantity of packaged foods, 32, 36
nitrates/nitrites, 70–71, 73, 87
noodles, 336
nut butters, 301
nutritional claims on foods, 32, 40–41, 416–17
nuts, 26, 373

oats, 180
  oatmeal, 251
oatcakes, 228
Official Secrets Acts, 66
oil, 11, 20, 37, 324–8
  blended, 327
  cold-pressed, 326
  high in polyunsaturates, 327
  olive, 11, 326
oil wells, 126
okara, 187
olive oil, 11, 326
O'Neill, Terry, 70

Index

Organic Farmers and Growers (OFG), 329
organic foods, 80, 328–33 and *passim*
  baby food, 141–2
  coffee, 216
  crispbread, 227
  fruit juices, 265–6
  meat, 311–12, 313
  standards of, 328–31
  vegetable juices, 268–9
  vegetables, 256
  wine, 419–20
Organic Growers Association, 330
'organoleptic experience', 64
'overconsumption malnutrition', 74
overweight, 15
oysters, 239

pasta, 333–6
pasteurization, 317
pastry, 337
pâté, 338–9
peanut butter, 339–42
penicillin, 59, 60
phytic acid, 164
pitta bread, 168
polyunsaturates, *see* fats
popcorn, 374–5
pork pies, 342
porridge, 180–81
potatoes, 25–6, 128–9
poultry, 314–15
prawns, 240
preservatives, 38, 50, 54, 70–71, 73, 78, 85–8, 103–5
pressure cookers, 127
processed foods, 16, 31
processing aids, 56–7
propellants, 54
protein, 12–13, 26, 41 and *passim*
  see also animal protein; vegetable protein
pulses, 24, 342–3
purines, 97

quiches, 245–6

ready meals, 343–53
  Alutrays, 347–8, 352–3
  canned, 349–50, 353
  dry mix, 349, 353
  for vegetarians, 344–50
release agents, 54
rice, 354–5
Royal College of Physicians, 69, 71–2, 73
rusks, 144–6
rye
  bread, 166
  flour, 251

saccharin, 29, 99, 393
safety tests, 66–8
Safeway supermarkets, 77–9, 401 and *passim*
Sainsbury's supermarkets, 80, 401–2 and *passim*
salad dressings, 305–8
salads, 25
salmonella, 82
salt, 16, 132–3, 140–41
  cutting down on, 22
  in breakfast cereals, 179
  low-salt products, 155, 179, 299 and *passim*
sandwich spreads, 355–6
sauces, 356–61
sausage rolls, 368
sausages, 361–8
  additive-free, 365
  choosing, 363–4
  Continental, 366–7
  cooking, 365
  for vegetarians, 367–8
  home-made, 366
scallops, 239
Schauss, Dr Alexander, 74
schizophrenia, 73
seeds, 374

Index

selenium, 176–7
'sell by' date, 34, 36
semolina, 250–51
sequestrants, 55
sheep's milk products, 321, 433
shellfish, 238–40
shopping, checklist for, 137–8
silicates, 96
Single European Act
    ('Harmonization'), 58
skimmed milk solids, 428
slimmers' foods, 41
smetana, 434
smoking and cancer, 69
snacks, 29, 368–76
    carob, 375–6
    crisps, 369–71, 372
    mixes, 375
    nuts, 373
    popcorn, 374–5
    seeds, 374
    tortilla/corn chips, 371–2
    see also cereal bars; fruit bars
soft drinks, 29
Soil Association, 329, 332–3
solvents, 55, 99, 115
sorbet, 376–7
sorbitans, 94
soups, 377–81
    additives in, 377–80
    miso cup, 380–81
soy sauce, 360–61
soya milk, 381–5, 433–4
    choosing, 382, 383–4
    dried, 384
    storing, 382–3
spaghetti sauces, 361
Spar group, 79
spreads
    dairy, 303–4
    for diabetics, 285
    low-fat, 301–2
    types of, 280–85
    see also under individual headings,
        e.g. jam; yeast extracts

squash, fruit, 263–4
stabilizers, 53, 89–91, 92–4, 106–8,
    109–11
steamers/steaming, 123, 130
stearates, 94
sterilization, 317–18
steroids, anabolic, 59
stock, 385–7
storage of food, 121
strokes, 16
stuffing, 387
sugar, 15, 28, 29, 140–41, 387–95
    brown, 388
    cutting down on, 19–20
    hidden, 157
    in breakfast cereals, 179–80
    low-sugar products, 155–6,
        179–80, 182, 281–2, 286–9 and
        passim
    naturally occurring, 390
    types of, 388–90
    unrefined, 389
sulphates/sulphites, 71, 86
sulphur dioxide, 37–8, 70, 79
Sunday Times, 68
sunflower spread, 342
Superdrug stores, 80, 403
supermarkets, 76–81, 395–404
    and freshness, 396
Superquinn supermarkets, 80, 402–3
surveys, 44–5, 61–2
Swann Report (1969), 59
sweet industry, 15
sweet tooth, development of, 142–3
sweeteners, artificial, 55, 91–2, 99,
    109, 115, 393–5
sweets, 29
syrups
    fruit, 263
    sugar, 390–91

tahini, 341–2
takeaways, 404–8
tartare sauce, 359
tartrazine, 61, 70, 71–2, 80

Index

tea, 28, 408–12
  alternatives to, 411–12
  decaffeinated, 410
  herb, 411–12
  types of, 409–10
Tesco supermarkets, 79, 403 and *passim*
thaumatin, 394
thickeners, 55, 89–91, 92–4, 106–8, 109–11
toast, 172
tofu, 186, 412–13
tomato ketchup, 357
tooth decay, 15
tortilla/corn chips, 371–2
trans fatty acids, 290–91, 295

UK Agriculture and Food Research Council, 58
unwrapped food, 39
USA, 71, 74, 75

vacuum packing, 51
vegans, *see* vegetarians
vegetable fats, 11
vegetable juice, 28–9, 268–9
vegetable protein, 13, 26
vegetables, 253–6
  canned, 193–5, 198–9
  cooking, 129–32
  frozen, 256
  organic, 256, 331, 332
vegetarians and vegans, 13, 80 and *passim*
  additive checklist for, 101–16
  burgers for, 186–90
  canned foods for, 349–50
  cheese for, 205, 207–8
  ready meals for, 344–50
  sausages for, 367–8
vinegar, 413–14
vitamins, 14 and *passim*
  and cooking, 129–31
  oil-soluble, 12
  'scheduled', 40

Waitrose supermarkets, 80, 403–4 and *passim*
water, 14, 414–17
  added to foods, 37
  and health claims, 416–17
  bottled, 415–17
weaning, 140
Weetabix products, 183
wholefood approach, 17, 62–3 and *passim*
wholemeal bread/flour, *see* bread; flour
wine, 39, 418–24
wine/liquor industry, 39–40
Worcestershire sauce, 359
World Health Organization (WHO), 58, 74

yeast extracts, 424–5
yoghurt, 425–35
  additives in, 426–7
  choosing, 429–30
  drinks, 430–31
  fat in, 427
  goat's milk, 432–3
  'live', 427–8
  natural, 28, 431
  sheep's milk, 433
  soya milk, 433–4
  strained, 220, 431–2
  types of, 427–9, 431–3